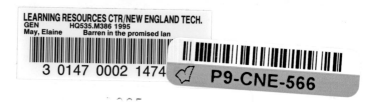

BARREN IN THE PROMISED LAND

Barren in the Promised Land

Childless Americans and the
★☆ Pursuit of Happiness

ELAINE TYLER MAY

BasicBooks

A Division of HarperCollins*Publishers*

Designed by Ellen Levine

Library of Congress Cataloging-in-Publication Data
May, Elaine Tyler.
    Barren in the promised land: childless Americans and the pursuit of
happiness / by Elaine Tyler May.
            p.   cm.
    Includes bibliographical references and index.
    ISBN 0–465–00609–4
    1. Childlessness—United States—History. I. Title.
HQ535.M386 1995
306.87—dc20   94–41427
                                                                        CIP

95 96 97 98 ❖/HC 9 8 7 6 5 4 3 2 1

In memory of my father
EDWARD TEITLEBAUM TYLER, M.D.

and for my mother
LILLIAN BASS TYLER, M.A.

*who dedicated their professional lives
to the cause of reproductive choice*

Contents

★☆

Preface

★☆

For as long as I can remember, people around me have been talking about childlessness. Although I am not childless myself, I grew up in a household where the subject was a central preoccupation. My father, an endocrinologist, devoted his medical practice to the study and treatment of infertility, prompted in large measure by the many years of childlessness he and my mother suffered before the first of their four children was born. From the 1940s until his death in 1975, he worked to advance reproductive medicine. He was among the clinical researchers who developed oral contraceptives as well as treatments for both male and female infertility. My mother, an art historian by training, forged a new career in partnership with my father, working in his clinic to counsel infertility patients through the emotional ups and downs of treatment and helping to establish free clinics in the Los Angeles area in which poor women and men could receive free reproductive health care. She became a major figure in her own right in the birth control movement.

Together, my parents dedicated their professional lives to the cause of reproductive choice. When I was still a young child, wondering what curing infertility had to do with birth control, they explained their philosophy to me: that every child should be a wanted child. It made perfect sense. Those who want children ought to be able to have them, and those who do not should be able to prevent having them. As I grew up, I traveled with them when they spoke at medical meetings, where dramatic new reproductive technologies were introduced. I worked in their clinics, typing and filing, and watched the anxious faces of the patients who came and went. I remember the grateful parents who named their children after my father, crediting him with their miracles. I remember boasting to my college friends in the 1960s that my father was one of the developers of the Pill. When they beamed and thanked him, he cringed; he believed in family planning, not sex outside marriage. Nevertheless, he and my mother were among those responsible for major advances in the effectiveness and availability of contraceptives and infertility treatments, which greatly improved the potential for reproductive self-determination.

When I became a historian, I never thought that I would become involved in the work of my parents. But on some level, this book is part of their legacy. I would not have embarked upon this project had I not grown up with the subject matter. My mother has been a source of insight and good suggestions as I have worked on this book. I have often wished that my father were here to give me his advice, too. I am sure that we would have had some good arguments, since I inherited much of his stubbornness but not all of his opinions. Nevertheless, his wisdom would have greatly enhanced this book. I was gratified to come across his articles as I did my research and found that I was still learning about the work he did and why he did it. Although he died twenty years ago, his influence on this work is evident in the endnotes.

Many others contributed to this project as well. Friends, family members, and several institutions provided essential help and support. I am grateful to the American Council of Learned Societies for a fellowship that enabled me to spend a sabbatical year working on this project. A Radcliffe Research Scholarship funded my research in the archives at Radcliffe and Harvard. The University of Minnesota generously provided a Graduate School Grant-in-Aid of Research, a Bush Sabbatical Supplement, a McKnight Summer Research Award, and a McKnight Research Fellowship. I also want to thank Deans Fred Lukermann, Craig Swan, and Julia Davis for their support of my research during my tour of duty in the deans' office at the University of Minnesota's College of Liberal Arts, as well as my fellow associate deans, Rus Menard and Rick Asher.

Archivists and curators helped me immensely in the detective work that this project entailed. I want to thank David Klaassen of the Social Welfare History Archives at the University of Minnesota; Richard Wolfe of the Rare Books and Manuscripts Archives at the Countway Library of Medicine at Harvard; all the helpful staff of the Murray Research Center and the Schlesinger Library at Radcliffe, especially Marty Mauzy, Nancy Cressin, and

Leslie Nitabach; and Ann Petter and the staff of the national headquarters of Resolve in Arlington, Massachusetts. The physicians at the Tyler Clinic in Los Angeles granted me access to files there, and the staff graciously tolerated my rummaging through the clinic's archives.

I could never have done this work without the creative, efficient, and energetic help of a group of extraordinary research assistants. My warmest thanks to Joy Barbre, Jane Cunningham, Jennifer Delton, Ginny Jelatis, Julia Mickenberg, Mary Lou Nemanic, Dan Pinkerton, Cynthia Richter, Andrea Rogers, and Csaba Toth.

Friends and colleagues contributed in a number of important ways. Bill Tuttle encouraged me to attempt an author's query and sent me all of his sample letters and publication lists. Amy Kaminsky, Cheri Register, and Naomi Scheman provided critical feedback in the conceptual stages of the project. Molly Ladd-Taylor and Margaret Marsh shared their ideas and insights, as well as their unpublished work in progress on similar topics. Specific contributions of many others are noted in the endnotes.

I was fortunate to have the benefit of critical readings of the entire manuscript from a number of distinguished scholars. Victoria Bissell Brown, Sara Evans, Estelle Freedman, Linda Gordon, Judith Walzer Leavitt, Lary May, Riv-Ellen Prell, Judith Smith, and Rickie Solinger all took time from their extremely busy lives to provide me with thoughtful criticisms and suggestions. The flaws that remain are due to my inability to measure up to their high standards of excellence.

A few people deserve to be singled out for dedication beyond the call of duty. Estelle Freedman provided a long-distance lifeline, bouncing ideas and extending support through phone calls, e-mail, and visits. Sara Evans and Riv-Ellen Prell read draft after raw draft of each chapter, patiently helping me to shape the argument and make sense of the data. In our weekly get-togethers over morning coffee, they provided sharp criticism, solid suggestions, enormous moral support, and constant encouragement. I cannot imagine life without the blessing of their friendship.

My superb editor at Basic Books, Steve Fraser, collaborated on this project from the time it was nothing more than a vague idea right down to the final draft. He helped to conceptualize the book and shape it along the way. Without his encouragement to take on the entire scope of childlessness, this book would have turned out very differently, or more likely, not turned out at all. Sandra Dijkstra, agent extraordinaire, had faith in this project long before I did, and her enthusiasm never waned. I am grateful for all the help she provided at every stage along the way.

Last but not least, I want to thank my family. Lary May has kept me going not just during this project but for a quarter of a century of shared endeavors. I could not have done this book without his careful, critical readings of my manuscript, his unwavering support of my work, his sharing of all household and professional tasks, his passion for ideas and for life, and his irrepressible playfulness. Our children, Michael, Daniel, and Sarah, helped in many ways and tolerated this project with their usual good humor. Although I have experienced neither the anguish of infertility nor the freedom of the voluntarily childless, my kids have enabled me to have empathy for both.

BARREN IN THE PROMISED LAND

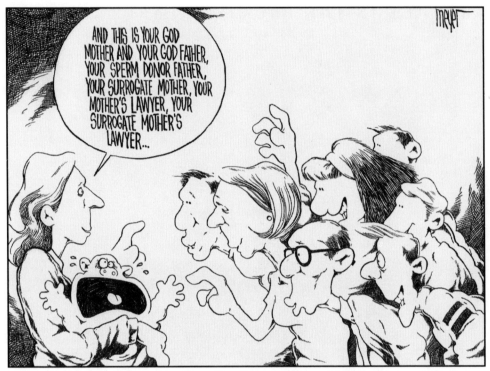

(Copyright © 1986 by Tom Meyer/San Francisco Chronicle. Used by permission.)

The Public and Private Stake in Reproduction
★☆

I was sterile, and sterile is a forever thing, with nothing to look forward to! . . . The hurt and the mind numbing pain . . . doesn't ever go away. . . . I felt guilty, because all our dreams for the future were gone. . . . I felt alienated from the rest of society. . . . I felt lost and knowing whatever I did it was never going to be ever good enough to replace the one thing I really wanted to be, a father to my own child!
—Dave Crenshaw, born 1941

We did not want to put up with a squalling brat all the time.
—Jason Domquist, born early 1940s

Being unable to conceive I think is the worst thing a woman can experience.
—Carol Hall, born 1955

Champagne, heady and sparkling, is how I describe my marriage without children.
—Lucy Bernard, born 1944

We are a nation obsessed with reproduction. From the media to the courtroom, from the clinic to the bedroom, Americans are preoccupied with their own and each other's procreative habits. The childless occupy the focus of much of this attention, for they inhabit a separate space on the margins of the mainstream. Yet there is no single experience of childlessness, as the foregoing statements by childless men and women suggest.

aspects of our lives—relationships with partners and kin, sexuality, and procreation—and the public life around us. It explores how the American preoccupation with reproduction emerged, what nourished its roots in our
historical past, and what in the national culture promoted it. Much more
than the majority who have children, the childless minority articulate the
tensions surrounding reproduction in this society and in the lives of individual women and men. By examining their experiences, we can understand
the changing culture of reproduction that permeates American Life. This
study of childlessness, then, is a study of us all.

To discover how the personal dimension of childlessness evolved over
time, I needed the voices of the childless themselves. I had no trouble
finding commentary on the subject from physicians, lawyers, clergy, popular advice writers, social workers, and a wide range of other experts and
professionals. It was much more difficult, however, to find out what childless individuals themselves thought, felt, and experienced. I decided to try
an author's query, which I sent to hundreds of newspapers and journals
across the country, asking childless people to write to me. I did not provide
a questionnaire; I wanted people to relate their stories in their own words,
with *their* concerns—not mine—at the center. I specifically asked for
responses from a wide range of people: young, old, women, men, gay,
straight, from all ethnic, racial, and religious groups. A Spanish version
went to Spanish-language journals; I invited tapes instead of letters for
those who preferred to speak instead of write; I sent letters specifically to
local ethnic newspapers, to the gay and lesbian press, and to urban and
rural publications all over the country. To my amazement, the response
was overwhelming. More than five hundred people wrote to me, and many
of them wrote twice or even three times. They ranged in age from twenty-
two to ninety-nine and included men and women from many different
ethnic and religious communities, from the arctic rim in Alaska to the tip
of Florida, and from a wide range of personal situations: married, divorced,
single, cohabiting, gay, lesbian, heterosexual, and celibate.[4]

The vast majority of the respondents were women. Like others who have
studied childlessness, I found that women were more likely than men to
express the pain and isolation of childlessness.[5] The women wrote more letters, and generally longer letters, than did the men. Margaret Lewis was one
of many wives who "wondered if this is purely a female experience. I am not
an ardent feminist and actually think of myself as apolitical, but I do feel
that it is much easier for a man to be who he is and show who he is through
his work. A woman is expected to express herself through her reproductive

The Public and Private Stake in Reproduction

★☆

I was sterile, and sterile is a forever thing, with nothing to look forward to! . . . The hurt and the mind numbing pain . . . doesn't ever go away. . . . I felt guilty, because all our dreams for the future were gone. . . . I felt alienated from the rest of society. . . . I felt lost and knowing whatever I did it was never going to be ever good enough to replace the one thing I really wanted to be, a father to my own child!
— Dave Crenshaw, born 1941

We did not want to put up with a squalling brat all the time.
— Jason Domquist, born early 1940s

Being unable to conceive I think is the worst thing a woman can experience.
— Carol Hall, born 1955

Champagne, heady and sparkling, is how I describe my marriage without children.
— Lucy Bernard, born 1944

We are a nation obsessed with reproduction. From the media to the courtroom, from the clinic to the bedroom, Americans are preoccupied with their own and each other's procreative habits. The childless occupy the focus of much of this attention, for they inhabit a separate space on the margins of the mainstream. Yet there is no single experience of childlessness, as the foregoing statements by childless men and women suggest.

Rather, people reconcile their desires, felt needs, inclinations, and biology with social norms and pressures in a wide variety of ways. In a society that expects most adults to have children, their feelings about their status as parents or nonparents are uniquely their own.

Although procreation is a profoundly private experience, reproductive behavior takes place in a society that is deeply concerned about who becomes a parent and under what circumstances. This concern is not new, but the public's stake in who has children and who does not has changed over time. In the preindustrial era, the survival of the community and economic well-being depended upon high fertility. Today, children no longer offer demographic or economic advantages, yet the expectation that American adults will become parents remains strong. Furthermore, despite the shift in the negative stigma surrounding childlessness as reproduction has become an increasingly private matter, the society still has a powerful interest in personal procreative behavior. This book examines the history of childlessness to understand the changing public and private stakes in reproduction.

I began thinking about this project several years ago in the midst of the notoriety surrounding "Baby M," the infant born of a "surrogate mother" who was hired by an infertile couple to bear a child for them. After the child was born, the surrogate mother decided that she wanted to keep the child, and a huge public controversy erupted. Hundreds of stories and editorials appeared in daily newspapers and popular magazines, several books and theses appeared on the topic, a television docudrama retold the story, the clergy took up the matter in their sermons, and people across the country took sides and argued passionately. What struck me about the case was not that some people sided with the woman who gave birth and others with the infertile couple or that feminists were divided on the issue. What I found interesting was the massive attention the case received and the way the media framed the issues.[1]

In the first place, the stories about Baby M suggested that surrogate motherhood was something new, a high-tech reproductive technology that emerged in recent years to solve a problem that also seemed to be newly discovered: infertility. But infertility is not new; it was around long before there were reproductive technologies to cure it. And it is not an ailment that primarily plagues career-oriented women who have delayed childbearing. Readers and viewers of the popular media would probably be surprised to know that for most of the twentieth century, the highest rate of infertility was among poor Blacks, not affluent Whites.[2] Nor is it true that surrogacy is a new or high-tech solution to childlessness. It is as old as biblical times, when

Sarah and Abraham turned to Hagar as a surrogate. The "new" innovation of using artificial insemination to achieve conception is at least a hundred years old. Nor is it a "medical technology," since anyone with a turkey baster and a willing volunteer can do it.

What also struck me about the Baby M story was how unprepared we were as a society to deal with the consequences of the baby quest. Physicians, lawyers, judges, clergy, social workers, and the general public puzzled over the case, but there were no guidelines or precedents to handle it. What did it mean that we live in a society where any single child may have up to five "real" parents: a genetic father, a genetic mother, a gestational mother, a social mother, and a social father? The question at the center of the Baby M debate, like the controversies surrounding the many other children who are claimed by multiple sets of parents, was not only who were the "real" parents, but who were the most "worthy." These public discussions reflect not so much a concern about children, but a preoccupation with parents: who should raise the nation's future citizens.

The Baby M case was only one of many infertility stories to hit the news in recent years. But it caught my attention because at the time, I was just completing a book about the American family during the cold-war era, when the baby boom was in full swing. In those early post–World War II years, virtually everyone was having children. The childless faced both pity and scorn, taunted as immature at best and subversive at worst. Parenthood conferred not only full adult status, but also evidence of socially sanctioned heterosexuality and patriotic citizenship. When both the baby boom and the cold-war mentality began to wane, the birthrate dropped, and childlessness, along with singleness, became respectable choices with a measure of social acceptance. The powerful ideology of domesticity gave way to the "sexual revolution," the new feminist movement, the gay and lesbian movements, and a range of domestic options—married, unmarried, same sex, opposite sex, childless, or with children—signaling a new emphasis on individual choice and a lessening of social pressures to conform to the ideal of the nuclear family comprised of breadwinner father, homemaker mother, and children.[3] It seemed that the bad old days were over, and life with or without children ought to be perfectly acceptable. So why, I wondered, did there seem to be this lingering—even heightening—obsession with reproduction?

To be sure, every society on earth is vitally interested in the procreation of its people. But each culture has its own history, beliefs, traditions, and values that influence the public and private stakes in reproduction. This book examines the American context: the intersections between the most private aspects of our lives—relationships with partners and kin, sexuality, and pro-creation—and the public life around us. It explores how the American pre-occupation with reproduction emerged, what nourished its roots in our historical past, and what in the national culture promoted it. Much more than the majority who have children, the childless minority articulate the tensions surrounding reproduction in this society and in the lives of individual women and men. By examining their experiences, we can understand the changing culture of reproduction that permeates American Life. This study of childlessness, then, is a study of us all.

To discover how the personal dimension of childlessness evolved over time, I needed the voices of the childless themselves. I had no trouble finding commentary on the subject from physicians, lawyers, clergy, popular advice writers, social workers, and a wide range of other experts and professionals. It was much more difficult, however, to find out what childless individuals themselves thought, felt, and experienced. I decided to try an author's query, which I sent to hundreds of newspapers and journals across the country, asking childless people to write to me. I did not provide a questionnaire; I wanted people to relate their stories in their own words, with *their* concerns—not mine—at the center. I specifically asked for responses from a wide range of people: young, old, women, men, gay, straight, from all ethnic, racial, and religious groups. A Spanish version went to Spanish-language journals; I invited tapes instead of letters for those who preferred to speak instead of write; I sent letters specifically to local ethnic newspapers, to the gay and lesbian press, and to urban and rural publications all over the country. To my amazement, the response was overwhelming. More than five hundred people wrote to me, and many of them wrote twice or even three times. They ranged in age from twenty-two to ninety-nine and included men and women from many different ethnic and religious communities, from the arctic rim in Alaska to the tip of Florida, and from a wide range of personal situations: married, divorced, single, cohabiting, gay, lesbian, heterosexual, and celibate.[4]

The vast majority of the respondents were women. Like others who have studied childlessness, I found that women were more likely than men to express the pain and isolation of childlessness.[5] The women wrote more letters, and generally longer letters, than did the men. Margaret Lewis was one of many wives who "wondered if this is purely a female experience. I am not an ardent feminist and actually think of myself as apolitical, but I do feel that it is much easier for a man to be who he is and show who he is through his work. A woman is expected to express herself through her reproductive ability." Nevertheless, the men who wrote made it clear that the stigma of childlessness affected them deeply and that reproductive decisions and the desire to have children are not the sole preserve of women.

That the majority of respondents were women was no surprise. What was surprising was that many single people, as well as gay men and lesbians, wrote about their struggles over the issue.[6] Not long ago, reproduction was so closely identified with marriage that those who had children outside wedlock faced automatic disgrace. For gay men and lesbians, until recently, coming out of the closet almost certainly ruled out parenthood unless they already had children. Since the 1960s, the tight connection between marriage and legitimate parenthood has weakened, partly because of the large number of single parents who have successfully raised children. But the weakening of this connection also reflects new attitudes about the family and about reproduction that have rendered parenthood an individual decision, regardless of marital status or sexual orientation.[7]

James Aronski felt this shift in his own life, and it affected his reproductive goals. When he divorced his wife, they had no children. At that time, he would have liked to be a father, but "children out of wedlock were out of the question." Later, as social mores began to shift, "my values changed. Children out of wedlock were an option." Although he has not remarried, he wrote, "I still harbor hopes of becoming a parent. . . . I am the last of my line. . . . Most importantly, I desire to be a parent. I want to teach and watch and perhaps influence in a small way the continuance of creation. . . . I would welcome the opportunity if it is God's will. And try not to feel empty if it isn't."

Many of the unmarried childless people who wrote to me decided that they wanted to have children only in a partnership. But the fact that they pondered the issue at all reflects a profound change in the cultural expectation of individual entitlement to parenthood. Rev. Joyce Fiedler is an ordained Episcopal minister who recently completed a four-year tour on active duty as a chaplain in the U.S. Navy. She considered but rejected single parenthood, not because she was opposed to the idea herself, but because it would have made it difficult for her to pursue her career. "Somewhere in the back of my mind, I always thought I could 'have it all,' but it has not worked that way. In order to function effectively in my stated profession, my life must be reflective of conventional morality—and the profession itself precluded having much of a social life." Carol Norton, who left her husband because he did not want children, was forty-nine and divorced by the time she discovered that she did not need a spouse to have a child. "I realize now that I could have had children, but did not make a decision to act. There was plenty of sperm out there. I could have used it, but I never made the decision to take it."

At least for some people, being outside the marital norm as single, divorced, gay, or lesbian did not automatically rule out the possibility of deliberate and legitimate parenthood. One self-described "leftie feminist Jewish lesbian" joked about how her colleagues at a Catholic college might react when her donor-insemination pregnancy began to show: "I will just tell them that, hey, they're Catholic, they should know a miracle when they see it. . . . "[8] Don Drummond noted that "being gay does not necessarily mean that one cannot have children." Tom Cummings, who has been openly gay since his late teens, wrote that his homosexuality did not prevent him from considering parenthood: "The idea of having children interested me a lot between the ages of 22 and 30 but then dropped away." Now, he thinks that in some ways he is more isolated as a nonparent than as a gay man: "My childlessness sets up certain barriers and inequalities," especially within his family.

Among the more interesting variations on this theme were the reproductive goals of Mitchell Brand and Andrea Moray, who are married to each other. He wants a child, she does not; he is gay, she is straight. They are "best friends now," but have not lived together for five years. Currently, they both have boyfriends. Andrea never wanted to have children, but Mitchell and his partner "would like to and are currently exploring our options." Andrea wrote that "Mitchell may still get his wish," since a friend recently asked him if he would father a child for her. "The woman [who wants his baby] is legally married to his lover." Andrea quipped at the end of her letter, "I'll bet you could do a study simply based on that paragraph alone. Anyway, I love being childless. It's normal for me."

Another unexpected outcome of the author's query was the enormous response from the voluntarily childless. Given the media attention to infertility and the relative inattention to voluntary childlessness, I expected most of the respondents to be infertile. I was wrong. About 60 percent of the people who wrote to me were childless by choice. Among the younger letter writers, those under age thirty-five, the majority were infertile. Of those over age fifty-five, who were of childbearing age during the baby-boom years when it was virtually unthinkable to be childless by choice, most were infertile or single. The majority of those in the middle, the group I would identify as "baby boomers," were childless by choice. They answered my author's query to express their frustration at the negative connotations attached to their choice. I had previously assumed that in recent years, voluntary childlessness had become a fully accepted reproductive choice with little stigma attached to it. I was unprepared for the outpouring from men and women who experienced overt hostility because of their choice.

How was it possible that in the same society, at the same point in time, some Americans were sacrificing their health, financial security, and daily routines in a desperate medical quest to conceive babies, while others were so certain that they did not ever want children that they were trying to convince their physicians to sterilize them? Suzanna Drew, age twenty-two, wrote, "Sometimes I feel as though I am less of a woman—somehow not complete." Yet Karen Boncelli wrote just the opposite: "I feel complete and whole without a child." Vanessa Allan found these contradictions ironic. At age twenty-five and newly married, she and her husband had to persuade their physician "that we had given sufficient thought to our intentions" before he would agree to a tubal ligation. At the same time, her best friend also went through surgery on her fallopian tubes—to clear them so she might become pregnant. Commenting on their vastly different reproductive goals, Vanessa wrote, "We wished we could trade 'plumbing!'" What were the cultural, individual, and historical circumstances that might have given rise to both these impulses?

Although Vanessa did not want children and her best friend did, they shared certain assumptions. They both assumed that the decision was theirs to make and that medical experts would assist them in achieving their goals. At the same time, they realized that the professionals upon whom they depended also held certain assumptions about who should have children and who should not. Vanessa's physician was reluctant to render her sterile because he believed that she and her husband should be parents. Her infertile friend's physician, presumably, agreed to provide treatment because she met the appropriate criteria: She (or her medical insurance) could pay for the service, and she appeared to be worthy of parenthood. These providers of medical services, like others in the "helping professions," made judgments, based on prevailing ideas about parental worthiness, in keeping with criteria developed in clinics, adoption agencies, and legal institutions.

One of the fundamental paradoxes of reproductive culture in late-twentieth-century America is that powerful beliefs about reproductive choice and the right of every individual to make that choice go hand in hand with widely held and institutionalized beliefs about who should and who should not become a parent, and under what circumstances. As a result, heated controversies have erupted over such issues as compulsory sterilization, access to birth control, abortion, voluntary sterilization, reproductive technologies, and adoption. The resulting policies do not always support individual reproductive goals, nor do they necessarily serve the best interests of children.

Kurt Shelly and his wife learned the hard way that institutionally defined qualifications for parenthood could outweigh what seemed to be the obvious needs of a child. They decided not to have biological children, assuming that as two professionals who had worked with children and who had a combined income of over $110,000 a year, "We could always adopt, right?" But the state agency would not allow them to adopt a particular older child they wanted. As the little girl waited for a home, they went through months of classes, interviews, and paperwork. Finally, the agency caseworker decided against them. Kurt explained, "With all of our education and experience with children of all ages, her determination was that 'since we didn't have any parenting experience, we wouldn't be able to adopt.' Our worker said that if we could 'borrow' a niece or nephew for 6 to 8 weeks, it would help." Since they did not have friends or relatives who were willing to lend them a child, they gave up. Devastated and disgusted with the state adoption system, Kurt wrote, "We do feel bad that the little girl . . . won't have the benefit of our love and commitment, and we hope that she gets it somewhere besides the [state] system."

For the childless, state, medical, and social service institutions are often the gatekeepers of parenthood, and they resent the fact that fertile people who want children do not need to pass similar scrutiny. Yet many of the childless themselves made judgments about parental worthiness. Some who asserted their own right to reproductive self-determination wished to deny the same right to those they believed to be undeserving. Mary Rodney wrote that she does not want children and finds it "discouraging to see the lack of requirements for raising a child. I think people should be at least 21 and demonstrate the necessary emotional, financial, and physical skills for raising children that are healthy physically, emotionally, intellectually, socially, etc. before they are allowed to be parents."

Donna Naples expressed similar views. Childless by choice, she "cannot think of one positive reason to have children." Although she hopes to marry, she has no intention of allowing her future spouse to be part of the decision. "When I find Mr. Right, he will be just that, Mr. Right. I want to spend my life with him. Not to be distracted by kids." But she does not think that this autonomous reproductive decision making should be available to everyone.

It really burns me when the welfare or no-income women keep having children. Since we, the taxpayers have to support them, I believe we also have the right to tell them they can't have any more children. Either by using a product like Norplant [a contraceptive implant] or to give them tubal ligations [sterilization surgery]. They forfeited their rights to make that decision when they became a burden on society. What about my rights? Why do I have to support their mistakes? Here I am, responsible about having kids, and they don't even care about their kids or the fact [that] they may have more of them.

Wrongly assuming that the children of the poor are unwanted "mistakes," Donna not only wished to prevent the poor from having children, but presumed to know their desires. Gina Sanborn, another woman who chose to be childless, agreed: "People that cannot support their children should be sterilized."

The writers of these letters saw no irony or contradiction in the sentiments they expressed. They articulated two powerful contemporary reproductive norms: that individuals have the right to reproductive choice and that society as a whole has a legitimate stake in who has children. Many believe that parenthood is a status that can be chosen but must also be deserved. These widely held beliefs suggest that many Americans consider parenthood to be a right, a privilege, and a duty. These values often come into conflict, and the childless feel caught in this conflict intensely.

As the wide-ranging responses to my author's query suggest, no single circumstance or experience characterizes childless Americans. In fact, as a group they share nothing other than not having children. Some are childless by chance, some by choice, and others by coercion. A huge gulf separates an affluent White professional who seeks infertility treatment from an impoverished woman of color who was sterilized without her knowledge or consent, and neither of them has much in common with those who are childless by choice. What they all share, however, is a marginal position in American society, where parenthood is a major marker of adulthood. Their personal desires to have or not to have children and their struggles to achieve their goals illuminate the tensions between public values and individual reproductive choices. Public values take concrete form in medical, legal, and social service policies and practices. For those who do not automatically become parents, institutional practices either support or hinder their efforts to achieve reproductive self-determination. Generally speaking, those who are White and affluent have found public institutions to be helpful if their goal was to have children, but hostile if they wished to remain childless. The poor and non-White have been less likely to gain access to infertility treatment and more likely to face involuntary sterilization. But even these patterns have changed over time.

In recent decades, it has become possible for most individuals to achieve their procreative goals in ways that were unimagined in the past. Effective contraception, legal abortion, and new medical advances in the treatment of infertility provide the expectation, if not always the reality, of reproductive self-determination. If this is the "promised land" that guarantees all citizens the right to the pursuit of happiness, then nothing should stand in their way—not social constraints, not legal barriers, not even the limitations of their own bodies. These difficulties have become hurdles to overcome, not circumstances to accept. In spite of fierce political battles over such issues as abortion, the vast majority of Americans support reproductive choice—the right to have children or not according to one's desires.[9] They also believe that their possibilities for human happiness depend upon that right. Ironically, the increasing legitimacy attached to a variety of reproductive options, along with the promise of technological fixes to help achieve individual goals, has increased pressures and heightened the social stakes in reproduction. As a result, Americans have become more, not less, preoccupied with their own reproductive fates—and everyone else's as well.

In recent decades, the historical connections among sex, marriage, and reproduction have unraveled. By the 1960s, the widespread use of effective contraception made it possible to have sex without reproduction and soon afterward, medical technologies, such as artificial insemination and in-vitro fertilization, made it possible to have reproduction without sex. But with or without sex, the marital imperative remained a powerful determinant of legitimate reproduction until recently. Now, even that connection has weakened, and reproduction can be accomplished all alone, without sex and without a partner.

This remarkable development did not come about over night, nor is it simply the result of medical advances. It is, rather, the culmination of two parallel trends: toward the increased privatization of parenthood and the increased manipulation of reproduction. It is tempting to point to the technological revolution for an explanation. After all, Americans have always been inventive, they have placed great faith in science and medicine, and now medical technologies exist that promise ultimate control over our reproductive fates. But there is nothing inevitable about these scientific developments and the ways they have been used.

It is well worth asking why so much scientific expertise and so many medical resources have been devoted to costly, risky, and painful procedures that may enable the infertile to procreate, at a time when so many other health problems need attention, such as the scandalously high infant

mortality rate in this country. Many of the children who have already been
born need better health care, and we certainly do not need more children.
Children rarely make economic contributions to their families; as everyone
knows, they are a significant economic drain.[10] And the nation surely does
not need more children to consume resources, strain the school system,
and pollute the environment. So why has so much energy been devoted to
enabling more people to have more children? It is also worth exploring why
so many people seem to be so vehemently against the idea of having any
children—and why these self-defined "childfree" Americans have to
defend their position against the still-powerful pronatalist norm. Although
there are many books on the subject, from psychological and sociological
studies to how-to books and personal testimonials, I found nothing that
helped me to understand how this entire phenomenon developed.[11] The
problem seemed to cry for historical investigation.

To understand how we ended up where we are today, we need to begin
before the days when people assumed family life to be private, before
there were widespread interventions into the reproductive process, when
childbearing and child rearing were the work of the community. The story
begins long before the infertile and the childfree; it begins with the barren. "Barren" is a term laden with historical weight. It carries negative
meanings: unproductive, sterile, bare, empty, stark, deficient, lacking,
wanting, destitute, devoid. It is the opposite of fertile, lavish, abounding,
productive. Today, we rarely hear the term in ordinary conversation; it is
more likely to be used as a literary, metaphorical term. But in the past, it
defined a childless woman. Until the mid-nineteenth century, men were
believed to be fertile if they were not impotent, so "barren" women carried the blame if a married couple did not have children. The term, like
the condition, suggested moral and spiritual failure, and words like
"blame," "fault," and "guilt" have attached to childlessness ever since.
Today the involuntarily childless are "infertile," a medical condition that
afflicts men as well as women, presumably free of gendered or moral connotations. Yet even today, a powerful stigma surrounds the childless—a
stigma that still falls more heavily on women.

Childlessness is measured in terms of women. I found no data on childlessness among men. Although childlessness has increased in recent
decades, the rates have fluctuated dramatically over the past two centuries. During most of the nineteenth century, there were low rates of
childlessness, especially among married women born in the 1830s and
1840s, who had the lowest rate on record (9 percent). Among ever-married

women aged forty to forty-four, childlessness increased from 10 percent in 1910 to 17 percent in 1940, peaking at 20 percent in 1950. Because of the dramatic decline in childlessness among younger women during the years of the baby boom, the rate dropped quickly to 14 percent in 1957 and decreased even further to 11 percent in 1990. Although we often hear that there is an "epidemic" of childlessness in the 1990s, the long-term trends suggest that this is not the case.

These trends, of course, reflect the rates of childlessness among women who were married at some point during their potentially fertile years. But the picture shifts when never-married women are included. Considering all women together, regardless of their marital status, the highest rate of life-time childlessness on record, 20 percent, was among women born in the first decade of the twentieth century, who were in their childbearing years during the 1920s and 1930s. The next generation, women born in the 1920s and 1930s who were of childbearing age during the postwar baby-boom era, cut the rate of childlessness in half, to below 10 percent.

If the trends are examined according to race, the picture shifts again. Until the 1960s, Black Americans had a much higher rate of childlessness than did Whites, owing to infertility caused by poverty, disease, and poor health care. After 1960, when health care improved, that pattern reversed, and Whites had higher rates of childlessness than did Blacks, probably as a result of higher levels of voluntary childlessness among Whites. Marital status also affected the rates of childlessness among different groups of women. In the twentieth century, single White women were more likely to be child-less than were single Black women, with the difference increasing over time. By 1990, among never-married women aged forty to forty-four, 80 percent of White women were childless, compared to 45 percent of women defined by the census as Hispanic and 36 percent of Black women. Thus, in 1990, one in five never-married White women, compared to close to half the never-married Hispanic women and nearly two-thirds of the never-married Black women, were mothers. These statistics indicate that motherhood has been much more closely connected to marriage among Whites than among Blacks and Hispanics. The overall rates of childlessness, regardless of marital status, were lowest among Hispanic women in 1990. When one considers class, however, the rates converge: Educated, affluent women of all racial backgrounds have similar rates of childlessness. These data suggest that rates of childlessness are related to a number of complex factors, including economic status, race, religion, health, marital status, and cultural beliefs.[12]

Regardless of the wide diversity among them and the many different reasons why they do not have children, the childless share the stigma and isolation of being nonparents in a pronatal society. Rude, intrusive questions and comments reflecting the parental norm infuriated many of the childless who wrote. Several agreed with Kathy Quell that "the most difficult part of being childless and infertile was the things that family, friends and strangers said to us." Dierdre Kearney was one among many who provided a list of frequently heard offensive remarks: "I really would like to write a book entitled, *What NOT to Say to Infertile Couples!* 'Just forget it and go on.' 'I don't think it would have bothered me if I couldn't have had children.' 'If you'll just stop trying so hard, it'll happen.' These make me so mad, I could scream!" Patricia Painter found intrusive questions excruciating.

> For a while I tried telling people, "Oh, we're trying." Oh God, people were chuckling or laughing and saying, "Oh, isn't that all the fun." Yeah, it's loads of fun going to the doctor all the time and spending tremendous amounts of money, and having all these painful tests, horrible things, and not being able to have sex normally, loads of fun, let me tell you how much fun I'm having. Anyway, it was terrible. Those comments were terrible.

Because reproduction usually (but not always) requires sexual intercourse, rude comments frequently included insinuations about sexual difficulties. Dorothy Norwich recalled friends asking her husband, "Do you want me to show you how to get her pregnant?" Kate Foley noted that acquaintances were "invasively questioning, rude, and almost brutal at times," offering unwanted advice about the "appropriate position or frequency of intercourse (like we didn't do it 'right')." Angela Carter was amazed "that people think our sex life becomes reason for open discussion and for some reason that is the root of our problem." Sharon Stoner and her husband resented rude remarks like, "'What's the problem, aren't you having good sex?' As if good sex has to do with procreation!"

Given the myths and stereotypes that plague those who are not parents, it is no wonder that many are sensitive about the language used to describe them. Although most of the respondents described themselves as "childless," some either embraced or rejected value-laden terms. Katie Bolter, who is infertile, described herself as barren: "I felt as if my womb was unfruitful." Many of the voluntarily childless used the term "childfree." Some of those who wrote objected to my using the word "barren," or even "childless." Sherry Alasi wrote, "Barren in the Promised Land. This title is offensive. It implies that the promise is breeding. This is only part of the promise; the other part is freedom from the burden of childbirth and child rearing." Kristen Lorner objected to the term "childless" and warned, "You are walking into the subject of your book with a conscious or unconscious bias—built in. ['Childless' implies] that the natural state of being is to have children and that to not have children is to be less than those who have chosen to have children."

Yet Kristen's story demonstrated the power of the very term to which she objected. She explained that she always assumed she would have children, but at the age of thirty "I was not in a relationship and I was certain that I would only consider being a parent with a mate. I consciously made the decision to let go of the idea of becoming a mother." The grieving process took her two years. By the time she met her future husband, she no longer wanted children. But he wanted three. Finally, she agreed to have one child because he was "father material . . . a nurturing, caring person . . . sensitive, soft, loving and kind. I realized I wouldn't have to do all the work." Once she agreed to have a child, they began a long and tortured journey. "Our sex life went through chaos trying to time when we made love. We were actively trying to conceive." She described their quest for a baby as a "roller coaster" that placed great stress on their relationship. She was reluctant to embark on infertility treatment because she had a low tolerance for pain. But she went ahead anyway. After excruciatingly painful tests, she found out that her tubes were scarred and that surgery would give her only a 20 percent chance of conception. Her physician told her, "All you can do is pray." When Kristen and her husband finally gave up treatment, she felt such deep disappointment that she could not even talk about it without crying. After all the pain and suffering she went through once she decided she wanted a child, she had to come to terms with being child*less*, whether she liked the term or not. Her own response to her infertility infused the word with meaning.

As Kristen's story suggests, there is often a thin line between "voluntary" and "involuntary" childlessness. Many men and women are both, often at different times in their lives. Marsha Montgomery explained, "For two decades, I was decidedly against having my own children. Now I am struggling with infertility. . . . It became an obsession." Corinne Gary decided against having children in her twenties, but at age thirty-two, she decided she wanted them: "I felt an emotional urge that was beyond any rationale." She and her husband went into infertility treatment, which turned the quest into an obsession. "When you start infertility treatment, the issue is no longer if you want to do it (be a parent), but more how are we going to make it happen. It was a monthly roller coaster ride: excited, try, wait, period, devastated, try again." After five years of surgeries, tests, and drug therapy, nothing worked. "The grief—the loss . . . I spent six years of my life trying to be a mom, and it was beyond my control. For a while I couldn't look ahead. I thought, how do I define myself if I don't do this? What am I if not a parent?" Finally, after months of recovery, she is "no longer feeling the biological time bomb. Sex is outstanding again." Corinne's quest illuminates the distinctions between the achievement of parenthood and the desire for children. After going through so much in an effort to become a parent, her decision not to pursue adoption sounds almost ironic: "Honestly, I never wanted children that bad."

Amanda Talley was also initially ambivalent about having children. But "once the decision was made, I was very gung-ho about it." She became "obsessed with getting pregnant." After two miscarriages, she was so drained and upset that she could not work effectively as a legal secretary: "There was no way I could possibly perform up to their standards. The reason that my work failed was because of all the stress and problems that I had been having with the infertility. And simply I did not give a damn anymore about my job." Amanda asked to be laid off and went back to the clinic for more treatment. "I was becoming more drained every day and couldn't really bear the pain of disappointment every month when I got my period. I literally was going out of my mind with grief and disappoint-ment." By the time she and her husband decided to try the grueling, risky, and expensive GIFT procedure [gamete intra-fallopian transfer], she was "really losing it." When that effort failed, "that was it. I couldn't take it any more. . . . I decided that it was time I started living my life again. I had given it all that I had. And I just couldn't go on like this." Although once she held a demanding job as a legal secretary and was ambivalent about having children, now her sense of self was shattered: "I find myself wandering [sic] every day about what I will do with my life and how I will fill this void in my soul. . . . I want to find fulfillment in something else one day, but for now I realize that I must first heal and grieve." For some-one who initially was not even sure that she wanted children, the agony, frustration, and obsession of infertility ultimately unraveled her entire life.

At a time when there are so many more options available to women than there were in the past, why has the baby quest taken on such urgency for so many? And why, throughout the twentieth century, have the stakes in having children increased, at the same time that the practical benefits of children have decreased? Emma Stein McCoy, who is childless by choice, described the overwhelming pressure to procreate that makes her feel out of synch with her peers. She had her tubes tied "just as my fellow baby-boomers and the media contracted a raging case of breedermania. . . . Movies and especially TV send out tremendous waves of breeder propaganda every day. I was really P.O.'d when Murphy Brown got pregnant, and I was *livid* when the delivery script ended with her singing 'You Make Me Feel Like a Natural Woman' to the newborn baby. Please!" The *Murphy Brown* episode provides powerful evidence that procreation, a profoundly private experience, is part of the public domain. The furor over Vice President Dan Quayle's criticism of the fictional Murphy Brown's single motherhood reflects the political and cultural meanings of individual reproductive behavior.

Murphy Brown's child was not at the center of the controversy; his mother's behavior was. Although no other adults competed for the baby and the child's financial security was assured, there was still the question of the mother's worthiness. In this respect, the controversy surrounding this fictional episode resembled the attention focused on real-life children, such as Baby M, who have been caught between competing sets of parents. Although enormous sympathy was expressed for the children in these cases, the national controversy revolved around the adults: Who were the most "deserving" of parenthood? It seemed as though everyone had a strong opinion about that. For the children in question, it was certainly a misfortune to be wanted by too many hopeful parents. But it is far worse to be wanted by none, and children who are not wanted do not seem to tear at the nation's heartstrings to the same extent.

These cases suggest that as a society, we are more concerned about reproduction and the status of parenthood than we are about children and their needs. Emma noted how children end up neglected by "a booming legal industry in cases of adoptive v. birth parents. A zillion doctors, lawyers, and parents pushing their own agendas, and precious few of them addressing what should be and rarely is the central issue: What's best for the kids? The kids! *The Kids!*" Our social policies bear this out: The United States lags far behind many other countries in using national resources to ensure the care and well-being of children. Given our lack of collective responsibility for the health and education of the young, it is clear that our society is hostile to children.

This collective hostility toward children makes the preoccupation with reproduction all the more curious. In recent decades, when the nation as a whole and individuals in particular have had little to gain and much to lose, in a material sense, by having children, the infertile have become more des-

perate and the voluntarily childless have become more defensive. This apparent paradox is one manifestation of the overall retreat from public life. As a result of this retreat, one's status as a parent and a life focused on the private realm provide the center of identity and fulfillment.

Marsha Montgomery explained her turn toward personal life and parenthood. Initially, she was childless by choice because of her pessimism about the future of the world. But eventually the very reasons that she avoided parenthood propelled her toward it. "It was this longing for closeness, for the love of a child, that balanced out my concerns for the greater world. I seem, in fact, to be increasingly fatalistic about the ill health of our planet. Everything in our world seems chaotic, such that people like myself retreat to the familiar, the comforting sources in life, such as home and family." This personal quest drove many of the voluntarily and involuntarily childless men and women who wrote to me to pursue fulfillment in private life. Through their letters, I discovered that whether they were childless by choice or infertile, they wanted the same things. They wanted control over their reproductive lives, to have or not have children according to their desires. And they expected to achieve their goals, with the help of social and medical institutions if necessary. Whether trying to have children or content without them, they wanted intimacy, love, a full and meaningful life at home, and enjoyment through consumerism and leisure pursuits.[13]

Although most of the respondents were members of the working- or middle class with at least a high school education,[14] other studies also have suggested that the desire for happiness through private life also motivates the reproductive decisions of the poor and less educated. Poor teenage parents, for example, who are frequently derided for being "irresponsible" and having "unwanted" babies, share many of the values of older and wealthier Americans. Studies of these young people indicate that their children are not necessarily unwanted or unplanned. Rather, in communities with few resources, children become a major source of pleasure and fulfillment, even if their presence makes the possibility of economic self-sufficiency and educational advancement much more difficult. When possibilities for fulfillment and status through participation in public life seem minimal at best, Americans of all ages, ethnic groups, and socioeconomic levels look to the one area in life that seems most within their control: their reproductive capacity.[15]

This intensely personal preoccupation represents a profound shift in American reproductive culture. Although childlessness has always carried a stigma, the stakes in having children have evolved over time. For centuries, the American national identity has been connected to its fertility. During the colonial era, childbearing was a matter of demographic survival and economic necessity. After the Revolution, it became a major source of national expansion and personal happiness. Manifest Destiny expressed the idea that the progeny of European settlers would move westward across the continent, "civilizing" the wilderness, cultivating the soil, and claiming the land inhabited by "savages" as rightfully theirs. Reproduction was no longer a matter of numbers alone; it was a question of propagating the *right* progeny. Only worthy parents were fit to bear and rear the nation's future citizens. This concern about proper procreation found expression in a number of experiments in reproductive engineering during the nineteenth century. Early treatments for infertility, expanding uses of contraception and abortion, and the dramatically declining birthrate attest to the fact that Victorian Americans manipulated reproduction to achieve not merely more, but better offspring. In this context, the meaning of childlessness changed from a matter of community survival to a question of civic virtue.

By 1900, a century of reproductive manipulation had succeeded in cutting the birthrate of White American Protestants in half. Suddenly millions of immigrants entered the country with much higher birthrates than the native-born Whites. Class, gender, and racial ideas infused the discussion of parental fitness. A panic over "race suicide" erupted, with eugenic reformers sounding the alarm that the nation would be overrun by the "unfit" and their progeny. Institutional and legislative attempts at reproductive engineering became much more powerful and systematic than were the incipient experiments of the nineteenth century. The Anglo-Saxon childless became more suspect in the face of "race suicide," and the fertility of the "masses" appeared more dangerous. The stigma surrounding childlessness intensified considerably as the eugenic movement gained momentum. For the first time, infertility emerged as a serious problem facing the nation, and voluntary childlessness became a crime against the citizenry.

But it was not until after World War II that reproduction became a national obsession, and childlessness a unique identity. This shift is rooted in the postwar turn toward private life as the only salvation for the nation and the self. With the onset of the cold war, the family surfaced as the ideological center of national culture, while public and community life declined. At the same time, a heightened faith in science and medicine gave rise to the belief that everyone should be able to control his or her private destiny with the help of professional experts. The fierce pronatalism of the baby-boom years marked infertility as profoundly tragic and voluntary childlessness as downright subversive. Although the parental imperative seemed to ease with the end of the baby boom and the challenges to the political and domestic ideology of the cold war, the preoccupation with private life continued to infuse the therapeutic culture of the 1960s and 1970s. The Reagan era of the 1980s extinguished the few remaining sparks of the New Deal spirit of public responsibility for the welfare of the country and breathed new life into private consumerism and personal indulgence among the nation's affluent.

In this atmosphere, the choice to have or not to have children became part of the lexicon of entitlements focused on private life. New developments in reproductive medicine bolstered the widely shared belief that the "worthy" should be in total control of their reproductive lives, at all costs to themselves and society. Along with that belief came the heightened resentment of the "unworthy" poor who "breed like rabbits" and make the taxpayers bear the burden. A sense of collective responsibility for the well-being of the nation's future citizens vanished in the process. As Americans turned further toward private satisfactions, they looked more to their own—and each other's—reproductive goals and less to a shared future. How that happened is the story that unfolds in the chapters that follow.

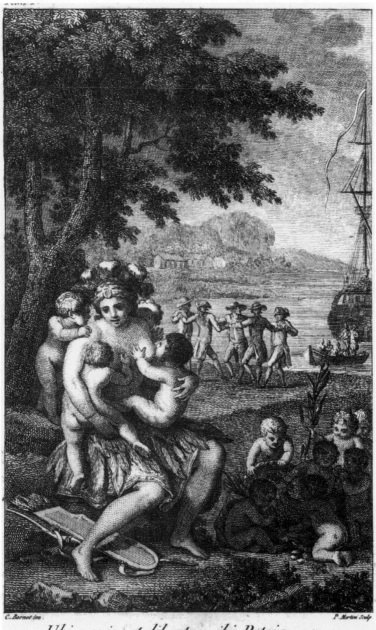

Ubi panis, et libertas, ibi Patria.

In this 1787 illustration of Manifest Destiny from Crèvecoeur's *Letters from an American Farmer*, fertility symbolizes European settlement and expansion. Note the men clearing the wilderness and the woman reproducing the white race. *(From the Rare Book and Special Collections Division, Library of Congress; also courtesy of Werner Sollors)*

CHAPTER 1

Barren to Infertile: Childlessness Before the Twentieth Century

★☆

Never may we write her Barren who is fruitful in good works, The orphans are her children, and their loins bless her in These—Sing O barren! thou that didst never bear! God's Grace and Spirit in thee is better than ten Sons. . . Fruitfulness can be but a Happiness, Compassion is a Virtue.
  —Reverend Benjamin Coleman, *The Duty and Honour of Aged Women*, 1711

What good man would prefer a country covered with forests and ranged by a few thousand savages to our extensive Republic, studded with cities, towns, and prosperous farms, embellished with all the improvements which art can devise or industry execute, occupied by more than 12,000,000 happy people, and filled with all the blessings of liberty, civilization, and religion?
  —President Andrew Jackson, Second Annual Message, 1830

In 1642, the poet Ann Bradstreet of Massachusetts Bay Colony prayed to God to bless her with a child. The English-born Bradstreet was one of the few early Americans who left a record of her feelings as a barren woman. Assuming that her sinful ways had brought the affliction upon her, she asked to be forgiven for her "Pride and Vanity" that had caused her to stray from God. She understood barrenness to be a test of her faith. Bradstreet searched her soul for the lapses in piety that might have caused God to punish her and confessed, "As I grew up to bee about 14 or 15 I found my heart more carnall, and sitting loose from God, vanity and the follyes of youth take hold of me." Her willful nature rose up again when she migrated to the colony with her husband. Although a good Puritan wife was to be submissive and obedient, Bradstreet chafed against life in the New World, where she found herself far from kin and community in an unfamiliar land: "After a short time I changed my condition and was marryed, and came into this Country, where I found a new world and new manners, at which my heart rose. . . . But after I was convinced it was the way of God, I submitted to it and joined to the church at Boston."[1]

Bradstreet believed that her sins rendered her barren and that only faith could cure her. As the Puritan minister Cotton Mather warned his female congregants, "Without your faith in Christ . . . No Good Fruit is to be expected from you, nor do I expect any good fruit" unless "you come to an Union with your Lord Redeemer."[2] Bradstreet took such warnings to heart, and apparently God forgave her: "It pleased God to keep me a long time without a child, which was a great greif to me, and cost mee many prayers and tears before I obtaind one, and after him gave mee many more, of whom I now take the care."[3]

Fertility was a blessing but not an easy one, as the poet wrote to her children years later: "As I have brought you into the world, and with great paines, weaknes, cares, and feares brought you to this, I now travail in birth again of you till Christ bee formed in you." The responsibility to care for her children became her calling in life, a task she welcomed in spite of its burdens. In 1656, Bradstreet wrote a verse about her pride and sense of accomplishment in rearing eight children:

I had eight birds hatcht in one nest,
Four cocks there were, and Hens the rest,
I nurst them up with pain and a care,
Nor cost, nor labour did I spare,
Till at the last they felt their wing
Mounted the Trees, and learn'd to sing.[4]

Bradstreet was lucky: her prayers were answered, her piety rewarded. Pride and satisfaction accompanied the successful bearing and rearing of colonial children. The colonists were eager to have many offspring, and they had a high rate of fertility. Prayer, laws that regulated sexual behavior, early marriage, basic medical principles, and folk wisdom all encouraged procreation. Although early Americans shared knowledge of contraceptive and abortion techniques that were used among Africans, Native Americans, and Europeans alike, all these communities valued high fertility, and aggressive intervention in the process of reproduction was rare.[5] It would be nearly two centuries before reproductive engineering began in earnest.

Fertility and Survival

For early Americans, having children was not simply a matter of personal happiness; fertility meant survival. Without children, households would be unable to function as economically productive units, and communities would wither and die. In the first century of European settlement in North America, all the inhabitants—African, European, and Native American— faced a potential fertility crisis. Native tribal communities suddenly encoun- tered the possibility of extinction as a consequence of the arrival of Europeans; wars and new diseases brought by the settlers killed a huge num- ber of people.

Africans who came to the colonies as indentured servants or slaves were at the mercy of their masters and experienced many difficulties try- ing to establish families. Before the plantation economy was established, most lived in relatively small households with limited space and resources. Because the masters had no use for unproductive mouths to feed, most of them discouraged the Africans from childbearing, or main- taining a family life in general. It was not until much later that slave own- ers began to encourage reproduction among their slaves, so in the early years, the population of Africans grew largely by importation, rather than by procreation.[6] Like Native Americans, the Africans struggled to form stable families and to survive amid the hostile atmosphere of European settlement.

For the European settlers, the group who would make the laws and dominate public institutions from then on, the demographic imperative to procreate was no less urgent. Reproduction was both a religious and an economic necessity. In New England, where the Puritans settled, religious motivations were particularly intense. It was incumbent upon the early settlers to "be fruitful and multiply," not only because God commanded it, but because material necessity required it. In this atmosphere, child- lessness was a serious problem. For the purpose of examining the intersec- tions of religious beliefs and material needs, New England provides a useful example.

Among New England settlers, fruitfulness itself conferred status. It was the production of children and their survival that counted. And counted they were—literally. As the historian Laurel Thatcher Ulrich noted, "To have 177 descendants was to achieve a crown on earth." Women tallied their life's achievements in terms of their progeny—not only the children they bore, but their children's children. Elizabeth Appleton, who grieved the deaths of dozens of children and grandchildren, nonetheless wrote with satisfaction in the last years of her life: "Here is an account of all my posterity. 6 sons and 3 daughters, 20 grand son and 20 grand daughters, 58 in all. 33 are gon before me. I hope I shall mett them all att Christ's rit hand among his sheep and lambs. I often look over this list with sorrow but with comfortable hopes that they which are gone are gon to rest and I desire they that survive may remember their creator in the days of thire youth, and fear God betimes."[7]

The concept of motherhood was closely tied to fertility, if not to the emotional or spiritual bond between mother and child. In a 1715 sermon entitled "Fruitful Mothers in Israel," Benjamin Coleman told his Boston congregation, "A mother with a train of children after her is one of the most admirable and lovely Sights in the visible Creation of God." Children were "among the Choice Favours and Gifts of Providence," another minister declared. Women had the responsibility, and the privilege, of bearing the children who would perpetuate the commonwealth. In the face of the dangers of childbirth and the high rates of infant mortality, knowledge of this divine purpose no doubt helped some women bear their burden. The wife of Thomas Clap, president of Yale College, bore six children and buried four of them before her own death at the age of twenty-four. In his eulogy at her funeral, Clap noted that although "She would Sometimes Say to me that Bearing tending and Burying Children was Hard work, and that She Had Done a great Deal of it for one of Her Age. . . . Yet [she] would Say it was the work She was made for, and what God in his providence Had Called Her to."[8]

With death so prevalent, families had a matter-of-fact and unsentimental view of children. Colonial children, like children in early modern Europe, were reared for the benefit of the community, not for the personal pleasure of their parents. As the historian Phillippe Ariès noted, "The family at that time was unable to nourish a profound existential attitude between parents and children. This did not mean that the parents did not love their children, but they cared about them less for themselves, for the affection they felt for them, than for the contribution those children could make to the common task."[9]

Although children were not sentimentalized, they were still highly valued—and the more of them, the better. The importance of having many children, as well as the absence of a romantic view of childhood, were both connected to the high rate of infant mortality in the colonies. To sustain the community, couples needed to have a large number of children. Most families experienced the death of at least one child. Early Americans accepted death in childbirth and infant mortality as part of a divine plan. But the numbers were devastating. Nearly one in four colonial infants died in the first year, and nearly half the children did not live to reach age ten. Martha Ballard, a successful New England midwife, lost three of her six children in fewer than ten days during a diphtheria epidemic in 1767–70, in which 12 percent of the county's population died. Most of the 144 who died were children aged two to fourteen. Martha's uncle and aunt lost eight of their eleven children in the same epidemic. Such heavy losses to families and kin groups were not uncommon.[10]

The high rate of death among children meant that a couple would need to bear twice as many children as they hoped to raise to adulthood. Infant mortality also affected the level of emotional investment that parents had for their children. Although there is much evidence to show that colonial parents loved their children, they mourned them with restrained sorrow and resignation, and accepted their deaths as a sad but expected part of life. As one man noted in 1776, "To lose a Child when first brought into Life is very hard but it is a Tax we must pay."[11]

Given the high level of infant mortality, early European settlers in New England took their duty to procreate seriously. Fertility rates were substantially higher in the colonies than in England. The average colonial woman gave birth to about eight children, a rate that would never again be matched in this country and that was higher than contemporary European birthrates. These high rates of fertility resulted not only from the desire for children, but largely from the even number of men and women in the population, early marriage, and the health of women. These conditions were not the same in all the colonies. Patterns of childbearing varied, depending upon economic and demographic circumstances. The New England colonies were among the healthiest, and most communities flourished in that region. But in every colony, population growth was necessary for building thriving settlements.[12]

"Sing O Barren!"

In a society so focused on procreation, childlessness was a heavy burden. Losing children was painful, but having none was even worse. Religious leaders, acknowledging the lack of possibilities for intervention into fertility, admonished barren women to accept their fate and find other ways to lead a godly life. If a woman did not bear children, it was her responsibility to demonstrate her piety and productivity. There were many ways that childless women could achieve respectability and contribute to the community because there were always children who needed caretaking. "Never may we write her Barren who is fruitful in good works," wrote the Reverend Benjamin Coleman in 1711. "The orphans are her children, and their loins bless her in These—Sing O barren! thou that didst never bear! God's Grace and Spirit in thee is better than ten Sons . . . Fruitfulness can be but a Happiness, Compassion is a Virtue."[13]

Cotton Mather echoed these sentiments in his treatise on "The Virtuous Mother." Young women should marry, and

> tis ordinarily expected, that they will bear Children when they marry. If a virtuous Wife be deny'd the Blessing of Children, her not Bearing is not a Trial that she cannot bear. She humbly addressed the God of Heaven, like Hannah, for that gracious and powerful Word of his which makes fruitful, remembering, That Children are an Heritage of the Lord, and the fruitful Womb is his Reward.

For the woman who remained barren, there were other avenues to salvation. She should not complain: "But she will not impatiently long like Rachel, Give me Children, or I die, lest she die by her having of those children" as God's punishment for her lack of submission and acceptance. Rather, she should "be more fruitful in all the good Works of Piety and Charity; more fruitful in her Endeavors otherwise to serve her Generation after the Will of God; more fruitful in all those Things whereby, The heavenly Father may be glorified: And she will consider with herself What Service of God, and His People, and my own Soul have I now a Leisure for?"[14]

Acceptance of one's fate was a central tenet of Puritan philosophy, and it meant that there was a place for everyone who lived a pious life, including the childless. It also meant that the community must not scorn those who did not procreate. "Do not despise the Neighbor who is not blessed" with children, wrote the Reverend Benjamin Coleman. In a society where children were counted as blessings, he also admonished those with few children "not to envy those with more."[15]

These messages suggest that barrenness was a problem of some magnitude, and that it was likely to spark frustration and envy among the childless and scorn or suspicion from those around them. Indeed, barren women comprised a noticeable minority in the population, and a group that was at risk of becoming further marginalized. Although most New England women bore several children, approximately one in twelve was barren.[16] Childless women did have some advantages. They were spared the dangers of childbirth, the sadness of having infants die, and the work of rearing those who lived. Yet women without children suffered from their inability to fulfill the biblical commandment and contribute progeny of their own to help the community thrive.

When reproductive efforts went awry, the woman was suspect. In the seventeenth and eighteenth centuries, women's procreative powers carried a certain awe and mystery. As bearers of children, healers, and midwives, women had life-giving powers not available to men. Because birth was attended by female friends and relatives, it was an important community ritual that excluded men. Early Americans both admired and feared women's exclusive powers to bring forth life. Not only barrenness, but any reproductive mishap might bring suspicion upon a woman.

In colonial New England, several women who defied the codes of proper womanly conduct gave birth to stillborn babies, which local authorities blamed upon the behavior of the women who carried them. Intellectual women who challenged church leaders were particularly vulnerable to such accusations. Perhaps the most well known was Anne Hutchinson, the bold and charismatic leader who challenged the authority of the local clergy and gained a huge following. For her Antinomian beliefs Hutchinson was ultimately banished from the colony. Her misdeeds included not only her religious teachings, but her violation of appropriate gender roles. The mother of thirteen children and a successful midwife as well, she had formidable reproductive abilities. Governor John Winthrop noted that as a respected healer, she "easily insinuated her selfe into the affections of many" because she was "a woman very helpfull in the times of child-birth, and other occasions of bodily infirmities." When Hutchinson miscarried at age forty-seven, minister Thomas Weld described the fetus as a monstrous offspring and claimed that she had brought forth as many as thirty monstrous births, none in human shape.[17]

Jane Hawkins, a follower of Hutchinson and also a midwife and lay physician, was similarly accused of heresy. Known for giving women oil of mandrake and other potions to cause conception, she was brought to court to answer for her religious beliefs, as well as her medical practices. Hawkins and Hutchinson were both present in 1638 when their good friend Mary Dyer, another of Hutchinson's followers, delivered a malformed, stillborn infant. Governor John Winthrop, Hutchinson's most powerful foe, claimed that when the fetus died two hours before birth, the bed shook, implying that it was a Devil child of Satan. A local minister explained Dyer's stillbirth by claiming that "as she had vented misshapen opinions, so she must bring forth deformed monsters." But the Reverend Thomas Weld gave more credit to God than to the Devil, claiming that "God himself was pleased to step in with his casting voice ... in causing the two fomenting women in the time of the height of the[ir] Opinions to produce out of their wombs, as before they had out of their braines, such monstrous births as no Chronicle (I think) hardly ever recorded the like." Nevertheless, it was widely rumored that these women had sold their souls to Satan and had become witches.[18]

In the vast majority of cases, witchcraft was considered a woman's crime, frequently associated with misdirected powers of fertility. Witches, it was thought, specialized in harming infants or young children or interfering with the reproductive process by preventing conception or causing miscarriages, deaths in childbirth, or "monstrous" (deformed) births. Those suspected of witchcraft were sometimes accused of destroying their own children, either in utero or after they were born, or of suckling evil spirits or the Devil instead of babies. They were also thought to cast spells on pubescent girls or to attack men in their beds at night in quasi-sexual assaults, beating, choking, or biting them; sitting or lying on them; smothering them; or otherwise sapping their strength.[19] The historian John Demos, in his study of the New England witch-hunts, noted, "Many witches were believed to have an inordinate, and envious, interest in infants and small children."[20]

Many women who were accused of witchcraft were, in fact, childless. Nearly one in six was barren—twice the rate of the female population at large. And those who did bear children had fewer than the norm. Out of a total of sixty-two married women who were accused of witchcraft in seventeenth-century New England, twenty-three had one or two children, thirty-two had three to five children, and only seven had six or more children. This is a low birthrate compared to the New England population at large at that time; 60–70 percent of all couples produced at least six offspring.[21]

As the sermons from the era make clear, married women who did not bear children needed to make extra efforts to prove their piety and worthiness. They were more likely to be accused of witchcraft if they failed to demonstrate appropriate submissiveness and virtue. Eunice Cole of Hampton County was a widow without children whose various misdeeds, coarse language, and vulgar behavior earned her a long-standing reputation for witchcraft. As a childless woman, she bore the burden of proof that her barrenness was not a sign of God's disfavor. In Cole's case, that proof was not apparent. Rather, her behavior offered additional evidence of her sinful nature. Cole was accused of witchcraft because she allegedly tried to "entice" young girls into evil ways. Demos suggested that there may have been some truth to the suspicion that Cole was inordinately focused on children: "Herself childless through many years of marriage, Eunice Cole may have sought in her widowhood to become a 'parent,' after all. It would be easy enough to understand her yearnings in this direction, given a culture which consistently affirmed childbearing as a central part of life." But colonial society looked less kindly upon Cole than did Demos, the twentieth-century historian who chronicled her world. Imprisoned and whipped several times, Cole finally died destitute and ostracized from the community.[22]

Most of the women who were accused of witchcraft were over age forty and were no longer performing their most important task, that of bearing children. A disproportionate number were of menopausal age, suggesting that colonists believed that women were susceptible to spiritual crises during this transitional phase in their lives. Witchcraft was also associated with a variety of sexual crimes, including fornication, adultery, illegitimacy, abortion, and infanticide. At least fourteen women who were suspected of witchcraft had been previously accused of these sins.[23]

Although most of those who were suspected of witchcraft were women, some men were accused as well. Jon Godfrey was single and had no children. That circumstance placed him on the margins of Puritan society, and, combined with his general unruliness, earned him a reputation as a witch. Men who were accused of witchcraft were also likely to be charged with interfering in the reproductive process. For example, William Graves of Stamford was charged with bewitching his married daughter at the time of childbearing, during a dispute over inheritance, so that her child died. William Brown of Gloucester was accused of a similar crime against his neighbor, Goodwife Prince, with whom he had a dispute. Although these men were not ultimately convicted of witchcraft, they were judged guilty of "diverse miscarriages."[24]

Community Child Rearing

To avoid suspicion, childless women and men had to prove themselves worthy in ways that their fertile neighbors did not. But they had many opportunities to do so. Most childless settlers participated in rearing and training the community's children by bringing youngsters into their homes. Economic and demographic survival depended upon the functioning of large and complex households, which often included both relatives and nonkin. Most children lost at least one parent before they reached adulthood, which meant that many orphans needed care. Along with young apprentices and servants, these orphans moved among households in which they were needed and would be reared. The children in any given family might or might not be the offspring of the head of the household, but they still received nurture, religious education, and discipline while participating in economic production.[25]

Women provided nurture not only to their own children but to other children in the household and community. Accordingly, barren wives were likely to participate in rearing the community's children. Whereas women had primary responsibility for the day-to-day care of youngsters, men were in charge of the discipline, religious training, and social behavior of their own offspring, as well as servants, apprentices, or orphans in their households. Childhood as an extended period free from responsibility was unknown in the seventeenth century. Children of both sexes began working as young as age six or seven in their own homes or as servants in other households.[26]

It was up to the parents to "break the will" of youngsters, so they would become adults who would sacrifice their personal desires for the good of the community. The colonists believed that individualism and personal ambition were negative character traits. They never described boys and girls as precious, adorable, or innocent. The innate sinfulness of children had to be controlled so they could function as useful adults as soon as possible. A seventeenth-century father remarked that "surely there is in all children, though not alike, a stubbornness, and stoutness of mind arising from natural pride, which must, in the first place, be broken and beaten down; that so the foundation of their education being laid in humility and tractableness, other virtues may, in their time, be built theron." Because the household was primarily an economic unit, child rearing involved physical care, religious training, and discipline rather than attention to children's unique psychological needs.[27]

Colonial families were not private, domestic retreats. Townspeople kept an

eye on their neighbors and reported any breaches of conduct, and the inter-
twining of household economies fostered this system of mutual surveillance.
Although households were primarily nuclear in structure, families blended
into one another as the needs of each economic unit changed. Childless
colonists had no legal means of adopting a child, but given the flexible household structure, such laws were not really necessary. Most adopters were childless couples who took in children of relatives to raise as their own. Unlike the
system of primogeniture in England, which rested on biological ties and birth
order, inheritance laws in New England allowed for de facto adoption. If a
father died, a child might be sent to another family, even if the mother was
alive. In 1658, at Plymouth Colony, William Peaks's wife testified that on his
deathbed, her husband bequeathed their youngest child to John Allin and his
wife, Ann. When the Allins asked how long they could keep the boy, the lad's
father replied, "for ever." When Andrew Hansonn died, leaving his wife with
four small children and pregnant with a fifth, the mother apprenticed her oldest son, who was nine years old, to Joseph Weeks "for his maintenance and
breedinge." Weeks would raise the boy as a member of his household until he
was twenty-one. These fluid and flexible arrangements suggest that child rearing was much more communal, less private, and less biologically or legally
defined than it would become in later centuries. Childless couples had many
opportunities to bring children into their homes and to participate in the care
and training of the community's young.[28]

Procreation and Marriage

Procreation was life-threatening; as many as one in five women died in
childbirth. But few colonial women remained single, and most of those who
married were eager to have children. Contraception, abortion, and infanticide were common in England and France at the time, but not in America.
Although there is evidence that women made efforts to space their children
using various birth control methods, deliberate family limitation was not
widespread in the colonies until the late eighteenth century. In a rare case,
Rebekah Chamblit, age twenty-seven, was executed for infanticide in
Boston in 1733. Before she died, she made a long confession and warned
others to avoid the sins and temptations that led to her downfall.[29]

The colonists believed that bearing children was women's natural lot, and
most women accepted the risks and dangers of reproduction as part of life.

Even the language reflected the centrality of reproductive labor: Words like "breeding" or "teeming" described pregnant women. These terms lingered in the vocabulary long after the colonial period, but their later use was limited to describing fertile slave women whose value was based solely on their reproductivity. Despite the fact that fertility was a blessing, women looked forward to the end of their childbearing days. As the eighteenth-century healer Elizabeth Drinker noted in her diary, "I have often thought that women who live to get over the time of Child-bareing, if other things are favourable to them, experience more comfort and satisfaction than at any other period of their lives."[30]

Although high fertility was a community goal, bearing children was not in itself a mark of virtue. Procreation had to take place in the appropriate familial context, within the covenant of marriage. The colonists did not believe that sexual virtue was natural in either men or women and thus rigorously enforced stringent codes regulating sexual behavior. Sexual encounters between betrothed men and women were treated lightly because they did not threaten the familial order, but wanton sexuality was not tolerated. If a woman's sexual misbehavior resulted in offspring who would become a burden to the community, the woman would be severely punished. Servant women who gave birth to illegitimate children were subject to fines or whippings and were often required to serve an extra twelve to twenty-four months to repay their masters for the "trouble of [their] house" and lost labor. A servant who became an unwed mother might also lose her child, since the courts would often bind such a child out for service at an early age. Thus, the incentives were high for a woman to marry the father of her child. And whereas fornication was routinely punished, adultery—the supreme violation of the familial order—was a capital crime. Although capital punishment was rarely carried out for adultery, at least three colonists were executed for this offense.[31]

Marital duties were legally enforced, and court records indicate that deliberate efforts to remain childless were grounds for divorce. When Abigail Emery in 1710 accused her husband of Onan's "abominable" sin (which might have been either masturbation or coitus interruptus), it was not so much the act itself that bothered her, but the fact that "he feared the charge of children." Similarly, Russell Knight stopped sleeping with his wife because he would not risk producing "a Parcel of young Children more to make him a Slave as long as he lived when she would not do anything to help him."[32] To avoid the responsibility of procreation was an affront to one's spouse, the community, and God.

The refusal to procreate was grounds for divorce, but barrenness was not, since a childless woman could still be a good wife and sexual partner to her husband. However, impotence was grounds for divorce because men were expected to provide sexual companionship, as well as procreation, in marriage. An impotent man could be neither husband nor father.[33] Katheren Ellenwood had her marriage annulled in June 1682 because "of her husband Ralph Ellenwood's insufficiency." Along with her testimony, fully seven other neighbors and acquaintances testified at the hearing. Most of them gave evidence that Katheren was "a woman of civil carriage in word and action," and a few were "ordered by the court to report upon Ellenwood's condition." One witness claimed that Ralph had told her at his house late one night that "he thought there were witches not far off." Whatever poor Ralph believed was the cause of his difficulty, his marriage was annulled.[34] Similarly, a Plymouth woman in 1665 gained a formal separation from her husband John Williams, Jr., because of his "insufficiency for converse with women," and another wife sued for divorce in 1686 because her husband was "always unable to perform the act of generation."[35] Thus, an impotent man was denied the opportunity to achieve the status that conferred manhood in colonial society: head of a household.

Medicine and Magic

With so much pressure placed on early Americans to "be fruitful and multiply," those who did not readily procreate turned to whatever means were available to help them. One possibility was prayer, and for some, like Anne Bradstreet, it apparently worked. Others turned to female lay healers and midwives or male physicians. Most of the routine healing was done by female midwives, who, along with delivering babies, also aided women who wished to achieve or avoid motherhood. These women may have kept their secrets from men. Even as learned and experienced a man as Benjamin Franklin had little scientific advice for a bachelor friend who was trying to remain childless but not celibate. Franklin encouraged him to marry, but added, "If you will not take this Counsel and persist in thinking a Commerce with the Sex inevitable, then I repeat my former Advice, that in all your Amours you should *prefer old Women to young ones* . . . Because there is no Hazard of Children, which irregularly produc'd may be attended with much inconvenience." A midwife might have had some other ideas as well for preventing conception, including various medicines, douches, potions, and barrier methods. But Franklin was probably correct that the surest way for a man to remain childless was to avoid intercourse with a fertile woman.[36]

Science merged with religion and folk wisdom in the practice of healing; there was little difference between medicine and magic. European medicine incorporated Indian and African cures, and an aura of magic, mystery, and power surrounded healers from these communities. "The Negro Caesar's Cure for Poison" was among the medicines used by the respected midwife Martha Ballard. Physicians gained some ascendancy in the late eighteenth century, but they offered little that was not provided by female healers. Both midwives and physicians were part of a broader medical community, but occupied different positions within it.[37]

Childless women and men often turned to midwives for help. Midwives, like most women in colonial towns, were active in the local economy and were well known among their neighbors. Martha Ballard, for example, had a thriving midwifery practice. Midwives did not use the invasive and aggressive techniques that physicians typically used to treat diseases. Ballard never used bleeding, for instance, and never trusted the procedure, even though it was standard practice among physicians. In addition, midwives did not use the strong medications and dramatic surgeries that male physicians routinely used.[38]

Healing practices were based upon the theory that the healthy and well-functioning body remained in balance and harmony with nature. Nicholas Culpeper's A Directory for Midwives, one of the most widely used medical texts in Europe, as well as in the colonies, addressed the matter of barrenness extensively. Culpeper defined "natural barrenness" as "that which causes Barrenness in a Woman; the instruments of Generation being perfect in both herself and her Husband, no Preposterous or Diabolical course used to cause it, yet the Woman remains naturally barren." He began by listing some reasons for barrenness, reflecting the holistic approach that characterized the healing arts of the time.

One cause he listed was "Want of love between man and wife . . . or when a woman hates her husband." He also warned against masturbation, or "Onan's sin." Another cause was "loss of carnal copulation. Men and women come to the School of Venus either not at all, or so frigidly, that as good never a whit, as never the better. This is perpetually caused of a cold Distemper, and must be cured by such things as heat and nourish." Culpeper's remedy for the lack of amorous feelings was far from painful:

"Let such eat and drink of the best. . . . Without good Meat and good Drink, Venus will be frozen to death. . . . Let the desire of Copulation come naturally, and not by provocation. The greater the Womans desire of Copulation is, the more subject is she to conceive. . . . Exercise your Body before you take counsel under the sheet; go to the School of Mars, before you go to the School of Venus." Not all cures were so pleasant, however. In a prescription geared primarily to men, Culpeper wrote, "Look in what part of the body the faculty which you would strengthen lies, and take the same part of the body of another Creature, in whom the Faculty is strong, as Medicines. For example, the Vertue procreative lies in the Testicles, therefore [take] Cock stones, etc., and Medicinal for this Disease. . . . The stones of a Fox dried to powder, and a dram taken every morning in Muskadel."

Like most of his contemporaries, and physicians for centuries to follow, Culpeper believed that barrenness was much more likely to be caused by a problem with the woman, "for in men there is nothing required but fruitful seed spent into a fruitful womb. But women besides the meeting of their own seed, must receive, retain, and nourish the mans; and afford matter for the forming of the child, in which divers accidents happen, and any of these will cause Barrenness." To keep the body healthy, Culpeper encouraged women to lead active and virtuous lives. Women should "give themselves to exercise" if they "would be fruitful," for "idleness is hateful to God, and destructive to the Creation; and thats the reason such women that laye idely (as most of our City Dames do) have so few children . . . whereas poor men and women that labour hard, have many Children usually, and they are strong and lusty." Culpeper continued with his diatribe against lazy city women who indulge in "apish education" and warned against "immoderate exercise (which is a thing our City Dames are utterly unacquainted with, unless it be Exercise of their tongues)."[39]

Colonial medicine, like medicine today, offered no guaranteed cures for childlessness. Nevertheless, the population boomed. By the eighteenth century, all the mainland colonies had high birthrates. In spite of persistent infant mortality, the colonies grew rapidly. Benjamin Franklin noted in 1751 that the American population (White, that is) doubled every twenty years, and Thomas Malthus, who derived his theories of population growth from his observations of North America, claimed that this rate of growth was "probably without parallel in history." This high fertility can be explained by the material and demographic conditions of life in America, the widespread availability of land, and the scarcity of labor. Franklin and Malthus offered this explanation, as have countless observers since. In addition, the political system was favorable to property ownership, and all children, not just the oldest male heir, could inherit property. American marriages also took place at an earlier age than did those in English agricultural communities. There is no question that these factors were conducive to high rates of fertility. Colonists even gave their children names that evoked fertility, such as Increase or Fruitful. The high rate of fertility impressed visitors to the colonies, and some settlers bragged, "Our Land free, our Men honest, and our Women fruitful."[40]

Early Americans used whatever means they had available to produce progeny. They prayed, did good works, married as early as was possible or practical, rarely used contraception or abortion, appreciated and enjoyed conjugal sex, and turned to healers of body and soul when their procreative desires were thwarted. They brought children into their homes and raised them as they would biological offspring. But they did not engage in large-scale reproductive engineering. In the communal society of early America, it was possible to build a family and to achieve the status of household patriarch or "goodwife" without having biological children. Child rearing was a community responsibility, and all adults—the fertile and the infertile alike—were expected to participate in the task.

This culture of reproduction changed dramatically in the early years of the new nation. By the end of the eighteenth century, in the expanding towns and cities, the economic functions of the household began to decline, and marital privacy began to replace the community surveillance that had functioned to regulate conjugal behavior in the early colonial era. As individual choice and romantic love became increasingly important in all sexual and reproductive matters, children took on new meaning and value. Procreation shifted from a matter of survival and necessity to a source of expansion, national identity, and personal happiness.[41]

The Pursuit of Happiness

In the early years of the republic, notions of progress, perfection, and happiness infused the national identity and gave new meaning to reproduction. Manifest Destiny, the guiding principle of expansion across the continent, called upon the descendants of European settlers to tame the wilderness and fill the land with their worthy, civilized progeny. In his

Fourth Annual Message to Congress in 1800, President John Adams described the fledgling country as "a great nation advancing with unexampled rapidity in arts, in commerce, in wealth, and in population."[42] The following year, in his First Inaugural Address, President Thomas Jefferson linked the westward expansion of "our descendants" to the nation's destiny: "Kindly separated by nature and a wide ocean from the exterminating havoc of one quarter of the globe; too high-minded to endure the degradations of the others; possessing a chosen country, with room enough for our descendants to the thousandth and thousandth generation . . . with all these blessings, what more is necessary to make us a happy and prosperous people?"[43]

President Andrew Jackson echoed these sentiments in 1830: "What good man would prefer a country covered with forests and ranged by a few thousand savages to our extensive Republic, studded with cities, towns, and prosperous farms, embellished with all the improvements which art can devise or industry execute, occupied by more than 12,000,000 happy people, and filled with all the blessings of liberty, civilization, and religion?"[44] In this vision of Manifest Destiny, the future of the nation depended not simply on high fertility, but on descendants of European settlers—rather than Native American "savages"—bearing and rearing future citizens.

For Americans of European descent, Manifest Destiny evoked metaphors of fertility and new birth. Fertile settlers, as well as fertile soil, would define the future of the nation. Those who settled what they believed to be a "virgin land" did so with the hope of achieving a perfect society. One representative image from the new republic accompanied J. Hector St. John de Crèvecoeur's *Letters from an American Farmer* in 1782. The frontispiece illustration, reproduced at the beginning of this chapter, personified American civilization as Mother Earth, nurturing two infants at her breasts while other children played with the fruits of the land harvested from the cultivated soil. In the background, the surrounding wilderness yielded to the conquering European men building houses and planting crops. In this new national vision, men were the builders of the nation, women the vessels of propagation, and children the hope of the future.[45]

Progeny became not only the source of progress, but the route to happiness. Beginning in the towns and cities among the middle and upper classes, economic endeavors moved out of the home into a separate place of work, leaving the family domain a private retreat from the cares of the world. A new ideology of domesticity emerged in the commercial centers, giving new meaning to family life as the training ground for citizenship.[46] Children in these homes were unlikely to go to work at a young age; rather, they were groomed and educated for the civic responsibilities they would assume as adults. With the privatization of the family came a new sentimentalized view of children. As early as 1797, the *American Spectator* waxed eloquent in this regard, articulating the "pursuit of happiness" in decidedly familial terms:

> Happy Americans! Whose free government, and fertile regions invite to Marriage, and promise the full reward of love. Here the corrupt maxims of the old world are little known. . . . Here Industry, crowned by the blessing of benignant Heaven, supplies the wants of all; and the blooming youth are seen in every dwelling, smiling around their parents, like blossoms on a fruitful tree. Health glows on the cheek, innocence and contentment sparkle in the eye, and the voice of Nature tells the traveller, "HAPPINESS DWELLS HERE."[47]

George Washington explained this new philosophy of domestic bliss in 1785: "In my estimation, more permanent and genuine happiness is to be found in the sequestered walks of connubial life, than in the giddy rounds of promiscuous pleasure, or the more tumultuous and imposing scenes of successful ambition." But the "father of our country" never had biological children of his own. When the future president married the young widow Martha Dandridge Custis in 1759, his wife's fertility was apparent. Martha had four children in eight years of marriage with her first husband, Daniel Park Custis, who died in 1757, leaving her a wealthy young widow with two surviving children. George Washington was already a hero of the Virginia militia, but public life was not sufficient to provide him with happiness and fulfillment. Although there was no provision for formal legal adoption, he immediately assumed the guardianship of his two stepchildren, on whom he lavished love and attention. He grieved deeply when both children followed their two siblings to an early death; Patsy died of epilepsy at age sixteen, and George Park Custis died as a young man from dysentery acquired during the American Revolution. Soon after these tragedies, Washington took in two children from his extended kinship network and raised them as his own.[48]

Although it seems obvious that Martha was abundantly fertile, George assumed that he was capable of producing offspring and that the problem, somehow, was Martha's. In 1786 he wrote to a nephew,

If Mrs. Washington should survive me there is moral certainty of my dying without issue, and should I be the longest liver, the matter in my opinion is almost as certain; for whilst I retain the reasoning faculties I shall never marry a girl and it is not probable that I should have children by a woman of an age suitable to my own should I be disposed to enter into a second marriage.[49]

Washington must have assumed, in accord with the medical wisdom of the day, that because he was not impotent, he was therefore fertile. But the evidence suggests otherwise. It is not clear what caused Washington's apparent sterility, but the many devastating illnesses he endured may have affected his reproductive capacity. Nevertheless, being father of his country was clearly not enough for Washington—he wanted to be father of his children as well—and he found ways to do so.[50] Washington's attachment to the children he raised, along with his love of family life, reflects the beginning of a new ideology of domesticity that marks a striking contrast to the colonial household. Although he lived on a busy plantation, Washington considered his home a refuge from the world and the children he reared as a major source of emotional pleasure.

Unlike the early colonists, who broke their children's wills to render them economically useful at a young age, middle-class parents in the new republic nurtured their "lovely children, to perpetuate our names; to enjoy the fruits of our honest industry, and to derive to us a sort of new existence. . . . Ye tender parents! say, what music in nature is equal to that which thrills through your delighted nerves when your little prattlers, with infant voice, first attempt to lisp your names!" In this sentimental view, rather than helping to support the family in tangible ways, children now served to warm their parents' hearts and consume "the fruits of [their parents'] honest industry." Even the task of child rearing became a source of joy: "Fond parents, with eyes swimming with delight, gaze on [their children] and on each other, filled with gratitude to Heaven for such precious treasures, and daily and gloriously employed in training them up to virtue and happiness. Delightful task! pleasure more than mortal!"[51]

These sentimental expressions of parental tenderness toward children reflect the emerging concept of romantic love as the basis for marriage and family life among nineteenth-century Victorians. According to the historian Karen Lystra, middle-class couples considered their offspring "love tokens." One woman described her daughter as a "little pledge" of her love for her husband, and another said their child was a "tie to both our hearts." An enraptured husband told his wife, "You are my life Darling, *and* I cannot look upon our baby, except through you. My love for him does not arise from consanguinity alone, [but has its] roots deepest in the soil of the love I bear my wife." The historian Anthony Rotundo noted that as "the purpose of sex was changing from procreation to intimacy, the purpose of procreation itself was changing from the embodiment of lineage to the embodiment of love."[52]

Parental Worthiness

If innocent children nurtured in private homes were to become the future citizens of the republic, society had a vested interest in their breeding and care. Only worthy parents could be trusted to fulfill this important task. Changes in the laws and practices surrounding custody and adoption reflect an increasing concern about parental worthiness. As the population became more diverse, particularly in the towns and cities where working-class immigrants began to arrive, middle-class reformers became concerned about the informal practices of the past that had allowed children to flow easily from one household to another. As future citizens, children needed the care and attention of virtuous—and prosperous—adults.[53]

Gradually the concept of the "best interest of the child" emerged as a corollary to beliefs about parental worthiness. As reformers endeavored to protect children from possible exploitation or neglect, the informal child-sharing practices of the past gave way to formalized laws of adoption. Under the new system, would-be parents faced new scrutiny of their fitness for child rearing. Massachusetts enacted the first adoption law in the United States in 1851, based largely upon a concern for children's welfare. Before then, state legislatures handled adoption requests on a case-by-case basis, a system in which adopted children had no particular rights. The goal of adoption reform was to make certain that adopted children would have the same legal rights as did biological children. To ensure the welfare of the child, the judge had to be satisfied that the adopters were "of sufficient ability to bring up the child." Often, biological parents had to prove their worthiness, not so much on the basis of the quality of care they provided, but on whether they would be able to offer the appropriate moral and material environment for their children. As a greater number of childless middle-class couples sought to adopt children, biological parents faced greater scrutiny and were vulnerable to having their children taken from them.[54]

Precedents for ascertaining parental worthiness came largely from custody cases in the early national period. In 1796, for example, the Connecticut appellate court ruled, in *Nickols v. Giles*, that a father forfeited his right to custody because he was a man of "very irregular . . . temper" with "very little property" and "no house." His child was "well taken care of" with the mother and maternal grandfather, and the court decided that the child was "not likely to be so [taken care of] by the father." A Pennsylvania case in 1810 went even further, deciding that the father was "an immoral man, and neglected to maintain his family" and that he was "destitute of a settled habitation" and spoke "profligate language, in the presence of his wife and daughter," which the court deemed "too indelicate to be repeated." But the mother was also a "disgusting" character, who kept house for a tavern keeper who was separated from his wife, and "there is every reason to believe they live in constant habits of adultery." Concerned with the "virtue and innocence" of the child, the court decided that she could not "be trusted with safety" to the custody of either parent and placed her with a relative "where her mind and morals [were] in the least danger of being corrupted."

Three years later, in *Commonwealth v. Addicks*, the Pennsylvania Supreme Court explicitly cited the best interest of the children when denying custody to a divorced woman who had married her lover. The court decided that the relationship "rendered it highly improper to permit [the children] to remain under her care." Although this case was presumably decided in accord with the best interests of the children, no evidence was presented that indicated what kind of care the children received from their mother and stepfather. The criteria used to determine the best interests of the child did not really focus on the children at all but, rather, on ideas about parental fitness. According to the historian Jamil Zainaldin, "Sexual roles, parental conduct, the image of childhood, and the age of the child were becoming important components in the newly invented abstractions of 'parental qualification' and 'welfare of the child.' The father's traditional common law claim to the custody of his legitimate child was being replaced by a vague but definite test for parenthood."[55]

The class and ethnic dynamics of adoption were apparent from the beginning. Most adopters were native-born, upwardly mobile Protestants, whereas most parents who gave up children for adoption were blue-collar immigrants. Poor families were more likely to suffer economic hardship when disrupted by death, divorce, separation, or dysfunction. Such circumstances made them vulnerable to charges that they were unable to care for their children properly. Rather than provide resources to help these families survive, agencies for the poor were likely to remove the children, often requiring the remaining parent to give up all parental rights. The Temporary Home for the Destitute in Boston operated on the assumption that unworthy parents should surrender their children to worthy ones who would nurture them properly. Its annual report of 1859 proclaimed: "The parents may drink; stay out of work; fill our almshouses; but they are beyond reform, and will be with us not tomorrow. But their children! Those prizes! The children are ours!"[56]

Cures for the Childless

In the decades ahead, as the American population became increasingly diverse and stratified by race and class, ideas about parental worthiness would become more important in determining the fate of the childless who turned to adoption agencies, medical institutions, and the courts in their efforts to achieve parenthood.[57] But in the early decades of the nineteenth century, even the "worthy" childless could not expect much help. Sally Bliss, a deeply religious woman who was married eight years, was despondent over her childlessness. She wrote in her diary in 1828, "My life has been spared one year more. . . . I feel as if God was saying let me alone this year and see if I shall bear fruit and if I should it would be well if not then cut it down for why should I cumber the ground[.] I feel as if I had not been so faithful the year past as I had ought to have been." Like the poet Ann Bradstreet nearly two centuries earlier, Bliss questioned her own faith and wondered if she had not been as "faithful . . . as I had ought to have been." But unlike Bradstreet, who prayed stoically and asked God to grant her children, Bliss depicted God as watching her, to see if she would be fruitful on her own. Bliss expressed a more powerful sense of individual will, as well as a greater degree of anguish. By the following year, she was suicidal. After mentioning the funeral of a man who had "cut his throat," she wondered, "I do not know how soon I may be left to do the same[.] I hope that God will keep me from all evil." Her despair did not lead her to suicide; she died in 1872 at the age of eighty-one. But as a married woman with no children in the early republic, she felt that her life was useless.[58]

Barren women like Bliss had little to gain by turning to medicine. One early medical text claimed that sterility in some individuals was part of nature's design: "It is a mistaken idea that nature has intended that all women should be mothers: for some have original imperfections in the uterine system, which cannot be remedied by any operation of art, and which remain often concealed till after death."[59] Although the spermatozoon was recognized as an essential element in reproduction during the 1820s, most medical practitioners still believed that barrenness was primarily a malady of women and largely an expression of women's moral condition. According to the historian Paul Starr, in the early national period, scientific medicine still "coexisted uneasily with moral views of misfortune."[60] One medical text claimed that barrenness resulted from "irregularity, excess, or luxury . . . and is very frequently occasioned merely by indolence." To achieve a cure, "let the lady restrain her passions, and keep her mind in tranquility; and she will soon be rewarded for these restraints by the blessing of numerous offspring, whose health, vigor, and perfect forms, will amply repay her for the sacrifices of high living and polite amusements." If virtuous and healthy living did not suffice, physicians might prescribe "astringent medicines, such as alum, dragon's blood, the chalybeate, and bark with the Spa, Bristol, or Pyrmont waters, and the use of the cold bath. . . . " But there was a limit to what medicine could do. "When sterility is occasioned by grief, anxiety, or other passions of the mind, the cure lies not with the physician; the friends of the patient must endeavor to administer comfort, the only remedy that can be offered; and the patient must call to her aid sense, reason, and religion."[61]

By the middle of the nineteenth century, in an effort to respond to the anguish and frustration of childless women like Bliss, physicians began to experiment with more aggressive ways to treat sterility. Medical theories moved away from organic notions of the balance of bodily fluids to mechanical models of the body as comprised of various separate parts. Surgical treatments for infertility became popular with physicians in the emerging field of gynecology. The physician J. Marion Sims routinely treated sterility by making incisions in the cervix because he believed that cervical obstructions blocked the passage of the sperm into the uterus. He performed hundreds of such surgeries without anesthesia, but there is no evidence that his patients ever became pregnant afterward.[62]

Sims and other physicians also experimented with artificial insemination, using a syringe and the semen of a woman's husband. This procedure was also largely unsuccessful, and Sims eventually gave it up. Other attempts to cure infertility included mechanical appliances to rearrange and support the reproductive organs. In some cases, barrenness resulted from vaginismus, a condition that caused extreme pain during intercourse. Sims used anesthetics to render these patients unconscious so their husbands could attempt to impregnate them.[63]

Throughout the nineteenth century, childless women and men increasingly turned to medicine, and physicians tried to provide them with effective treatments. These efforts represent one aspect of the growing trend toward greater control over reproduction. A new faith in science, combined with the powerful desire of Victorian Americans to control their own destinies, their bodies, their sexuality, and even the natural world around them, fostered a number of experiments in reproductive engineering. In their attempts to bear and rear children who would expand and build the nation, middle-class Americans endeavored to have children wisely and deliberately. But an unintended result of thousands of individual women and men engaged in prudent procreation was the drastic decline in the birthrate.

Reproductive Engineering

Manifest Destiny contained some internal contradictions. Although citizens were expected to populate the continent with "worthy" offspring, the obligatory care and nurture of precious children meant that parents—particularly women—would need to devote themselves wholeheartedly to each individual child. With an emphasis on the quality, rather than the quantity, of children, married couples tried to limit the size of their families. In 1800, the average married couple had seven children. By 1850, the number had declined to five or six and by 1900, to only three or four. The overall decline in the fertility of White Americans was driven largely by the dramatic drop in the birthrate among the urban middle class. Fertility declined to a lesser extent in rural areas, where it remained essential for families to have enough children to keep their farms going, but not too many for the land that was available.[64]

The declining birthrate of White Americans represents the first large-scale effort at reproductive engineering. Part of the decline resulted from demographic shifts. As the age of first marriage increased, women spent fewer of their fertile years married and therefore had fewer children. But married couples also limited the size of their families by using contraception, including coitus interruptus (withdrawal), condoms, cervical caps and diaphragms, douching, and abortion. The decline in the birthrate represents a deliberate effort by a large number of Americans to gain control over their reproductive fates.[65]

Much of the impetus for the declining birthrate came from women, who risked their health in pregnancy and childbirth and carried the major responsibility for child rearing. The ideology of domesticity increased women's stature and autonomy within the home, enhancing their ability to persuade their husbands to practice birth control and to limit sexual intercourse. Yet women were not the only ones with a desire to limit the size of their families. Men also faced the economic pressures of providing for large families and recognized that fewer children meant greater possibilities for upward mobility.

Some men were clearly ambivalent about having children, even though fatherhood was expected of Victorian husbands. The late-nineteenth-century writer and social critic Henry Adams never had children of his own. While he was "a believer in the necessity of propagating our kind," he was happy to leave that task to "all my able-bodied friends and relations devoting themselves to this end." As for Adams himself, "Nothing can reconcile me to the position of head of a family. . . . I have myself never cared enough about children to be unhappy either at having or not having them." Adams was, however, deeply devoted to his nieces, and to his writings, which he often described as his "offspring."[66]

Victorian sexual ideology also fostered family-limitation practices in the nineteenth century. New ideas about sex encouraged marital restraint by defining women as "passionless" and men as at risk of wasting their productive energy in too much sexual indulgence. The idea of "passionless" women emerged to distinguish women from men, who were believed to be much more driven by their passions, and to distinguish White women from Black women, who were believed to be inherently lascivious.[67] There is ample evidence to suggest that nineteenth-century White women were not "passionless," but that their attitude toward reproduction was undoubtedly ambivalent. Many women died in childbirth, and those who lived were likely to experience pain, illness, and disability as a result of their childbearing. The historian Ellen Rothman, in her study of nineteenth-century courtship, found that young middle-class men and women expressed their love for one another in passionate, sexual terms. But she also found that some women attempted to avoid sexual intercourse and to postpone marriage largely to delay childbearing. Others became concerned about the dangers of childbirth after marriage or the birth of their first child and tried to avoid frequent pregnancies.[68] "Passionlessness" gave women some power within the marital relationship and provided a rationale for them to limit their pregnancies by limiting sex—a goal that men were expected to share. According to prevailing middle-class norms, sexual excess was unhealthy for men, as well as for women. In women, a strong sex drive was evidence of illness; "nymphomania" was defined as a disease with medical cures ranging from total sexual abstinence to surgery. For men, "male continence" was the corollary to "passionlessness." According to the theory of "male continence," infrequent intercourse conserves strength, whereas "excessive indulgence frequently causes general debility, weakness, and lameness of the back, dyspepsia, impotency, and [a] predisposition to almost innumerable diseases."[69]

Contraception and Abortion

Sexual restraint was one way to limit offspring, but it was not the only way. The increasing use of contraception and abortion suggests that continence was not necessarily the preferred method of controlling fertility. In fact, information on birth control became widely available between the 1830s and the 1870s, in spite of efforts to repress it. Radical thinkers advocated contraception as a way to enhance sexual enjoyment and to reduce the risk of pregnancy. The first treatise on the subject in the United States, by the utopian socialist Robert Dale Owen, appeared in 1831. In regard to the sexual instinct, Owen asked, "Is it desirable, that it should never be gratified without an increase to population? Or, is it desirable, that, in gratifying it, man shall be able to say whether offspring shall be the result or not?"

Owen believed that sex had two purposes, reproduction and enjoyment, and argued that it should be possible to separate the two. He advocated withdrawal (coitus interruptus) as the best and most effective method of birth control. "As for the sacrifice, shall a trifling (and it is but a very trifling) diminution of physical enjoyment be suffered to outweigh the most important considerations connected with the permanent welfare of those who are nearest and dearest to us?" Although some medical writers condemned the practice of withdrawal as harmful to both men and women, Owen believed that it was preferable to either abstinence or celibacy, which he called "a mortification of the affections, a violence done to the social feelings, sometimes a sacrifice even of the health."[70]

The year following the publication of Owen's tract, Charles Knowlton, a graduate of Dartmouth medical college, wrote a book that advocated the use of birth control on medical, economic, and social grounds. The fact that Knowlton was prosecuted, fined, and sentenced to three months in jail did nothing to dampen the popularity of his book, which went through nine American editions. By the late nineteenth century, the book was selling over 250,000 copies a year. Knowlton's book explained the use and effectiveness of a number of birth control methods, including withdrawal, the "baudrache" (apparently a device like a condom), sponges, and douches. After Knowlton's book came at least a dozen more, which provided information and advice on contraceptive methods, including "The Wife's Protector" (a diaphragm patented in 1846), pessaries, sponges, condoms, and syringes for douching.[71]

Abortions also increased throughout the nineteenth century among all groups of women. At the beginning of the nineteenth century, abortion was legal everywhere in the United States. Although exact figures are not available, reformers estimated that in the first three decades of the nineteenth century, one abortion occurred for every twenty-five to thirty live births. By mid-century, estimates were as high as one abortion for every five or six live births. In the early years, according to observers at the time, abortion was most likely to be the last resort of single young women "who have been deceived and ensnared by the seducer." But later in the century, abortions were most common among married women. A Michigan Board of Health report in 1878 estimated that one-third of all pregnancies in that state ended in abortion and that most abortions were obtained by "prosperous and otherwise respectable married women."[72]

In the first half of the nineteenth century, abortion was not condemned if it occurred before "quickening," or the time when the woman could feel the fetus moving inside her body, usually in about the fourth month of pregnancy. Laws at the time reflected the prevailing religious belief that life began at "quickening." Medical books described cures for "obstructed menses" and mentioned the causes of miscarriages, so it was easy to discover how to terminate a pregnancy by following the examples.

Methods of achieving abortion circulated in the folk culture, as well as in the commercial society. Patent medicines became widely available and were advertised in newspapers and magazines. Native American midwives and healers used roots and herbs, as did Black women. Most of these remedies involved ingesting various substances that caused miscarriages.[73]

Surgical abortions were also performed by practitioners, or pregnant women themselves, by inserting instruments into the uterus. Sometimes these methods resulted in severe illness or death. But most abortions were effective and caused no long-term health problems. It was not until the late nineteenth century, when the influx of immigrants and the declining Anglo-Saxon birthrate caused alarm, that the practice was widely condemned. As an increasing number of middle-class married women turned to abortion, legislators, physicians, and other professionals began to consider it a social problem. Although there were no laws against abortion in 1800, from 1860 to 1890, forty states and territories enacted antiabortion laws, limiting access and transferring legal authority for abortion from women to physicians. By 1900, abortion was a criminal offense in virtually every jurisdiction. These statutes, along with the Comstock Law passed in 1873, which prohibited the dissemination of birth control devices or information through the mails, made it more difficult to gain access to the means for controlling reproduction. Nevertheless, the birthrate continued to decline.[74]

Single and Childless

As the nineteenth century advanced, more and more women and men chose a single life. In a curious way, the Victorian ideology of domesticity actually encouraged this trend. The evolution of the home from a unit of production to a place of nurture accompanied a larger cultural transformation that repositioned women in society. Early leaders of the nation puzzled over what the role of women should be in the new republic. According to the historian Linda K. Kerber, a new concept of "republican motherhood" emerged to provide a place for women in the democratic state. Women would still be prohibited from owning property, voting, and acting as citizens in other vital ways. But they would now be vested with the responsibility for bearing and rearing future citizens, which meant that they would need to be educated to fulfill that vital role. White middle-class women in the towns and cities embraced the role of republican mother, for it conferred new status on women and gave them an important political function. It would be this role, as the educators of future citizens and the moral guardians of society, that would soon provide the rationale for women reformers, who moved beyond the domestic realm to improve society more directly.[75]

Ironically, the ideology of republican motherhood actually made room for women without children. If women were naturally suited to be the moral guardians of the society, they could provide that function whether or not they had biological offspring. Single women could therefore earn respected positions in society by providing maternal functions in the civic arena. The educator Catherine Beecher, one of the foremost theorists of nineteenth-century female domesticity, was nevertheless single and childless. She claimed that the woman who exercised her maternal influence in the larger society was even more virtuous than was the mother in the home, and argued that unmarried women "of superior mind and acquirements have risen to a more enlarged and comprehensive boundary of exertion, and by their talents and influence have accomplished what, in a more circum-scribed sphere of action, would have been impossible."[76]

Some of the most powerful advocates of Victorian motherhood were childless. Like Catherine Beecher, Lydia Marie Child was one of the mid-dle-class reformers who advocated new child-rearing principles. In 1828, at age twenty-six, she married against her parents' wishes. Although she never had children, she wrote *The Mother's Book*—an advice manual ded-icated "to American mothers on whose intelligence and discretion the safety and prosperity of our republic so much depend." The advice that Child gave mothers was a far cry from the stern philosophy of her Calvin-ist ancestors: "It is important that children, even when babes, should never be spectators of anger, or any evil passion. They come to us from heaven, with their little souls full of innocence and peace; and, as far as possible, a mother's influence should not interfere with the influence of angels."[77]

Such advice might seem puzzling coming from childless women. But the belief in women's innate maternal potential actually empowered sin-gle and childless women to be active republican mothers in the broader world. Many women realized that they could not do the work they believed was their "calling" if they had children. In most cases, they were right. When sisters Sarah and Angelina Grimke became abolitionists, they were both single. When Angelina married Theodore Weld, her colleague in the reform movement, childbirth and child rearing ruined her health and precluded her participation in the movement. It even inhibited her sister's public activities because Sarah was needed to help in the Weld household. Similarly, the unmarried Susan B. Anthony chided her married comrade in the suffrage movement, Elizabeth Cady Stanton, to free herself from the constant tasks of child rearing so she could participate more fully in the cause.[78]

Singleness was also increasingly respectable for men. With the decline of the man's role as family patriarch in charge of rearing the children, men in the home became breadwinners with much less day-to-day involvement in their children's training. At the same time, nineteenth-century ideas that valued independence and industry made the life of a single man attractive to some. Some men resisted the yoke of matrimony and family life, turning instead to the many clubs, lodges, and taverns that provided an alternative source of comfort and camaraderie. In 1851, Ik Marvel wrote in *Reveries of a Bachelor*, "Shall a man who has been free to chase his fancies over the wide-world, without lett or hindrance, shut himself up to marriage-ship, within four walls called Home, that are to claim him, his time, his trouble, and his tears, thenceforward forever more, without doubts thick, and thick-coming as Smoke?"[79]

Although republican motherhood provided ideological space for childless women to be civic moral guardians, not all single women were motivated by the desire for a more expansive maternal role. Some, like their male peers, embraced the new ideal of independence. Many Americans in the early republic were no doubt familiar with the ideas of the English women's rights radical Mary Wollstonecraft, who wrote, "It is a happy thing . . . to be able to pursue one's own whims, where they lead, without having a husband and half a hundred children at hand to tease and control a poor woman who wishes to be free."[80] If a colonial woman had such a thought, she would dare not express it. But in the nineteenth century, many women actively chose a single life without children. The writer Louisa May Alcott spoke for those "busy, useful, independent spinsters" like herself who chose to be single, "for liberty is a better husband than love to many of us."[81]

Some single women believed that raising children was a distraction from what they considered to be more important work. An unmarried sculptress wrote, "Even if so inclined, an artist has no business to marry. For a man, it may be well enough, but for a woman, on whom the matrimonial duties and cares weigh more heavily, it is a moral wrong, I think, for she must either neglect her profession or her family, becoming neither a good wife and mother nor a good artist." A young woman teaching at a boarding school hardly disguised her disdain when her aunt, who had important responsibilities at the school, became pregnant: "Such scrapes are very inconvenient. I think people might have more consideration than to get into them, when there is such a poor way of getting out, but I suppose . . . they are willing to make sacrifices 'for the sake of replenishing the earth.' Very dubious! They deserve sympathy for their benevolent enterprise."[82]

Singleness became increasingly popular throughout the nineteenth century. The proportion of never-married women increased from 7.3 percent among those born in the 1830s to 11 percent among those born in the decade following the Civil War. Although spinsters faced a negative stigma, a "cult of single blessedness" countered that image with a positive one. Many spinsters considered an active and independent life to be a "higher calling" than marriage. One claimed that "the best women, the brightest women, the noblest women are the very ones to whom [housework] is most irksome." Others sought to avoid the "ordeal," "painful drudgery," "severe anguish" or "appalling suffering" involved in bearing and rearing children. With so many women suffering illness, disability, or even death from the many risks of motherhood, it is no wonder that an increasing number of them would avoid it. As Susan B. Anthony, the unmarried advocate of women's suffrage, sadly remarked to her mother after the death of her cousin in childbirth, "It is rather tough business, is it not Mother?"[83]

As these examples suggest, numerous men and women gladly left the business of "replenishing the earth" to others. Although there were many reasons, then as now, for not getting married, remaining single was one form of reproductive self-determination. Since marriage was almost certain to include childbearing, unless the couple was infertile, singleness represented the earliest large-scale manifestation of voluntary childlessness. Although contraception and abortion within marriage provided other means of reproductive engineering, some people found neither option to their liking. Dozens of utopian communities emerged that offered alternatives to the norm of marriage, sex, and procreation. Most of the nineteenth-century utopian communities were grounded in religious principles, and nearly all of them included experiments in sex and procreation. They also provided opportunities for people who wanted some form of family and community life without the burdens and dangers of childbearing. Because of their visibility and the controversies they sparked, the utopian experiments had an impact far beyond the number of individuals who actually joined them.

Childless in Utopia

For those who wanted families, but did not want children, the Shakers offered an ideal situation: They prohibited sex. The Shakers established celibate communities in which men and women were strictly segregated. Their *Orders Concerning Intercourse Between the Sexes* articulated the rules of celibacy: "The gospel of Christ's Second Appearing, strictly forbids all private union between the two sexes, in any case, place, or under any circumstances, in doors or out." Private talks were not allowed, nor were men and women permitted to be alone together. "Neither should brethren and sisters touch each other unnecessarily." The Shakers prospered in their settlements, providing material security, religious devotion, and familial love for their members. By adopting children, they sustained their communities for many years. Although their numbers declined in the late nineteenth century, the Shakers continued their communities well into the twentieth century.[84]

The Mormons were another religious group that experimented with an alternative to the nuclear family. Among the Mormons, who practiced polygamy in the nineteenth century, plural wives meant that the community would "be fruitful and multiply." According to Mormon law, the justification for the practice was biblical: "Again, let us look at Sarah's peculiar position in regard to Abraham. She understood the whole matter . . . and longed for Abraham to have seed. And when she saw that she was old, and fearing that she should not have the privilege of raising up seed, she gave to Abraham, Hagar. . . . " Plural marriage guaranteed that progeny "may become as numerous as the sand upon the seashore." The presence of multiple wives, however, also meant that some women might have the benefits of marriage without the rigors of childbearing. Some Mormon wives never lived with their husbands, remained childless, and led active lives in the community. One such woman was a childless wife of Brigham Young, Eliza R. Snow, who was an important leader among the Mormons. Other Mormon plural wives, like Ellen Whittaker, never had children but helped to raise those of her co-wives. For an infertile woman like Whittaker, polygamy offered the possibility of child rearing that monogamy precluded.[85]

In terms of reproductive engineering, perhaps the most ambitious utopian experiment was that of the Oneida Perfectionists, under the leadership of John Humphrey Noyes. Noyes was the first to put into practice a eugenic program of selective breeding for the purpose of "improving the race." He established a system of "complex marriage," in which all the men were married to all the women in the community. Outsiders derided the practice as "free love," but members engaged in a rigorously controlled system called "stirpiculture." Intercourse was permitted only by mutual consent and with the requirement of "male continence," which meant that men were not permitted to ejaculate during intercourse. The practice reinforced ideas of male sexual self-control as healthy, while providing contraception. It also contained the radical notion of female sexual pleasure, although the extent to which the system worked in women's favor is still a matter of historical debate. Nevertheless, if a couple wished to have a child, they had to request permission from Noyes, the group's leader, who decided on the basis of eugenic principles whether the couple was worthy of procreating. Any children born in this way were raised communally. As one community member said in defense of the eugenic practice, "Millions are spent upon improving the breed of domestic animals, but men and women permit themselves to be influenced by the most sordid motives, such as position in society or financial considerations, oblivious of their liability to produce either genius or idiocy, health or disease." Under the system of stirpiculture, most of the Oneida Perfectionists remained childless.[86]

For all the idealization of the home and motherhood that permeated Victorian America, most radical reformers were deeply critical of the nuclear family. It is no accident that nearly every utopian community experimented with new sexual, gender, and family arrangements and that many of them explicitly or implicitly endorsed childlessness as a legitimate option. Social reformers outside the religious utopian communities were also critical of the institution of marriage. Many considered it to be exploitative of women, particularly in terms of sex and reproduction. From "free love" advocates like Victoria Woodhull to supporters of temperance and suffrage, reformers called for greater autonomy for women within the home.

One important crusade to emerge from the late-nineteenth-century movement for women's rights was the campaign for "voluntary motherhood." As a precursor to the birth control movement, it called for a single standard of sexual morality based on the female model of chastity. Its proponents argued that sexual intercourse was for procreation only and that women should be able to determine when and how often they would become mothers. The means for this control would be sexual restraint within marriage, and men were expected to cooperate. Along with calls for reform of the divorce laws, the voluntary-motherhood campaign was an effort to empower women within marriage and to elevate motherhood to a higher status. It probably had a greater impact than did the utopian experiments because it conformed to the prevailing gender ideology and contributed to the increasing acceptance of reproductive manipulation and intervention.[87]

The Grim Legacy of Slave Breeding

Infertility treatment, male continence, stirpiculture, plural marriage, singlehood, voluntary motherhood, and the declining birthrate reflected the changing culture of reproduction among middle-class Whites in the nineteenth century. But by far the most ambitious large-scale effort at reproductive manipulation was the experiment in human breeding that took place within slavery. Slave breeding emerged gradually. Slave owners were surprisingly slow to realize the value of slave women's reproductive potential, but by the middle of the eighteenth century, they were aware of the benefits. After Congress outlawed the overseas slave trade in 1807, slave holders realized the profit potential in slave breeding and exploited and manipulated female slaves' sexual relations. The economic value of female slaves depended upon the women's presumed fecundity. If the women were barren, their value decreased and they were likely to be sold away from their families. Most slaves were sold before age 25, so early childbearing was critical. Couples tried to have children quickly, to minimize the chance that they would be sold away from each other.[88]

Slave breeding was a deliberate, systematic practice of reproductive engineering. Within slavery, childless women were extremely vulnerable. One Southerner noted, "Planters command their girls and women (married or unmarried) to have children; and I have known a great many negro girls to be sold off, because they did not have children. A breeding woman is worth from one-sixth to one-fourth more than one that does not breed." Traders advertised female slaves in terms of their procreative potential. An advertisement in the Charleston *Mercury* of May 16, 1838, read: "A GIRL about 20 years of age. . . . She is remarkably strong and healthy.

... She is very prolific in her generating qualities, and affords a rare opportunity for any person who wishes to raise a family of strong and healthy servants. . . . " An auctioneer in New Orleans said, of a pregnant 16-year-old girl who already had an infant, "She'll no doubt be the mother of a great many children . . . and that is a consideration to a purchaser who wants to raise a fine young stock."[89]

Although childlessness rendered slave women vulnerable to the harshest aspects of slavery, some slave women resisted the system by refusing to serve as "breeders." It is difficult to know the extent to which slave women practiced birth control and abortion, although they definitely practiced both. A Georgia physician reported in 1849 that abortion and miscarriage occurred much more frequently among slave women than among free White women. The cause was either the harshness of slave labor or, as the slave owners believed, "the blacks are possessed of a secret by which they destroy the fetus at an early stage of gestation." Physicians were aware of the planters' frequent complaints about the "unnatural tendency in the African female to destroy her offspring. . . . Whole families of women . . . fail to have any children." Another physician said that slave women used "medicine," "violent exercise," and "external and internal manipulation" to achieve abortion.[90]

For those who took the risk, childlessness was an active form of resistance. Slave women exerted as much control over their reproductive lives as they could. One who was sold as "unsound" and barren in 1857 had three children after emancipation. In another case, a slave woman refused to have children because her owner forced her to marry someone she did not like. After she was sold and chose her own partner, she had ten children. Another woman recalled that her mother was forced to remarry when her father was sold away to another plantation. "Mama said she would never marry a man and have children so she married my step-father Trattle Barber, because she knew he had a disease and could not be a father." The knowledge of bringing a slave child into the world, possibly to be sold or abused, must have added to the slave women's ambivalence about having children. Some slave women even killed their children to protect them from the horrors of slavery, but the extent of infanticide is unknown. It is likely that many babies died because of poor health care and nutrition. Infant mortality among slaves was twice as high as among White newborns.[91]

Resisting the breeding system could be extremely dangerous for slave women. One former slave named Rose recounted her futile efforts to thwart her master's designs. When she was sold, "de auction man say . . .

She's never been 'bused and will make de good breeder." Initially, she was grateful to her new master because he bought her with her parents, to keep the family together. But when he forced sixteen-year-old Rose to live with Rufus "'gainst my wants," she refused. Rufus found an unwilling partner when he crawled into her bunk. "'Git out,' I's told him, and I puts de feet 'gainst him and give him a shove and out he go on de floor." When she complained to her mistress, she learned that her master wanted to breed her with Rufus. But she still refused: "Dat night when him come in de cabin, I grabs de poker and sits on de bench and says, 'Git 'way from me, nigger, 'fore I busts yous brains out and stomp on dem.' He say nothin' and git out."

But the next day, her master came to Rose and told her, "Woman, I's pay big money for you and I's done dat for de cause I wants you to raise me chillens. I's put yous to live with Rufus for dat purpose. Now, if you doesn't want whippin' at de stake, yous do what I wants." She considered her situation, remembering her master's initial kindness and the danger she now faced: "I thinks 'bout massa buyin' me offen de block and savin' me from bein' sep'rated from my folks and 'bout bein whipped at de stake. Dere it am. What am I's to do? So I 'cides to do as de massa wish and so I yields." Later, after emancipation, she stayed on the plantation to sharecrop the land with her parents until they died. But "I never marries, 'cause one 'sperience am 'nough for dis nigger. After what I does for de massa, I's never wants no truck with any man. De Lawd forgive dis cullud woman, but he have to 'scuse me and look for some others for to 'plenish de earth."[92]

By refusing to bear children, some women were able to gain some minimal control over their lives under slavery. But as Rose's story indicates, resisting the system was fraught with risks. Others managed to use their reproductive potential in different ways to take advantage of the system. By becoming pregnant, or even feigning pregnancy, it was possible for some women to mitigate the harshness of slavery. Childbearing gave slave women some privileges and protection because they were likely to receive better care if they produced children. The *American Cotton Planter* urged that slave mothers be "well treated and cared for, and moderately worked . . . their natural increase becomes a source of great profit to their owner. Whatever therefore tends to promote their health and render them prolific is worthy of his [the owner's] attention." Alabama planter John Calhoun explained, "Over-work produces premature old age, bodily deformity and debility of constitution, and checks the increase of females." Pregnant slave women were especially well cared for, and slave women who bore and reared many children were rewarded with extra food or clothes. The rice planter P. C. Weston pronounced that "women with six children alive at any one time are allowed all Saturday to themselves."[93]

Some slave women took advantage of the privileges their reproductive potential would allow. For example, pregnant slave women often claimed to be ill to avoid hard labor in the fields. One slave woman obviously feigned pregnancy for two months, as she stayed in bed eleven months before delivering her child. Childless slave women could not get these privileges and were likely to have a much harder life. Nevertheless, having children did not always mitigate the harshness of slavery and sometimes even made it worse, since children were frequently sold away from their parents. As one slave wrote to her husband in a rare surviving letter between slaves, "I write you a letter to let you know my distress my master has sold albert to a trader on Monday court day and myself and other child is for sale also . . . a man buy the name of brady bought albert and is gone I don't know where. . . . I am quite heartsick."[94]

The harsh conditions of slavery also made childbearing more grueling for slaves, even with privileges and better treatment. One Southern mistress, Frances Anne Kemble, was sympathetic to the plight of the women slaves on her plantation. She noted in her journal that a group of pregnant women came to

> entreat of me to have the sentence (what else can I call it?) modified which condemns them to resume their labor of hoeing in the fields three weeks after their confinement. Their principal spokeswoman . . . appealed to my own experience; and while she spoke of my babies, and my carefully tended, delicately nursed, and tenderly watched confinement and convalescence, and implored me to have a kind of labor given to them less exhausting during the month after their confinement, I held the table before me so hard in order not to cry that I think my fingers ought to have left a mark on it.[95]

But there was nothing she could do to help them, because her husband was intent upon maximizing production in the fields.

Race and Worthy Parents

After slavery ended, White Americans no longer had a stake in the high fertility of Black women, and the birthrate of Blacks began to decline, along with that of Whites. As the nation's population became increasingly diverse, largely as a result of the huge influx of immigrants from southern and east-ern Europe, Anglo-Saxon Protestant reformers became alarmed at the rela-tively low birthrate of their own kind. They considered immigrants, Black people, and Native Americans to be "unfit" to bear and rear the nation's future citizens and the high fertility of these groups a danger to "the race."

Early genetic theories of fitness, based largely, though loosely, on the work of Charles Darwin, competed with widely held beliefs that even the children of "inferior" peoples might be properly reared to make a contribution to society. As a result, the reformers looked for opportunities to remove chil-dren from what they considered to be the evil influences of unworthy par-ents and raise them according to middle-class Victorian values. In tune with these dubious child-saving strategies, many poor immigrant families lost their children to adoption agencies, which turned over these families' off-spring to affluent childless couples or sent them to rural areas, where they would be removed from the allegedly corrupting influences of the city.

The most blatant example of the racial and ethnic criteria for "parental worthiness" was the government's wholesale removal of Native American children from their parents, all of whom were deemed "unworthy" by virtue of their tribal cultures. From the late nineteenth century well into the twen-tieth, agents of the U.S. Government invited, cajoled, and even kidnapped Native American children and placed them in federally funded schools, where they would be "civilized." These schools required the children to cut their hair; wear mainstream, middle-class clothing; and speak English. Prac-ticing tribal religion or speaking Native American languages was forbidden and harshly punished. Often children were kept from their parents and com-munities for years at a time; many died from the harsh and unhealthy condi-tions at the schools, never seeing their parents again.[96] The removal of Native American children from their parents and the transfer of poor immi-grant children to middle-class Protestant couples are examples of the power of mainstream social institutions to determine who would be parents and who would not.

Backdrop to the Twentieth Century

The public and private stakes in reproduction changed dramatically from the early days of colonial settlement to the end of the nineteenth century. In the preindustrial era, economic and demographic survival depended upon high fertility. Childlessness was a misfortune for the individual as well as the community, but there was little for barren women to do other than pray, accept their fate, and participate in communal productive and child-rearing endeavors. Informal child-sharing arrangements provided both for the care of orphans and for the needs of childless households. These seventeenth- and eighteenth-century practices declined in the early national period, especially in the commercial towns and cities, where the importance of children shifted from quantity to quality. Childlessness became a new kind of problem in the nineteenth century, when personal happiness, as well as the future of the citizenry, depended upon the bearing and rearing of carefully nurtured offspring. Now the childless could turn not only to prayer, but to medicine or the law in their efforts to bear or adopt children.

The many experiments in reproductive manipulation that emerged in the nineteenth century represent an unprecedented public intervention into private procreative behavior. Driving much of the experimentation was a powerful belief in progress, bolstered by a new faith in science and the professionalization of medicine. As American society became increasingly diverse, social reformers tried to regulate access to parenthood. In this atmosphere, childlessness among the "worthy" became a matter not only of personal concern, but of political consequence. In the years ahead, all the tools and theories of reproductive engineering would be marshaled to enable and encourage the "best stock" to procreate. Voluntary childlessness would be met with increasing suspicion. Childless Americans who were deemed worthy of parenthood would find the institutions of society at their service. If they were judged unworthy, however, they might find their road to reproductive self-determination blocked. On the eve of the twentieth century, reproductive manipulation was already woven into the fabric of social and institutional life. From this point on, childlessness would take on new public, as well as private, meaning.

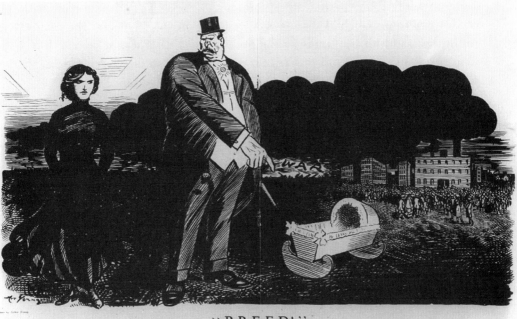

"BREED!"

"Breed!" by Arthur Young: A radical protest against the eugenics campaign, from *The Masses*, December 1915. *(Courtesy of the Tamiment Institute Library, New York University)*

CHAPTER 2

The "Race Suicide" Panic: Eugenics and the Pressure to Procreate

★☆

When home ties are loosened; when men and women cease to regard a worthy family life . . . as the life best worth living; then evil days for the commonwealth are at hand. There are regions in our own land, and classes of our population, where the birth rate has sunk below the death rate. Surely it should need no demonstration to show that wilful sterility is, from the standpoint of the nation, from the standpoint of the human race, the one sin for which the penalty is national death, race death; a sin for which there is no atonement; a sin which is the more dreadful exactly in proportion as the men and women guilty thereof are in other respects, in character, and bodily and mental powers, those whom for the sake of the state it would be well to see the fathers and mothers of many healthy children, well brought up in homes made happy by their presence. No man, no woman, can shirk the primary duties of life, whether for love of ease and pleasure, or for any other cause, and retain his or her self-respect.

— President Theodore Roosevelt, "Sixth Annual Message to Congress," December 3, 1903

Now, gentlemen, You Who Rule Us, we are your "wage slaves," my husband and I. . . . You can refuse us any certainty of work, wages or provision for old age. We cannot help ourselves. But there is one thing you cannot do. You cannot use me to breed food for your factories.

— Anonymous childless working-class woman, the *Independent*, April 1907

I n 1903, the president of the United States placed reproduction at the center of the national reform agenda when he announced that Americans were committing "race suicide." Theodore Roosevelt's worries had nothing to do with the declining population in the country, for indeed, the population was increasing. The problem was that the increase was coming from the "wrong" sources: immigrants pouring into the nation and then having more children than the American-born middle class. Although Roosevelt was not the first to warn against race suicide, he helped to fuel a powerful eugenics movement, the first systematic and large-scale crusade to achieve reproductive engineering in the United States. Unlike the individual efforts of Victorians to control their fertility and the various small-scale experiments in human breeding that emerged in the nineteenth century, the eugenics movement of the early twentieth century resulted in political, institutional, medical, and legislative measures that encouraged some Americans to become parents but prevented others from doing so. As part of their campaign, crusaders for eugenics launched the first major attack against the childless, who, in President Roosevelt's words, were shirking their duty to the nation through "wilful sterility." While urging the "best stock" of Americans to procreate, Roosevelt vilified those who avoided procreation as "criminal against the race . . . the object of contemptuous abhorrence by healthy people." Directing his remarks to female citizens, he compared women's reproductive obligation to the noble male sacrifice of military service and condemned the "viciousness, coldness, shallow-heartedness" of any woman who avoided "her duty."[1]

Roosevelt's military metaphors reflect the sentiments of many reformers at the turn of the century who waged war against internal enemies. The increasing diversity of American society, along with major changes taking place in the rapidly industrializing and urbanizing cities, filled many middle-class Americans with alarm. Vice zones and amusement centers drew more and more young White Americans into public spaces, where they mingled with the others of the opposite sex and of different classes and races. Women began to participate in a "moral revolution" that prompted at least one observer to proclaim that "sex o'clock" had struck in America. Many feared that if foreigners outnumbered "old stock" Americans, the social fabric of democracy would unravel and the nation would collapse. For those who held these views, childless Anglo-Saxons were as dangerous to "the race" as were the prolific immigrants.

Nearly all eugenicists considered childlessness, whether voluntary or involuntary, to be caused by bad decisions. If not willfully chosen, childlessness was presumably the result of unhealthy activities that caused sterility or bad choices of spouses or sexual partners. For women, dysgenic activities included almost anything that challenged time-honored gender arrangements, such as remaining single, pursuing jobs or careers, going to college, crusading for women's rights, using birth control, having abortions, or participating in the moral revolution. Reformers also blamed men for the increase in childlessness, noting the epidemic of venereal disease and the large number of men and women who were rendered sterile by gonorrheal infection. Observers considered sexual degeneracy to be one of several symptoms of the decline of American manhood. Roosevelt advocated the "strenuous life" for men who were becoming "soft." The rise of large organizations that employed an increasing number of middle-class men undercut the entrepreneurial tradition and struck a blow to masculine independence. The declining Anglo-Saxon birthrate and the increase in childlessness reinforced fears that the American middle class was losing both its vitality and its hegemony.

Although White Anglo-Saxon Protestants still controlled most of the major institutions in the society, many newcomers clearly challenged their ability to infuse urban society with their moral values and codes of behavior. In a widespread xenophobic panic, they blamed the newcomers for what they perceived as problems in their midst: new amusements, vice districts, moral experimentation, class and racial mixing, and challenges to Victorian gender roles. Some also blamed the immigrants for the poverty, overcrowding, and absence of sanitation they suffered, even though these problems resulted from the lack of decent jobs and housing. Rather than address these concerns at the level of social policy by providing more opportunities for economic security, many reformers looked to the family to solve the nation's woes. It was a pattern that would repeat itself many times throughout the twentieth century.

Eugenics offered an appealing solution for many who worried about race suicide. Turn-of-the-century eugenic theorists correctly observed that the American birthrate had been declining steadily for more than a century and that the birthrate among immigrant women was twice that of American-born women. To make matters worse, many potential "worthy" mothers were not even getting married. The rate of lifelong singleness among women peaked at 10 percent in the late nineteenth century before declining to half that level by 1965. At the same time, the proportion of childless American-born wives was increasing, from 14 percent in 1910 to 21 percent in 1940. Among foreign-born wives, the rates of childlessness were much lower: rising from 11 percent in 1910 to only 13 percent in 1940. Worse still, according to the eugenicists, the most highly educated groups in the society appeared to be reproducing at the lowest rate. A physician writing in the *Ladies Home Journal* warned that "Race Suicide among the rich is only one phase of the diminishing birth rate."[2]

Those who were concerned about the low birthrate offered little tangible help to struggling families. Rather, they resorted to gimmicks to encourage high-quality procreation. Biologist Charles B. Davenport, a follower of Mendel's theories of inheritance, became the nation's leading eugenicist. As director of the Eugenic Record Office in Cold Spring Harbor, New York, he raised large sums of money that funded scholarships for scientists who came to study heredity there. In an effort to involve ordinary citizens in the eugenic project, he invited people to fill out "Records of Family Traits" and send them to his center to register their family pedigrees. Thousands of couples responded.[3]

At the same time, the American Eugenics Society sponsored Better Babies and Fitter Families contests at state fairs around the country, starting at the Kansas Free Fair in Topeka in 1920. Any healthy family could enter these "human stock" competitions if it had evidence of medical examinations, Wassermann tests, psychiatric assessments, and intelligence tests, along with a eugenic family history. An exhibit at a Philadelphia fair read, "How long are we Americans to be so careful for the pedigree of our pigs and chickens and cattle—and then leave the *ancestry of our children* to chance or to 'blind' sentiment?" The society also sponsored a contest with a $1,000 prize for the best essay on the causes of the decline in "Nordic" fertility.[4]

With publicity stunts such as these, the American Eugenics Society hoped to encourage those with pride in their heritage to marry carefully selected mates and have plenty of children. In an effort to encourage reproductive impulses among college-educated women at a time when half the graduates of women's colleges remained single, *Good Housekeeping* published a two-page photograph captioned "A College Baby Crop" depicting thirty-nine well-dressed alumnae of Pennsylvania State College and their babies. Others hoped that coeducation would "urge the good to marry" and procreate.[5] Even the U.S. government got into the act. In what may have been the most powerful symbolic response to the sagging enthusiasm for motherhood, a 1914 joint resolution of Congress established Mother's Day "as a public expression of our love and reverence for the mothers of our country."[6] But none of these gimmicks was effective in turning around the declining birthrate, and eugenicists continued to wring their hands over the fate of "the race."

Eugenics and Donor Insemination

Emboldened by the enthusiasm for eugenics and the panic over race suicide, Dr. Addison Davis Hard decided to reveal an experiment conducted as
a cure for infertility that he had kept secret for over two decades. Actually,
the experiment did not "cure" infertility, but it did enable a childless Anglo-
Saxon wife to bear a child. The 1909 publication of Hard's article in the
Medical World unleashed the first of what would become many raging controversies over the highly charged subject of "artificial reproduction." Hard
wrote that he had witnessed the first human conception by a procedure he
called "artificial impregnation."[7] In 1884, when he was a medical student, an
affluent infertile couple sought out the assistance of one of Philadelphia's
most prominent physicians, William Pancoast. The forty-one-year-old husband was a successful merchant, and his thirty-one-year-old wife was from a
wealthy Quaker family—traits that qualified them as "worthy" of parenthood according to prevailing eugenic ideas.

Initially, Pancoast found no apparent cause for the couple's difficulty.
Since the husband did not suffer from impotence, he was presumed to be
fertile, so Pancoast decided to examine the wife first. Victorian delicacy did
not prevent him and his six students from conducting a thorough examination. Hard, who was among the students present, described the examination
as "very complete, almost as perfect as an army examination." Pancoast
found no physiological impediments to impregnation. He also claimed that
the examination provided evidence to prove a widely held theory about
reproduction: that female orgasm facilitated conception. Although it is not
clear precisely how the examination proved this theory, Hard noted that
"during this examination was discovered for the first time, as far as I know,
the suction function of the uterus, which takes place during orgasm."[8]

Since the examination revealed no physiological abnormality, the woman
was spared the treatments for sterility available at the time, such as surgery,
bleeding of the cervix with leeches, the application of electricity, and the use
of various mechanical appliances to rearrange the reproductive organs. She
was also spared the typical behavioral prescriptions, such as the regime recommended by one contemporary physician: infrequent coitus, pure air, qui-
etude of mind, temperance in food, drink, and sleep, and the "cultivation of
correct habits of mind and body."[9] But she was not spared the indignities of
the examination. Next Pancoast examined her husband and found no physical defect. But when he studied the semen under the microscope, he found
that it contained absolutely no sperm. Pancoast informed the man of his

findings and suggested that the problem probably was the result of an early bout of gonorrhea, contracted in his youth. Pancoast then began a course of treatment that he assumed would remedy the problem.

After two months of treatment, however, the husband showed no sign of improvement. At this point, one of the students in the class allegedly remarked jokingly that "the only solution of this problem is to call in the hired man." Although made in jest, the remark gave Pancoast an idea that led to an unusual plan of action. Pancoast anesthetized the woman with chloroform. While she was unconscious, he selected the "best-looking member of the class" to provide semen for the experiment. Thus began a long tradition of using medical students as sperm donors for artificial insemination. Using a rubber syringe, Pancoast inserted the semen of the student into the woman's uterus.

Pancoast was undoubtedly familiar with the work of J. Marion Sims, who, in the mid-nineteenth century, was apparently among the first to use an "impregnator" tool, a syringe device, to facilitate conception. In cases in which sperm did not travel adequately to fertilize the egg, Sims used the tool to deposit the semen of the husband directly into the uterus of the wife. It was not a successful form of treatment. Sims used the syringe fifty-five times, but only one pregnancy resulted, so he ultimately gave up the practice. But other physicians continued to experiment with the technique. For example, according to the historian Victoria Bissell Brown, Harry Haldeman, the physician-husband of Alice Addams Haldeman, the sister of the reformer Jane Addams, may well have artificially inseminated his wife with his own semen; they had been married for a decade before she finally became pregnant in the late 1880s.[10] Pancoast's novel innovation was the use of a sperm donor. As it turned out, the woman became pregnant.

At this point, according to Hard, Pancoast became a bit nervous. He had neither asked permission nor even informed the woman or her husband of the procedure before doing it, and now the woman was expecting a child. Reluctantly, Pancoast informed the husband (although not the wife) of what he had done. Fortunately for Pancoast, the man was pleased. His only request was for absolute secrecy, so that nobody should ever know what happened, not even his wife. He preferred that she should remain ignorant of his early bout of gonorrhea, as well as the method of her impregnation. Pancoast agreed and pledged the six students who witnessed the event to absolute secrecy.

Nine months later, the woman gave birth to a healthy son, who grew up to follow in his father's footsteps. By age twenty-five, the son had moved to New York and become a successful businessman. Nobody ever knew about

the peculiar means of his conception. But Hard—most likely the sperm donor himself—maintained a lifelong interest in the case. Twenty-five years after the child's birth, Pancoast was no longer alive, and Hard was a general practitioner in Marshall, Minnesota. To satisfy his curiosity, he traveled to New York to see the young man (whom in all likelihood he had sired) and "shook his hand."

When Hard finally disclosed the event in his 1909 article, he did so to advocate artificial insemination not so much as a miracle treatment for infertile couples, but rather as a tool for eugenic reproduction and a cure for race suicide. He wrote:

> Artificial impregnation offers valuable advantages. . . . Persons of the worst possible promise of good and healthy offspring are being lawfully united in marriage every day. Marriage is a proposition which is not submitted to good judgement or even common sense, as a rule. . . . Artificial impregnation by carefully selected seed, alone will solve the problem. [It should] become recognized as a race-uplifting procedure.

The case was the first recorded artificial insemination by donor (AID) in the United States, but it was not necessarily the first that occurred. Artificial impregnation required no complicated medical technology or specialized expertise, only a rubber syringe and a willing donor. Virtually anyone could do it, and there is no way to be sure that it had not been done in the past without medical intervention. Yet, Hard claimed the procedure as a medical innovation, and the offspring born by this method were the first to acquire the misnomer "test-tube babies." For nearly a century after Pancoast performed his experiment, artificial insemination, as it came to be called, remained largely under the control of the medical profession. AID performed by physicians offered the advantages of confidentiality, screening of donors, and anonymity that many couples desired. But this first published account emphasized the advantages to society over the advantages to infertile couples.

The reaction to Hard's article ranged from outrage to applause. The introduction of the sperm donor into the process of reproduction was intriguing to eugenicists and appalling to moralists. The ensuing controversy revealed the wide range of opinions within the medical profession at that time. Most of the physicians who responded to the article were horrified. One refused to believe that a respected physician would do such a thing and called the story a

chimera of a disordered brain. . . . Dr. Pancoast was a gentleman, and would not countenance the raping of a patient under anesthetic. . . . In the first place it is an impossible story that a wealthy merchant should present himself and wife for a "private and confidential examination," with a "section of the class" of medical students to "assist." The story of taking the gentleman's seminal fluid to be examined by the students to see if it contained any "spermatozooans" is a flight of fancy. . . . Accusing the professor of raping his patient with the semen of "the best looking member of the class," a preposterous crime, is certainly going a little.

Some agreed that the event was "ridiculously criminal," not because of the syringe but because of the donor. "The deed of your professor was neither honest nor moral," wrote another, shocked by the deception perpetrated on the woman. "It would have been a thousand fold better and more honorable had your professor seduced that woman while conscious; or, if you please, just as honorable had he had intercourse with her while unconscious."

Others, however, responded with enthusiasm and paid scant attention to the dishonest treatment of the wife. One had "personally used the impregnator with success on mares that were apparently steril (sic)" with good results and claimed that if "from a commercial standpoint, it be a paying process in the animal kingdom, why would not its influence be many times greater in the human family?" Another wrote that although "it was bad taste to tell this story on a dead confrere," he endorsed the procedure: "If Dr. Pancoast had permission from the woman in the first place and the husband in the second place, then whose biznes (sic) is it to find fault?" Of course, no such permission was requested or granted.[11]

After months of controversy, Hard finally responded to the many letters his article had sparked. He backed off from his strident advocacy of artificial insemination by donor.

> Bless my critics. I would not wish to own a child that was bred with a hard-rubber syringe. And I do not care to think that my child bears toward the millennium no traces of his father's personality, humble tho it be. I am a firm disciple of impregnation in the good old orthodox manner, with all its esthetic (sic) features and risks of evil.[12]

The reactions to Hard's article reveal a great deal about the social tensions in American society at that time. When Hard published his account in the *Medical World*, the controversy remained within the medical commu-

nity. Public discussion of donor insemination did not emerge until the 1930s, when its use became more common. In 1909, artificial impregnation pleased those physicians who believed that science could and should further the goal of increasing the "best" class of people. But others objected to interfering with the "natural" means of reproduction and were offended by the challenge to traditional beliefs about marriage, the family, sex, and reproduction. They found the idea of artificial insemination socially repugnant, religiously unacceptable, and morally outrageous. The debate foreshadowed many that would surround later discussions of birth control, abortion, and various forms of artificial reproduction.

Most striking about the controversy, however, is that few physicians who responded expressed concern for the deceived woman. Twenty-five years had passed since the event took place, years of tremendous agitation in the area of women's rights. Except for the writer who mistakenly assumed that the couple had granted permission for the procedure and the other who likened the event to rape, no other respondent made reference to the enormous deception perpetrated on the wife. After the fact, the physician, the husband, and the students who witnessed the insemination all conspired to keep the woman ignorant of what happened. In the 1909 controversy, the respondents paid a great deal of attention to the matter of the donor and the rubber syringe, but little to the woman who had been so impregnated.

Women's Rights and Maternal Duties

At a time when women's rights were at the top of the reform agenda, this neglect seems peculiar. The woman in the story seems to have been nothing more than a vessel of propagation—an idea that even the Victorians rejected. At the same time, however, neither the Victorians nor the Progressives had abandoned the notion that women's most exalted role in life was motherhood. After all, the woman in question came to the physician for medical assistance because she wanted a child, and bore a child as a result of the treatment she received. Although she never knew the source of her impregnation, she was no doubt happy to become a mother. Most feminists at the time would have been appalled at the means, but would have cheered the outcome: motherhood. Even the most radical advocates of women's rights argued that motherhood conferred upon women the moral superiority that was the foundation of their public activism.

Charlotte Perkins Gilman, a socialist and a feminist, advocated collectivized housework and child care to enable women to pursue their professional lives. Although she bore only one child herself, she believed that it was women's "patriotic duty" to bear children and endorsed eugenic principles:

> The business of the female, as such, is not only the reproduction but the improvement of species. . . . It is her duty to bear children. . . . This means citizenship in the highest sense. If her race is decreasing, all patriotic duty should call for a higher birth rate. . . . Biologically, politically, economically and ethically, women should face their special work of regulating and improving the race. An active sense of social motherhood is desperately needed among the women of today, if we are to put a stop to war, to cease producing defectives, and to begin the conscious improvement of our stock.[13]

Other feminist activists shared these sentiments. In a book dedicated to Theodore Roosevelt, "who first aroused the nation to the danger of 'race suicide,'" the feminist, trade unionist, and peace activist Lydia Kingsmill Commander called upon "intelligent Americans" to have six children each because the American nation "is not a handful of loosely united, crude savages, content to hunt and fish, war with neighboring tribes." She advocated governmental incentives to encourage the better classes to procreate, instead of "soldiers, imbeciles, and cripples, three classes with which we might well dispense."[14]

Appealing to the Progressives' faith in science and the potential for social improvement, the eugenics movement caught on among radicals and conservatives alike. The call to elevate motherhood resonated with White middle-class feminists, beginning in the nineteenth century. As the historian Linda Gordon noted, "This concern with eugenics was characteristic of nearly all feminists in the late nineteenth century."[15] Some of the most vigorous supporters of positive eugenics were social radicals like Victoria Woodhull, presidential candidate in 1872. Woodhull was among the Victorian proponents of "free love" and "voluntary motherhood" who advocated control over reproduction. Although they opposed contraception and abortion and believed instead in sexual control, they argued that women should be the ones to decide when and how many children should be born. But they did not approve of separating reproduction from sexual intercourse. Later activists, including the birth control pioneer Margaret Sanger and the anarchist Emma Goldman, encouraged that separation, advocating sexual pleasure for its own sake. They also called for better health care and a reduction in maternal and infant mortality. Overall, they honored and exalted motherhood in the name of providing benefits to women as mothers who were responsible for the improvement of the "race."[16]

Hard's arguments in favor of artificial impregnation were not necessarily incompatible with those of women's rights advocates and sex radicals who supported "artificial" birth control. Although feminists would have opposed vehemently the deception perpetrated on the woman in Pancoast's case, they might have agreed that any procedure that enabled an involuntarily childless woman of the "best stock" to become a mother was in the woman's, as well as society's, best interests.

Taken to its logical conclusion, however, voluntary motherhood and the rights of women led to another, more dangerous right: the right of a woman not to be a mother at all. It was this concern that struck panic in the eugenic crusaders and their many allies at the time. Even noted women reformers like Gilman argued that motherhood was a duty central to women's identity. Yet there was some irony in these exhortations. These eugenic advocates—mostly White, affluent, and well educated—did not necessarily practice what they preached. Many were single, and those who were married rarely had large families. Their own social activism in some ways absolved them of the requirement to procreate abundantly, since they were furthering the cause of motherhood on a societal rather than a personal level, as their Victorian predecessors had done. They realized, as did many of their less-famous sisters, that it was virtually impossible to combine any sort of work outside the home with motherhood.

To make matters worse for the eugenicists, many of the nation's most famous and respected women were unmarried and therefore childless. Among the women listed in *Who's Who in America* of 1913–14, few had children.[17] Women like Jane Addams and other professional reformers never married and lived their lives with other women, often in deeply committed "Boston marriages." A few single professional women, like the prison reformer Miriam Van Waters, adopted children, giving further evidence of their charitable and nurturing natures. But most did not have children. These women were childless because they opted not to marry, not because they refused to have children. Many were considered maternal, even though they were not mothers themselves. If these women could be motherly without bearing children, so might others who looked up to them as role models. But when ordinary women made similar choices, they set off a national alarm.[18]

Although single women were numerous and visible, over 90 percent of all women married. It was the childless wives who bore the brunt of the eugenic crusaders' ire. Some of these women eagerly wanted children, but others were content without them. These women were not flocking to physicians to cure their sterility. Hard suggested that artificial impregnation would help to "improve the race" by enabling worthy women to conceive, but the procedure was useless if the childless did not seek help. Before medical intervention could be effective, reluctant potential parents had to be persuaded that having children was a good idea. As the eugenic movement gained momentum, the popular press suddenly exhorted White Anglo-Saxon women to have babies and scorned those who did not.

Race, Class, and Eugenic Reform

The class and racial dimensions of the race-suicide panic were evident from the outset. Dark, lusty outsiders, as well as "restless" White women, were equally vilified. According to George B. H. Swayze, a contemporary obstetrician,

> The patriotic enterprise of recruiting [the] American population with the blood of American citizenship is being gradually shifted to the lusty sexual output of foreign breeders. . . . The Jew, the Russian, the Hungarian, the Italian complexion is to-day darkly outshading the Americanized descendants of the English, the Irish, and Scotch, the German and Swede . . . This backward lapse of national progress hinges on the fact that our educated, restless, esthetic American women have preached to womanhood the subtleties of emulating manhood in the guise of worldly spheres, and have developed among the masses an ethical, almost a constitutional reluctance to pregnancy.

Because American women were shirking their duty in their ill-advised efforts to gain equal rights, the nation would soon be overrun by "the unrestricted progeny of the underfed ignorant toilers, the underrated 'mudsill' grade of population, the encroaching offspring of the prolific Negro, of the stoic foreign representatives of recent immigration more and more profusely encumbering our shores." [19]

For the first time ever in the United States, experts from a wide range of fields began to accuse affluent and educated women of deliberately avoiding motherhood and causing a "national decline." G. Stanley Hall, the psychologist and president of Clark University, raised the specter of race and immigration when he pointed to "the yellow and Oriental peril" and warned native-born White women to procreate early and often: "The future belongs to those people who bear the most and best children and bring them to fullest maturity. They will in the end wield all the accumulated resources of civilization, and infertile races will fade before them." One physician writing in 1919 returned to the old myth that education destroys women's reproductive organs and offered prevention as the best cure: "Prevent young girls from over-studying."[20] His opinion had long been supported in the popular press. The *Independent* editorialized:

> The Harvard graduate has on an average seven-tenths of a son, the Vassar graduate one-half of a daughter; and these figures are representative of the entire educated or so-called intellectual class in America. . . . The common belief is that this decline of the birth rate is caused by voluntary prevention, and is attributable to luxury, selfishness, and love of ease. . . . [But in fact] it is very largely a result of sheer physiological failure, an actual loss of reproductive power [that is due to] the substitution of the school for the home as the chief educational institution. . . . It is probably not an exaggeration to say that to the average cost of each girl's education thru [sic] the high school must be added one unborn child.[21]

In 1901, even before President Roosevelt called attention to race suicide, Dr. George Engelmann wrote an article in the *Journal of the American Medical Association* expressing alarm over "The Increasing Sterility of American Women." Noting that the highest rate of sterility was among college graduates, "of whom comparatively few marry, and a large proportion of those who do marry are barren," he claimed that his statistics "clearly show the influence of college work and nerve exhaustion . . . over-pressure in schools." He also blamed the use of contraceptives and abortions: "Too often the young wife enters the sacred bonds with the distinct understanding that she desires no offspring, and does so because of the inconvenience it would give her." He found that 9 percent to 12 percent of "Americans" had conceived but never carried a child to full term, compared to only 3 percent to 6 percent of "foreigners." Claiming that "barrenness, in the large majority of instances, is independent of physical causes," he condemned women who "willingly avoid conception" and concluded that "the main causes are moral; therefore, the treatment does not fall strictly within the sphere of the gynecologist." Nevertheless, physicians should take heed: "This is an important subject, for the lack of fertility has invariably been the precursor of national decline."[22]

Although Engelmann was a physician writing in a medical journal, his views did not represent the entire medical profession. Several physicians responded to Engelmann's article, and many disagreed with him. One agreed that contraceptives were to blame because they fostered "that worst of all vices, marital fornication." But others defended educated women and blamed their husbands: "It is not because these girls have graduated from Vassar that they are sterile. . . . Men contaminate their wives" with venereal disease and render them sterile. Dr. M. K. McCoy wrote that

> college graduates should not be held responsible for the decreasing family. . . . However, the women of America have no encouragement to become mothers. What protection has she or her children? Confronting gonorrhea, the saloon on one side, the brothel on the other, and back of it all the abortionist, it is a wonder that any children are born.[23]

Dr. A. J. Rongy spoke for many eugenic reformers when he denounced the sexual behavior of single young men who consorted with lower-class women and prostitutes. The "average youth finds a ready outlet for his sexual desires, bringing back to his future home and wife the affliction which such acts frequently entail." The "ready outlet" for the wayward youth's sexual desires was rarely his future wife. Claims about the spread of venereal disease were alarming. One study in 1914 estimated that half the men in the country had contracted gonorrhea, and most observers blamed prostitution and "promiscuity" for the epidemic. Rongy asserted that "the greatest single factor in the production of sterility is gonorrhea and its complications. . . . It is absolutely certain that nearly 60 percent of women who suffer from primary sterility give evidence of gonorrheal infection." Rongy also pointed to other vices, including both male and female masturbation. Female masturbators "are not amenable to treatment and the prognosis is very poor, notwithstanding any effort at a cure. They are usually very anemic, in poor health, highly nervous, and very unsatisfactory subjects for treatment." They suffer from "cirrhosis of the ovaries. . . . The vaginal vault presented a hard shriveled appearance."[24]

There is no doubt that the spread of venereal disease was a major cause of sterility in these years, especially because antibiotics were not yet available. In their efforts to combat the problem at the source, physicians warned men of the dangers of promiscuity and prostitution. Although men took the blame for sterility caused by venereal disease, women continued to be held responsible for much of the childlessness, allegedly because of their reluctance to become mothers. Education, careers, contraception, and abortion were presumably the follies that led to childlessness. Physicians believed that much of the sterility was due to "failures of volition" in American women.[25]

The Infertile

There were, of course, many women and men who were involuntarily childless. Eugenic reformers, mostly White and middle-class themselves, were primarily concerned with the fertility of their own group. Few realized that the most alarming rate of sterility was among Black Americans, and it was getting worse. Childlessness rose among ever-married Black women from 16 percent in 1910 to 26 percent in 1940. By the mid-1940s, the rate was more than twice as high for Black women as for White women, owing to poverty, disease, and poor health care.[26] Women's rights activists, who were campaigning for measures that would improve maternal and child health, worried about poor women who were living in rural areas without access to adequate health care. But they were unable to achieve any substantial legislation that would have addressed the problem. Most eugenicists were unconcerned with infertility among the poor. They were much more worried about the fact that the overall birthrate of Black women, along with other people of color and immigrants, was higher than that of Anglo-Saxons.[27]

Given the demographics of fertility, eugenic-minded physicians began to consider that infertility among affluent American-born Whites was one of the factors that was contributing to race suicide. Their social concerns converged with their genuine interest in helping their childless patients achieve parenthood. Even practitioners who believed that the trouble resulted from some early and unwise folly, such as the use of contraceptives or abortion, hoped to restore their patients' fertility. As one physician explained, it was "the duty of the physician to persist" in treating any woman who had avoided pregnancy in the past, provided she "relented of . . . the nefarious practices of [her] early married years," gave up "her selfish life of egotism, and with the best instincts of woman aroused now longs for the joys of motherhood."[28]

Then as now, however, infertility treatment was an imperfect art. In the early twentieth century, few effective cures were available. The ovarian cycle was not plotted until the 1920s, and it was only in the 1930s that it

was generally understood by physicians in the United States. Hard's pro-
posal for artificial insemination with donor semen, which might cure
childlessness although it did not cure infertility, did not catch on until
the 1930s.[29] Physicians did everything in their power to help their
patients, but the most common treatment remained surgery, which had a
low rate of success and a high risk of complications. Most surgeries were
attempts to open passages that were presumed to be blocked. Physicians
tried many different surgical remedies, from reshaping the cervix to ovarian transplants.[30]

Women remained the focus of attention in the treatment of infertility,
even though by the 1920s the function of sperm was well understood. In
what would become a common refrain among specialists in reproductive
medicine, one physician reminded his colleagues, "In practice, it must
not be forgotten that the fertility of the husband should always be ascer-
tained at the outset and certainly before any operative treatment is
undertaken" on the wife.[31] According to another, "There is still, I am sorry
to say, a tendency on the part of many general practitioners to recommend a little 'stretching and scraping' to every disappointed bride who
consults them."[32]

Some practitioners began to question the value of surgery, even though
few other treatment methods were available. In 1924, one physician
bemoaned the fact that "recent literature offers little that is new concerning the causes or treatment of sterility in women." He found the lack of
progress distressing, not only because of the medical problem that needed
attention, but because of the costs of infertility to society:

> The subject of increasing sterility among highly civilized peoples has now
> become so important as to be regarded as a sociological problem of the
> first order. Throughout the world the birth rate appears to be in direct
> inverse ratio to the material prosperity and intellectual advancement of
> the races under consideration, so that it is now estimated that among the
> foremost peoples of the earth one marriage in every ten is childless.[33]

Even though there were few reliable cures for sterility, both the public
and private stakes in childlessness were evident. In 1925, for example, in
response to a desperate childless man who was hoping for "the wonderful
blessing and joy of parenthood," the editor of *Hygeia* replied, "The question
of having a family is not alone a problem for the individual but also concerns
the nation at large."[34] Another physician echoed, "Probably no question is of

such sociological significance to the gynecologist as that of sterility. Homes are wrecked, lives are sacrificed, and fortunes lost, all because of the inability of a woman to conceive or to successfully bring forth the fruits of her conception."[35]

In spite of the obvious concern of reformers and professionals, the treatment of infertility remained hampered by lingering Victorian reticence and misconceptions about gender and sexuality. While some physicians urged openness about matters of sex and reproduction to serve their patients' needs, others hindered effective treatment by their own attitudes and discomfort with the subject. Dr. Edward Reynolds, writing in the *Journal of the American Medical Association* in 1913, noted that "the physiology of coitus and impregnation have been subjected for obvious reasons to but little direct observation." But he did not advocate openness between physicians and patients: "The discussion of such a subject with women is distasteful and must necessarily be brief." Reynolds argued that moderation and gentleness were the keys to successful procreative sex, defining frequent intercourse or female sexual aggressiveness as "abnormal." He gave an example of an excitable woman who tamed her inappropriate desires for sex and came to accept her husband's gentleness. When her desire lessened to an appropriate level, she conceived. Reynolds's theories about the "appropriate regulation of intercourse" did not represent a consensus among physicians at the time. But his ideas were sufficiently persuasive to reach the pages of the nation's premier medical journal.[36]

In spite of the efforts of many physicians to improve the treatment of infertility, childless couples who turned to them for help in the early years of the century were likely to be disappointed. As Mrs. B. R. G. lamented in *Good Housekeeping* in 1911, "Suppose you want children with all your heart; suppose you are told by physicians there is no physical impediment . . . and still there are no children to bless your union—what are you going to do about it?" Another woman wrote, "There has not been a year of my married life when I would not gladly have welcomed a child."[37] Infertile people like these had few places to turn for advice and help. Adoption was a possibility for some, but as early as 1910 there was a shortage of available infants. The vast majority of children in institutions had relatives who would not allow them to be adopted. There were at least twice as many hopeful parents for each available child, and those who applied for adoption had to pass careful scrutiny to be approved as worthy parents.[38]

Some who wanted children turned to the U.S. Children's Bureau. Mrs. D. O. from New Mexico wrote to the bureau in 1921, "Please send me a medecine and an advice so I can give birth to children. I was married 20 yrs ago, and I have never give birth to children. I never have had a baby nor a miscarriage in all my life and I feel sick always. . . . Please ans as soon as you can. Yours truly." Mrs. E. M. of Indiana wrote in 1925, "I am a strong woman and are 32 years of age and has always wanted children in my home of my own, and hasn't any. I have taken all kinds of medican but have failed to get the kind that would do me any good. And I kindly ask that you advise me what I should do that would be a help to me in that Respict." Mrs. F. S. from Cincinnati wrote remorsefully that she had an abortion because her pregnancy was making her violently ill. "I have regretted the day I ever went to that doctor. . . . Now I am afraid I can never have any more children. My hubby and I are just crazy to have a baby. But I am afraid I cannot, please tell me if I can ever be a mother or not. . . . My only goal in life is to be a mother." The Children's Bureau representative who responded encouraged her to see a "good physician" and added that "nature is usually very kind and she does not always punish by depriving women of children when they have destroyed only one child."

In her letter to the bureau, Mrs. E. B. from Mississippi addressed "Mr. Stork." She asked, "Have you any babies to spare? We won't one. We live at ———. Will you please bring us one? We won't a girl. Bring her and put her on the bed. If you haven't any, please write me and tell me were I can get one." These letters suggest the despair felt by many infertile women in the early decades of the century, as well as the limited resources available to help them. Many of these women lived in remote rural areas where most of the childlessness was the result of infertility. They had little access to medical care. Even if they had, physicians had little to offer the infertile at that time.[39]

The "Shirkers"

Although infertility received relatively little attention outside the medical community, voluntary childlessness became the focus of national concern. Numerous articles in the popular press called upon women to procreate for the national good. Ida M. Tarbell, noted for her muckraking journalism, wrote that the "militant woman" who does "a man's business" finds that "society regards her as one who shirked the task of life, and who, therefore, should not be honored as the woman who has stood up to the *common burden.*" It was "nature's plan" for the "normal woman" to have children. Using a loaded term that implied childlessness, Tarbell insisted that the career woman "must be made to realize the essential *barrenness* of her triumph, its lack of the savor and tang of life . . . the lack of the great adventure of natural living." Harking back to the theme of republican motherhood, she argued that to "make real democrats . . . we must begin with the mother."[40]

Writers like Tarbell appealed to potential parents' sense of duty. As early as the turn of the century, H. C. Potter wrote in *Harper's Monthly Magazine* that "the Founders of the Republic bred great offspring because, though burdened beyond the conception even of modern mothers, the women gave themselves, first of all and before all, to the rearing of their children." At the same time, Potter made a derogatory remark about those who shirked their duty: "We are in danger, some of us, of getting a little too fine for that."[41]

Although most of these articles were geared toward women, who faced the greatest risks and sacrifices, men also had to be convinced to take on the burden of supporting children. E. S. Martin addressed men in a 1904 article in *Harper's Weekly*. Since the rewards of parenthood were few and the sacrifices were great, he offered a classic Victorian answer: Parenthood builds character. Men needed children to give purpose to their lives.

> The natural, ordinary man needs the spur of necessity or strong obligation. . . . Natural man profits by family cares. . . . Children are a mighty incentive to other virtues besides industry and thrift. They have enormous influence on the parental conduct. . . . Only the duty of serving the public can rival [having children] in weight of obligation and in richness of reward. . . . Nor can he do better by society than by leaving behind him worthy and valuable living representatives of his labors on earth.[42]

But such exhortations to men were rare.

Career women and feminists received the lion's share of criticism. Although women's rights activists had actually done a great deal to exalt motherhood, *Living Age* unfairly blamed "the feminist movement over the last thirty years" for "The Refusal to Multiply." The writer nonetheless correctly observed "that the duties and privileges of motherhood and family life are incompatible with the calls of certain careers, and with the temptation to seek an apparently larger sphere of immediate action and influence in the rough and tumble of industrial, social and political life."

Others blamed career women for "the Extinction of the Upper Classes."[43]

These alarmists called upon women to sacrifice for a cause. According to an editorial in the *Independent*:

> The first duty to posterity is to have posterity, and to pass down an improved human race to the succeeding generations. . . . And yet from lack of courage, or from a greed for pleasure or money, a herd of cowardly celibates threatens us with hastening ills where wealth accumulates and men decay. . . . [We must] prove that our nation has a collective will to live. The soldier risks his life for his country. Every true man and woman will have the true soldier spirit, ready to toil or suffer for his country; and his country means the next generation.[44]

But the "true soldier spirit" appeared to be lacking. It is unlikely that an ambivalent woman would be moved to have children by reading that "no woman can really live until she has suffered the pangs of child-birth, and learned the joy of sacrificing herself for the good of her children."[45]

Messages like these were not likely to motivate the childless to procreate. Nevertheless, writers assumed that women had to be convinced to have children. Indeed, many women did need convincing. Even though reformers and professionals in a wide range of fields and across the political spectrum embraced eugenics, it never succeeded as a popular movement. The general public did not rally to the cry. The birthrate continued to decline, and childlessness increased steadily for the first four decades of the century.

The reasons for this decline were many. As the nation urbanized, the advantages of large families dwindled. Increasingly, children were sources of expenditure rather than investments. In the towns and cities where the birthrate declined the fastest, children were rarely economic assets. Middle-class parents normally did not expect their children to work to help support their families, and long years of schooling extended the children's economic dependence. At the same time, many of the reformers who jumped on the eugenic bandwagon also clamored for child labor laws, which effectively cut off a major source of income for many low-income working-class families who depended on the wages of everyone in the family just to survive. So the material incentives for having children shrank just as the reformers tried to persuade American-born couples to have more offspring. These economic pressures intensified as the nation sank into the depression of the 1930s. Given the financial implications of having children, it is not surprising that the birthrate dropped to an all-time low and childlessness rose to an all-time high during that period.[46]

But there were other reasons for the lower birthrate. Especially for women, not having children opened up other possibilities for life's work. Women who worked outside the home faced many obstacles to having children. Not only was child care a difficult problem, but motherhood also excluded women from a number of careers. Teachers, for example, were routinely fired if they became pregnant. These policies were intended to keep mothers home with children, but they often had the opposite effect. Ironically, at the height of the eugenics movement, such policies actually forced some women to remain childless to keep their jobs. These women may have wanted children, but they could not afford to give up their jobs. And teachers were likely to be the educated, middle-class women who the eugenicists hoped would have large families. With such obstacles, there were few material incentives to encourage women to have children. Most of the encouragement came in the form of moral suasion, which did not seem to be particularly effective.

Not only were there few positive incentives for having children, but there were powerful and frightening negative incentives. Maternal death rates were high and rising in the early twentieth century; one out of every thirty American women died in childbirth. The rates for women of color were nearly twice that of White women, and there was no improvement until the 1930s.[47] To risk death and disability to bear a child who would then become a drain on the family's resources and energy may have seemed a heavy price to pay.

Those who tried to counter such negative incentives called upon potential parents to see the material advantages of having children. One strategy was to suggest that children were consumer goods, "investments," rather than expenses:

> What luxury is comparable to the luxury of having all the children that you want? . . . To deny oneself other luxuries in order to raise them is not self-denial at all, but merely an intelligent choice of investment. . . . Let us think of children more as luxuries, and somewhat less as objects of expense.

Although raising children involved "a good deal of drudgery," the effort was worth the reward: "The good times you have had with contemporary playmates . . . do not constitute a very substantial basis for future happiness."[48]

Even in the depth of the depression, there were those who argued that childbearing would ease rather than aggravate economic woes. Louis I. Dublin, vice-president of Metropolitan Life Insurance Company, claimed that babies were good for business: "There are two ways of looking at a baby. One is the sentimental attitude. . . . The other is the practical attitude of businessmen, who see in each newborn child a consumer of automobiles and handkerchiefs, electricity and sugar-cured hams, fountain pens and woolen blankets."[49] But few potential parents resonated to these views.

The Childless Strike Back

The attack upon the childless prompted some nonparents to strike back. The voluntarily childless women and men of the early decades of the century represented the large and quiet underground resistance to the pronatalist cultural elite. In the first public defense of their choice, a few dared to proclaim that being childless was not such a terrible thing. In 1911, an "Old Subscriber" wrote a letter to *Good Housekeeping*, in which she stated, "Without any shame or hesitation . . . I have been married seven years and have deliberately avoided having children. I have seen many women look horrified at such an admission. . . . Then these same women go on to tell of their difficulties in making ends meet." This twenty-eight-year-old wife wrote that her marriage was "a pure love match, an affair of many years' standing, and we did not consider [that] marriage was necessarily for reproduction." Without children, "my husband won't be worried to death how to make ends meet and keep his wife his cheerful, constant companion."[50]

Clearly, this woman treasured her private life and her romantic relationship with her husband. She may have been slightly ahead of her time. By the 1920s, however, popular movies were filled with modern married couples enjoying life together—without children. A new youth culture emerged, focused largely on a young, couple-centered marriage. During this period, the stories, films, and advice about how to achieve a fun-filled, leisure-oriented home that pervaded the popular culture rarely mentioned children.[51] Accordingly, the twenties was a decade of more and younger marriages, but fewer children and higher levels of childlessness. Old Subscriber and her husband fit the new model of the modern couple. In contrast to her happy life, she described the fate of her friends who became young mothers: "One of the dear girls is now resting in her grave after the third child, another looks like an old hag with three," and most ruined their health and their social lives, "trying

to have children on a young man's salary and go out even a very, very little." Unlike these worn and struggling parents, Old Subscriber and her husband were determined to "enjoy each other's companionship."

The letter from Old Subscriber sparked such a barrage of correspondence that *Good Housekeeping* asked author Laura Richards to comment upon the original letter and the many responses to it. Richards was the daughter of Julia Ward Howe, a eugenics-minded feminist who believed that motherhood guaranteed a woman an "unlimited part in the future of her race. . . . She has learned the sweetness of self-sacrifice." Although Howe believed that some women have "a gift and callings" that justify their childlessness on behalf of other contributions to society, it was the selfish women "not yet weaned from the vanity of girlhood" that troubled her: "If this great blessing of maternity shall visit you . . . do not whine at its fatigues and troubles."[52]

Richards echoed her mother's sentiments and condemned the Old Subscriber for her selfishness and vanity. As a mother of seven and a grandmother of several "growing up in strength and beauty," Richards felt sorry for this woman "who so deliberately stultifies her being." Sounding the eugenic alarm, Richards warned, "I might remind her that while she and—I fear— many other intelligent and educated women postpone or refuse motherhood . . . the ignorant, the feeble, the vicious, bring forth their young at Nature's call, and add their thousands yearly to the ranks of the defective and criminal population." Like so many others who called women to motherhood, she used the military analogy: "The woman who refuses child-bearing is as a soldier who skulks in the trenches when the bugle sounds, and sees the army go shouting past him to battle and to victory."

Other respondents chafed at Old Subscriber's disparaging remarks about mothers. A mother of six seethed:

> I can see the "hags" (no true mother could ever have used such a cruel word) develop into happy middle age; and I can see the women . . . who have had the leisure to massage away the wrinkles of expression and to preserve the slender figure of their youth, but who cannot get rid of those little lines of selfishness that persist in settling about the mouth, or of that hard look in the eyes that comes from thwarting the deepest instinct of their natures [and causing] incalculable harm to the whole human race.

One young mother wrote that her marriage was also "a pure love match, and during our ten years of life together, my husband has become more and more of a lover. So I know whereof I speak, when I say that woman does not reach her full stature of womanhood until she becomes a mother." Another wrote that Old Subscriber should "hide her head with shame."

Finally "A Childless Father" wrote, complaining that he was a "home-loving man" whose wife "positively refused to have children." Although she was a "fresh, healthy-looking, gay spirited girl" when they met, she "loved the glare of the ballroom, indulged in a gay life, and her nerves were pretty well shot to pieces when we married. . . . I have often tried to show her the empty coming years, but she will not listen. I have hoped that she would some day soften, but it seems a disappointment." Although the Childless Father apparently kept hoping his wife would change her mind, other men in similar situations divorced their wives. Women who resisted motherhood or who had abortions against their husbands' wishes were judged "guilty" in the divorce court. One such woman was Margaret Linganfield, whose husband Lorimer complained in 1920 that the alluring flapper he had wed refused to have sexual intercourse with him, claiming that she did not want any "dirty little brats around her." The judge was sympathetic to him, and Lorimer was granted a divorce.[53]

Letters against the Old Subscriber continued for a full year. Only one respondent was sympathetic to the cause of voluntary childlessness. As she endured her fourth pregnancy in six years of marriage, she complained bitterly that "pregnancy is one miserable drag of illness. I can afford no help. . . . All this misery, agony, and horror is unnecessary." After each birth she hovered on the edge of death,

> then for several months afterward a slow gathering of strength to go over it all again. If these calamity howlers against race suicide would place their misdirected energies into a worthier channel . . . in order to find an easier path to our crown of motherhood, they would do more good. The increase in the birth rate would be as sudden and complete as the rise of a balloon when the restraining ropes are cut.[54]

Besides the Old Subscriber and her one supporter, there were other voices of protest. Some were more political and offered a radical critique of the politics and economics of reproduction. Arguing that crusaders for eugenics wanted to exploit women's bodies to produce laborers for factories and soldiers for wars, one working-class wife, writing in 1907, gave "A Woman's Reason" for not having children. Profoundly critical of American capitalism, she wrote, "Now, my husband earns $60 a month, the amount of our household expenses. This leaves us nothing for clothes, furniture, medical attendance, carfare, travel, reading matter or amusements, and it leaves us not a cent to save. It is my earnings which cover the latter." After a long and detailed accounting of their earnings and expenses, she asked:

> Can I afford to have a child? I want a child. I want it very much. I have wanted it for years—first, because I love my husband, and, then, because my maternal instincts are strong. . . . My husband and I have talked of that baby; that baby we have never had. We have discussed its possibilities, its education, its future. But we have never dared to have it.

It would be impossible for this woman and her husband to survive if she gave up her job, even temporarily. Like other reformers, socialists, and radicals who called for mothers' pensions, paid maternity leaves, and other supports for parents, she argued:

> Society would have to pay me my salary at least eighteen months if it desired me to bear and rear a child for its benefit. . . . I really think that society would get the worth of its money were it to make me that compensation. My services have commanded a good salary for quite a number of years. Yet a man could do the work I do as well. I ought to be doing something better. But society demands that I incur heavy expenses and heavy loss of income in order to render it a superior service.

This woman's concern was not the low birthrate of the educated elite, but the reproductive habits of the American-born working class. Noting that 12 percent of the people owned 71 percent of the wealth, she pointed out that "the American wage earner is ceasing to have children. There's the rub. The 88 percent of the population in whose hands rests that other 29 percent of the wealth is ceasing to turn out big families, and we begin to hear of race suicide. Our statesmen presume to rebuke American women for not doing their duty." Criticizing the immigrants for having large families, she continued, "Rather than bring children into the world as the women of our foreign quarters do, without one chance or hope for a decent start in life, destined from birth for wage slavery and exploitation or worse, I would commit suicide."

In a stinging retort to eugenicists, she continued, "Are the bodies of women to be regarded merely as baby machines, to supply the losses which civilization creates by its foul mismanagement? If society wants more children let it go save some of those already born before it calls on me for more." She closed with a taunt to the pronatalist elite: "Now, gentlemen, You Who Rule Us, we are your 'wage slaves,' my husband and I. . . . You can refuse us any certainty of work, wages or provision for old age. We cannot help ourselves. But there is one thing you cannot do. You cannot use me to breed food for your factories."[55]

The response to such concerns was feeble, at best. The most that reformers in the field of maternal and infant health could achieve was the Sheppard-Towner Act of 1921, which until its repeal in 1929 provided meager resources for maternal education but no funds for health care or nutrition. Child care centers and parental leaves were not even on the agenda. The only bow to women's economic concerns was the "family wage," which would allegedly enable a man to support his family so his wife and children did not have to work outside the home. Women were never expected to earn a family wage, and the concept actually served to keep women dependent at home or disadvantaged in the workplace. The family wage also remained out of reach for countless working men who were trying to support their families on meager earnings.[56]

Gradually, other voices came forward to challenge the pronatalist sentiments of the eugenic reformers. In 1916, Leta S. Hollingworth, a childless psychologist married to a physician, wrote an article in the *American Journal of Sociology*. She used intellectual arguments to refute the widely held belief that all "normal" women were born with a "maternal instinct." At the time, most experts agreed that "love of offspring is in man a cultivated emotion; in women an instinct. There are women lacking the instinct as there are calves born with two heads, but for the purpose of generalization these exceptions may be ignored."[57] Hollingworth argued that this was a myth: "We should consent to clear our minds of the sentimental conception of motherhood and to look at facts." She noted that children were no longer necessary for economic and demographic survival, quoting Sumner to support her claim:

> Children add to the weight of the struggle for existence of their parents. The relation of parent to child is one of sacrifice. The interests of parents and children are antagonistic. . . . if procreation had not been put under the dominion of great passion, it would have been caused to cease by the burdens it entails.

Writing at the height of the pacifist movement on the eve of the United States' entry into World War I, Hollingworth compared the sacrifices of mothers to those of soldiers. But unlike the eugenicists who glorified them both, she explained that motherhood "means great sacrifice of personal advantage; it involves danger and suffering, and, in a certain percentage of cases, the actual loss of life." Because there is "no verifiable evidence to show that a maternal instinct exists in women of such all-consuming strength and fervor as to impel them voluntarily to seek the pain, danger, and exacting labor involved in maintaining a high birth rate," the "maternal instinct" must be constructed and enforced by "those in control of society" who "invent and employ devices for impelling women to maintain a birth rate sufficient to insure enough increase in the population to offset the wastage of war and disease." If there were such a thing as a maternal instinct that was universal and equally powerful in all women, she asked, then why would there be a need for laws against abortion, birth control, infanticide, and the desertion of infants? Although Hollingworth was one of the few professionals in any field to question the existence of the maternal instinct, her ideas seemed to fit popular sentiment and behavior more closely than did those of the eugenicists. The rate of childlessness continued to climb, reaching an all-time high in the 1920s and 1930s.[58] As an attempt to reverse the declining birthrate among native-born Americans, the eugenics movement was a dismal failure.

The Contented Childless

While some of the childless defended themselves publicly against the pronatalist norms, others simply accepted their fate. And, of course, there were those who wanted children and pursued infertility treatment or adoption, but neither route guaranteed parenthood. Reproductive medicine was still in its infancy, and adoption was difficult. In the Progressive era of the early twentieth century, many reformers brought to their work a more compassionate view of the poor. A number of social service agencies abandoned their earlier practice of removing children from poor families and now tried to keep the families of the "worthy poor" intact. As a result, fewer children were available for adoption; in some places, the demand far exceeded the supply, and the first major "baby shortage" emerged.[59] Under these circumstances, those who were childless did not necessarily expect that medical or social service institutions would enable them to become parents. By the 1920s and 1930s, when childlessness was at an all-time high, many nonparents lived contented lives. Whether they were childless by choice or by circumstance, many discovered that there were advantages to not having children.

In spite of the intense pressures to procreate, childless couples found their circumstances reflected in the popular media of the 1920s and 1930s. The crusaders for eugenics permeated the popular magazines, professional journals, and prescriptive literature, but they did not have a huge impact on Hollywood. In stories of real-life Hollywood couples like Douglas Fairbanks and Mary Pickford or the cinematic dramas of Cecil B. DeMille, fans watched glamorous stars forge happy, modern, childless marriages. Popular movies featured romantic marriages between fun-loving flappers and their youthful, athletic mates in which children rarely appeared.[60] Childless men and women no doubt found validation and reassurance from these genres that life without children need not be empty or unhappy. The stories of a few such women and men indicate that whether they were from the working class or the middle class, infertile or childless by choice, childless Americans between the wars were able to resist or ignore pronatalist pressures.

Thomas Arkle Clark, for example, was involuntarily childless. Writing in 1925 at age sixty-five, he wrote as a member of the Victorian middle class who was looking back at his life from the vantage point of the 1920s. From the moment they married in the late nineteenth century, he and his wife were "both completely sold on the idea of having a good-sized family," but the hoped-for children never arrived. There is no evidence that they sought a cure; they simply accepted the situation. Although they faced "a good deal of pity and condescension" because of their childlessness, Clark insisted that "childless couples need not lead dreary lives." He had worked closely with young people all his life in his capacity as dean of men at the University of Illinois and felt great satisfaction from these relationships. Besides, he observed, there are those who "get really very little comfort or pleasure out of their children." One friend had wonderful children, which made him feel he had "missed something very beautiful and very precious. . . . I could imagine how it would feel to have their soft little arms about my neck, to have their bright curly heads snuggling down against my breast, and their sweet warm lips upon my cheek, and to realize that they were mine—bone of my bone and flesh of my flesh." On the other hand, he had friends with unpleasant children: "Their boy is stupid and lazy . . . a burden and a worry to both his father and mother. The girl is extravagant, disrespectful, extreme in her dress and vulgar in her manners." These children persuaded him that "we have missed nothing but responsibility and sorrow and trouble in not having children like these." Children were "not always a comfort," he concluded.

The visibility of the childless in the 1920s may have encouraged Clark to publish his thoughts on the subject. He listed all the disadvantages of having children: the lack of any guarantee that they would take care of their elderly parents, the intrusions into a peaceful life, the expense, and the toll on a marriage. "Children do not always strengthen the love between husband and wife," he noted. Although his article was intended to help the childless lead full lives and not feel sorry for themselves, it contained another powerful message: There were actual advantages to being childless. "The childless pair growing old together have many compensations for their failure to have children. Having only each other, if true love has brought them together, the lack of children draws them still closer." Clark endorsed the romantic ideal of the companionate marriage that was touted in the popular culture of the 1920s. But he also articulated the Victorian belief that personal fulfillment could be found in civic endeavors, as well as in family life, an idea grounded in the political culture of the nineteenth century:

> Since the responsibilities of home are not so exacting as if there were children in it [childless couples] have had more freedom; they have been able to give more to society, to the church, to the service of others. Having fewer responsibilities in the home, they have been able to assume more in the community. And out of these responsibilities and this service they have found happiness.[61]

Delores Taylor was also involuntarily but not unhappily childless in the 1920s. Younger than Clark, she was born at the end of the nineteenth century and came of age during the height of the eugenics movement. As an American-born woman of the working class, she dutifully tried to have children, but had three miscarriages instead. "I am about as childless as anyone can be," she noted, since she had no nieces or nephews and most of her friends were childless. "So I am not even a proxy aunt." Delores remembered two peers who "were sort of wild; they both married several times and had abortions before and after they were married." Even so, she and her infertile friends "all tried to have children but nature and our bodies didn't cooperate." At first she "felt awful" about it. "It wasn't because of any maternal instinct. I thought having babies was what women were for and it was my duty to reproduce, and I felt guilty." But she did not feel pressured. "Fortunately, my husband didn't care one way or another. Also, none of our parents liked kids so they never ragged us to give them grandchildren."

In the long run, Delores was glad. Writing in 1993 at the age of ninety-nine, she confessed,

I wouldn't admit this to anyone I know because it would sound either selfish or like sour grapes, but now that I'm old, it's a relief to not have children and grandchildren to worry about. I honestly never missed them. . . . We have had an unusually happy marriage and I think it's partly because we've never had to spat over what one of us wanted to do for the kids. . . . I can truthfully say we have never become bored with life or each other.

Delores and her husband both came from the working class, in which they remained all their lives. Her father insisted that she contribute to her own support. "He'd say, 'By god, if you were a boy I'd have you down on the corner selling the *Saturday Evening Post* so you could buy your own shoes.' Then he changed it to 'By god, if you were a boy I'd put you in the Navy.' He'd say, 'A man is a horses ass to tie himself down with kids.'" In her only passing reference to eugenics, she quipped, "Once he called me a horses ass but I didn't dare say anything about genetics. . . . " Her father did teach her many skills, however. "Oddly, I adored him and I was ecstatic when he had me up on the roofs of his rentals helping to put on new roofs. I helped build a garage and I used to paint the rentals." At the same time, "I learned that there are no free rides, and I became very independent."

This independence served her well. "I was willing to work at anything. I labeled bottles in a distillery, worked in a curtain factory and a zipper factory. During the war I got a good job in an electronics plant and was soon made a forelady. It was the only time I ever made any money." She stayed on the job for many years after her marriage, "but I always thought of it as a job not a career. I'm very much the domestic type, and, of course, I took for granted I would have children." When she did not have children, she continued happily with her work, as did her husband, a self-taught carpenter, plumber, and clock repairer who also defied traditional gender roles. "My husband knows how to do everything except cook; he's a lousy cook," but "he can even sew." They used their modest incomes to live comfortably and travel: "We haven't seen the whole world, but we sure have seen the parts we wanted to see, and we got to go there before we were too old and decrepit to enjoy ourselves. We could never have afforded it with kids." Looking back on her century-long adventure with life, she concluded, "When I think of the past, I wonder how I managed to be so happy and normal. . . . I was always a happy kid. Still am."

Anecdotal evidence drawn from the stories of childless women and men during the depression era suggest that the economic situation was only partially responsible for the declining birthrate. Undoubtedly, some people postponed marriage or remained single and had fewer or no children because they lacked the economic security and resources to establish families. But there were other reasons as well. The rise in childlessness resulted in part from the depression, in part from an easing of pronatalist pressures and fears of race suicide after the passage of immigration-restriction laws in 1917, 1921, and 1924, and in part from the availability of other sources of fulfillment for both women and men. In other words, in the years before World War II, childlessness was not simply a tragedy or a sacrifice; for many it was also an opportunity.

Like Delores, Bonnie Dwayne also had no children and no regrets. But Bonnie was childless by choice. Born in 1915, she was slightly younger than Delores. After "three marriages and quite a quantity of affairs," friends warned her that her lack of a settled life and children would make her "'a very lonely old woman.' Well, I'm not," declared the former teacher and journalist. Many observers claim that truly voluntary childlessness was not possible (unless one remained single and celibate) until the postwar years when effective forms of birth control were available, but this was not the case. The lack of totally effective contraceptives was not an insurmountable problem for those who were determined not to reproduce. Like Bonnie, they made use of the available reproductive strategies—contraceptive devices and abortion—to remain childless. Estimates of illegal abortions during these years ranged from 250,000 to 1 million per year. Alfred C. Kinsey reported that among his sample, fully 24 percent of the wives had abortions by the time they were 40, and almost 90 percent of nonmarital pregnancies were aborted.[62] Among the fertile childless respondents to my study who came of age before World War II, fully one-third mentioned abortions in their letters, and the majority of them terminated more than one pregnancy.[63]

Bonnie's story was fairly typical. In 1934, as a young married woman in her freshman year at college, she became pregnant. She "got an abortion for $25 and never had any after-effects, either physical or emotional, and never a moment's regret." But she recalled that it was "illegal, painful and difficult to obtain. . . . The woman who did it gave me a shot for pain" then sent her home, and Bonnie "never missed a lick in school or work." Bonnie's decision to remain childless had nothing to do with hard times. Her first husband left her, "partly, I suppose, because he started cheering for parenthood and I wasn't having it." In her second marriage, "I got myself pregnant again. Both times, I may add, the pregnancy was a failure of contraception. I was very conscientious about using a diaphragm, but they aren't 100 percent effective—obviously."

When Bonnie got pregnant in 1940, she again had to "hunt up an abortionist; one can always find someone who knows someone, who knows someone—I used to quip that when one moved to a different city the things to do were to find a good butcher shop, a reliable mechanic and a decent abortionist." Her second abortion was "somewhat more expensive"—around $100—but "the operator was less skillful and less conscientious." She survived the second operation, but it did not go well. The abortionist perforated the placenta, "gave no painkiller, and thus, of course, produced a rather painful and messy miscarriage. Never mind, it got the job done. Had no lasting physical, and no emotional, consequences, and never regretted it for a moment." In her late seventies, Bonnie looked back on her childless life with plenty of satisfaction and no regrets.

Sarah Cohen also chose to remain childless in the 1930s. Like many of her peers, she decided to have a career instead of children. "I could have married, but during my marriageable years, with marriage came children. It was expected. I did not want children so I opted not to marry." Sarah became a registered nurse, "unusual for someone with a Jewish background 50 years ago," and was comfortable with her decision to remain childless. As a single and respected professional, she pursued a dynamic career, moving from nursing to hospital administration and "wound up my career as a pioneer in HMO development." Although Sarah remained a virgin until she was thirty-two, she did not live a celibate life, and she became pregnant twice in her thirties. Like Bonnie and many other women of her day, abortion was a major part of her contraceptive strategy. "As a nurse I had no difficulty having an abortion each time. Never, ever, did I consider marrying the father or having the child. . . . And to this day, I do not regret that was my choice."

Childless Americans in the early decades of the century, like Thomas Arkle Clark, Delores Taylor, Bonnie Dwayne, and Sarah Cohen, came from different backgrounds and had different reasons for being childless. But they all resisted the alarmist cries of race suicide and lived contented childless lives. Eugenics never became a mass movement. The passion of eugenic reformers never took hold among the population at large. If the American people did not respond to pronatalist moral suasion, little could be done to boost the birthrate of the "best stock." With few material incentives and virtually no public policies that eased the burdens of parents, the crusade for positive eugenics failed. But there was another side to the movement: negative eugenics, geared toward preventing the "unfit" from becoming parents.

Although it was impossible to coerce the "worthy" to procreate, it was possible to prevent at least some of the "unworthy" from reproducing. Negative eugenics, in the form of compulsory sterilization, was much more successful in manipulating the reproductive lives of many thousands of Americans—those deemed unworthy of parenthood.

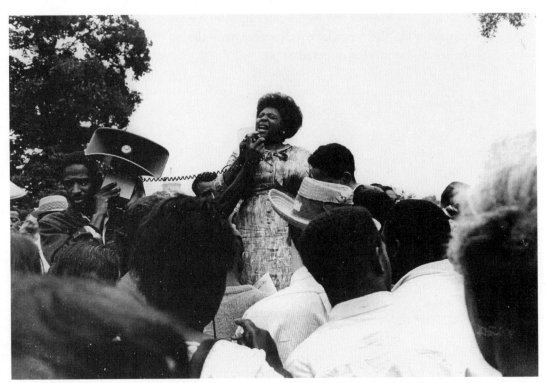

Civil rights leader Fanny Lou Hamer was sterilized without her knowledge or consent in 1961. *(Courtesy of AP/Wide World Photos)*

CHAPTER 3

Unfit for Parenthood: Class, Race, and Compulsory Sterilization
★☆

It is better for all the world if, instead of waiting to execute degenerate offspring for crime, or to let them starve for their imbecility, society can prevent those who are manifestly unfit from continuing their kind. The principle that sustains compulsory vaccination is broad enough to cover cutting the Fallopian tubes. . . . Three generations of imbeciles is enough.
—Justice Oliver Wendell Holmes, "Opinion of the Supreme Court of the United States," *Buck v. Bell*, May 2, 1927

If he was going to give that sort of operation, then he should have told me. I would have loved to have children. I went to the doctor who did that to me and I asked him, Why? Why had he done that to me? He didn't have to say nothing—and he didn't.
—Civil rights leader Fanny Lou Hamer, who was sterilized without her knowledge or consent in 1961, quoted in Kay Mills, *This Little Light of Mine: The Life of Fanny Lou Hamer*

Nowhere is the public stake in reproduction more evident and more powerful than in the successful campaign for compulsory sterilization in the first half of the twentieth century. While some crusaders for eugenics tried to persuade "worthy" Anglo-Saxon Americans to lift their sagging birthrate, others turned their attention to eliminating childbirth among the "unworthy." A century had passed since Thomas Jefferson's optimistic proclamation that the nation had room for "our descendants to the thousandth and thousandth generation," and already the population had extended across the western frontier and "our descendants" were being outnumbered. Along with the huge influx of immigrants came challenges to the values, moral codes, and social order of the Protestant elite. Anxieties over changing gender behavior and sexual mores, fears of racial mixing, and worries about the increasing number of poor immigrants who were entering the nation fueled a particularly reactionary wing of Progressive reform. Many middle-class Americans blamed the "undesirables" in their midst for crime, poverty, and a host of other social ills. The advocates of compulsory sterilization believed that preventing the "unfit" from reproducing would be the most efficient and cost-effective way to solve social problems. From the turn of the century onward, childlessness became not just a matter of personal circumstance, but a function of public policy.

The movement for compulsory sterilization began at the turn of the century with a few zealous crusaders in a few states who held positions of authority in state institutions for the mentally defective. Within the next few decades, they had mobilized enough political support to enact compulsory sterilization laws in dozens of states across the country. In 1927, the U.S. Supreme Court declared these laws to be constitutional. By the middle of the century, tens of thousands of Americans had been forcibly sterilized. Although compulsory sterilization never lived up to the grandiose designs of its proponents, the movement achieved remarkable legislative success and had a powerful and lasting impact. It empowered professionals and experts with the authority to render fertile individuals sterile. It fostered an approach to solving social problems like poverty by manipulating individual behavior, rather than by addressing structural flaws. And it had a profound impact on the lives of countless women and men who were sterilized against their will.[1]

Involuntary sterilization was directed against the poor. Because the wealthy could usually avoid state institutions and rarely needed to turn to public agencies for assistance, they more easily protected their private lives from state intervention. The poor were vulnerable not only because they were more likely to come into contact with coercive state institutions, but because their very poverty marked them as "unfit." Furthermore, the taxpayers' ire was easily aroused, then as now, over the use of public funds to support the poor and their offspring. So crusaders for eugenics could draw on a number of widely shared attitudes when campaigning for their cause.

Eugenic sterilization began long before it was officially sanctioned in state laws. It was first applied around the turn of the century in institutions for the "feebleminded"—an imprecise term used to describe those people believed to be mentally ill, mentally retarded, or of low intelligence. Initially, more men than women were sterilized, but within a few decades women became the primary victims. By 1960, over 60,000 eugenic sterilizations had been performed in state institutions throughout the country. This number includes only those individuals who were residents of state institutions for the mentally ill or mentally retarded. At best, only a few of these individuals consented. Most of the operations were performed on women who were never told that they were sterilized, many of whom thought they had received appendectomies. The average rate of reported sterilization was 83 per 100,000 people, or one person in 1,200. The number increased until World War II, then decreased during the war, and increased again after the war. Research suggests that these operations were underreported; one study followed 270 patients who were sterilized in Pennsylvania, even though Pennsylvania had no sterilization law. Many more legal as well as illegal sterilizations, especially on noninstitutionalized individuals, were never officially counted.

By the middle of the century, involuntary sterilization had shifted from institutionalized to noninstitutionalized people, from west to south, and from "feebleminded" White women to poor women of color on public assistance. The number of operations remained high, although accurate statistics are difficult to find. The abuse of sterilization did not begin to decline until the 1970s, when feminist activists called attention to the issue, initiated a number of highly publicized court cases, and demanded safeguards for informed consent. By that time, hundreds of thousands of poor women had been sterilized against their will.[2]

Most of those who were sterilized without their consent or knowledge left no records of their thoughts or feelings. The few who did expressed the enormous anguish they suffered. Their experiences add a human dimension to the political debates and cold statistics. One such woman was Mrs. P., who was sterilized in 1929 at the age of twenty. In 1941, she wrote to the birth control pioneer Margaret Sanger begging for help. She may not have known that Sanger, along with many other advocates of birth control, supported eugenics by the 1920s. Sanger did not favor sterilization, but hoped that the use of birth control among the poor would "stop the multiplication of the unfit." Nevertheless, by the 1940s the birth control movement had shifted its emphasis to planned parenthood and began to include services for infertility. It was undoubtedly this focus that prompted Mrs. P.'s physician to suggest that she write to Sanger to help her overcome the effects of her involuntary sterilization.[3]

"If you can help me find my heart's desire," Mrs. P. wrote to Margaret Sanger,

> I will be indebted to you the rest of my life. Darling Margaret about 12 years ago I was operated on for appendicitis and they took out my ovary tubes. They said a aunt of mine said Just as well take them out then she will never be bothered with children. Well when I learned of this both myself and my husband allmost cryed our eys out. To this day we have never gotten over it. I made up my mind I'd never give up until I got in the family way, and I've tryed every thing there is to try. I've sent off for medcine took and took so I could become pregnant but did no good, I'd go to Drs one after the other thinking one would help me. . . . Well time went on, dear Margaret I'm going to tell you something I never told anyone not even my husband. . . . please keep this secret will you. I actually swallowed the mess after we'd have intercourse never did hurt me but I thot if it got down into my stomach it might touch the germ from my ovary's without the tubes but that did no good I kno I was foolish but only any one wanting a baby as badly as I do could understand.

Mrs. P.'s desperation sent her on a quest for miracle cures:

> Dear margaret I read in true Story Magazine about Test Tube Baby. . . . Darling Margaret can you do any thing for me if you can please please will you help me. . . . We are just common people but could make a happy home for a baby. My husband is in perfect health and will do any thing for me that will make me happy he wants a baby so bad to.

Margaret Sanger read the letter "with great interest and sympathy" and sent it on to Abraham Stone, medical director of the Margaret Sanger Research Center. Stone replied that he would need to know more before he could give any definite advice, but he was not optimistic. "I must tell you that if the tubes have actually been removed there is no way at all of introducing the egg cell into the uterus directly." He went on to explain that a "test-tube baby" referred at the time to artificial insemination (it would much later be used to describe in-vitro fertilization). "Here the sperm of the man is introduced into the womb of the woman and then conception takes place in a natural manner, but if the egg cannot get to the womb from the ovary, there is no way of producing a conception." Stone then suggested that she try to adopt a baby.

But Mrs. P. did not give up. She wrote again to Sanger with an idea that was not so much "foolish" as it was decades ahead of its time: She actually imagined the possibility of egg donation and in-vitro fertilization.

> I'm asking you this can you fix me up by introducing the egg from another woman when it comes down, into my womb? I don't want any one woman to suffer on my acc't but please will you try this for me. . . . I will stand for all conquenciences [sic] if it should kill me no one is to blame I want a baby so bad. My tubes were removed by the record at the hospital. Could this be fixed up in a tube some way and introduced into my womb? My Dr. said he would do this for me if you say their might be a possible chance, to find a woman similar of my type and if you can and find a woman may God bless you and this woman until the day you pass away. Please Dear Margaret don't say no say you will I'll stand everything. . . . I may be wrong but if another woman will furnish me a egg cell my husband will do the rest. Please don't call me foolish for I've figured and studied and I want to try. Love Mrs. Dan P.

In 1941, this idea must have sounded preposterous. When she received no response, Mrs. P. wrote her third and final letter to Sanger: "I'm willing to go thru anything I need some help. Please write me soon please don't think I'm foolish because this is my greatest desire on earth. May God Bless You. Resp. Mrs. Dan P." There is no evidence that her last letter was answered. In later decades, in-vitro fertilization might have offered this woman some hope, provided that she could afford the expensive and often unsuccessful procedure. But in 1941, nothing could be done for a woman like Mrs. P. who was sterilized against her will.[4]

The "Feebleminded"

The sterilization of Mrs. P. was performed without her knowledge or consent, at the whim of a physician with the alleged consent of a relative. But this outrage was probably legal. By 1929, compulsory sterilization was legal in many states and was sanctioned by the Supreme Court. It is unclear what prompted the physician to rob her of her fertility during surgery for appendicitis, but the criteria for such decisions were vague. Most of the women who were sterilized during the first half of the twentieth century were judged to be "feebleminded." Authorities based their judgments upon crude definitions of the "unfit," drawn from dubious genetic theories, distortions of Darwin's ideas, and class and racial stereotypes.[5]

Advocates of compulsory sterilization believed that poverty, criminality, and immorality resulted from inherited traits. They differed from the feminists and social reformers of the late nineteenth century who believed in "race better-ment."[6] These reformers saw no contradiction between environmentalism and hereditarianism and advocated improving the "race" by improving social condi-tions. But conservative eugenicists who favored compulsory sterilization believed that changing the environment would not eradicate antisocial traits. They argued just the opposite: that the environment would continue to degen-erate because the propagation of "inferior" people would lead to more crime, poverty, and vice.

The debate over compulsory sterilization began well over a decade before Indiana passed the first state law in 1907. The controversy focused largely on "feeblemindedness," a catch-all category that included a wide range of allegedly inherited traits. Although both men and women were labeled fee-bleminded, much of the professional literature focused on women. The diagnosis of feeblemindedness was frequently based on behavior, particu-larly sexual behavior. And although the language centered on the nebulous category of race, the more salient issue was actually class. Using unsubstanti-ated and erroneous "facts" of hereditary racial, mental, or moral characteris-tics as their justification, officials incarcerated and sterilized women who they deemed feebleminded because they were poor, single, and sexually active, regardless of race, intelligence, or health.

Advocates of compulsory sterilization were preoccupied with matters of sexuality. Some argued that feebleminded men were oversexed, whereas others argued that they were undersexed. But these advocates did not disagree about the sexual proclivities of feebleminded women, all of whom were considered to be sources of debauchery, licentiousness, and illegitimacy. Feeblemindedness was almost universally associated with lower-class, sexually adventurous women. In 1896, E. P. Bicknell, the secretary of the Indiana State Board of Charities, articulated the common wisdom regarding feeblemindedness: "In the feeble-minded person the animal passions are usually present and are often abnormally developed, while will and reason, which should control and repress them, are absent. The feeble-minded woman, thus lacking the protection which should be her birth-right, falls easily into vice."[7] Walter Fernald, a physi-cian and superintendent of the Massachusetts School for Feeble-minded Chil-dren, agreed:

The tendency to lead dissolute lives is especially noticeable in the females. A feeble-minded girl is exposed as no other girl in the world is exposed. She has not sense enough to protect herself from the perils to which women are subjected. Often bright and attractive, if at large they either marry and bring forth in geometrical ratio a new generation of defectives and dependents, or become irresponsible sources of corruption and debauchery in the communities where they live.[8]

It is curious that Fernald described "feebleminded" girls as often "bright," suggesting that sexuality, rather than "dullness" or low intelligence, was the essential criterion. The historian Daniel Kevles noted that "the attention given eroticism, the denunciation of feminism, and the genital attack implicit in sterilization all suggest the possibility that mainline eugenics was driven in part by the psychic energy of a repressed discomfort with sexuality." Women were often incarcerated, in prisons or in institutions for the feebleminded, for no other reason than their nonmarital sexual behavior. Many of these women had become pregnant out of wedlock; others were prostitutes or simply "promiscuous." Men faced incarceration for sex crimes, such as rape, but only women were imprisoned for fornication, prostitution, or illegitimacy. Many women were segregated in institutions for the feebleminded for the sole purpose of preventing them from becoming pregnant. According to R. A. Mott, the physician and director of the Minnesota Institution for Defectives in 1890, "the fertility of the feebleminded is proverbial." The 1890 census's indication of the dramatic increase in the number of "idiots and imbeciles" gave rise to calls for solutions other than incarceration, since institutional space was limited. Sterilization was an alternative to segregation.[9]

The problem was not that these feebleminded women were easy prey for men who were looking for sex. Rather, it was that the women were the aggressors who snared unsuspecting, otherwise innocent men. "Many have been the instances in which the presence of a feeble-minded woman or girl in a village or country neighborhood has been a veritable curse to the community. Unable to control her debasing propensities, she has become a source of temptation and corruption to young men and boys, who otherwise would not have been led into vicious habits." The women's promiscuity was both evidence of and the effect of their feeblemindedness, which professionals deemed incurable and inherited.[10]

We know from the work of many scholars, including Christine Stansell and Kathy Peiss, that sexual experimentation as well as casual prostitution were not uncommon among young working-class women throughout the nineteenth and early twentieth centuries. These women were likely later to marry and lead "respectable" lives.[11] But according to the eugenic reformers, their behaviors were evidence of innate characteristics that marked them and their progeny as inferior. Although some of the women who were targeted for involuntary sterilization may well have been mentally retarded or of low intelligence, others were working-class or poor women who were incarcerated for "sexual delinquency." In Missouri, for example, the medical superintendent of the Independence State Hospital said that he sterilized all feebleminded women who he believed to be sexually promiscuous.[12]

One study of eighty-nine "tubectomized girls" in the Sonoma State Home for the Feebleminded concluded that "many of the girls had been guilty of promiscuity and wanted to convince the staff that they would not be repeaters if released. Of 433 feebleminded girls who were committed to California institutions, 9 in 12 had been sex delinquents, but follow-ups after their sterilization and release showed 1 in 12 delinquent." The study claimed that sterilization cured these women of promiscuity, but an equally plausible explanation is that the women curbed their behavior to avoid being incarcerated again. Even more alarming was the claim by C. C. Hawke, medical director of the State Training School in Winfield, Kansas, that he "used castration . . . extensively, though only on the vicious cases who made trouble with quarrels or homosexual attacks." Two hundred young people were reportedly castrated "for behavior difficulties—boys that were bullying the younger children and making trouble in the wards; girls that wandered round the wards all night looking for homosexual adventures."[13]

Race and Class

When eugenicists advocated "racial" improvement, they referred not only to color. Often, the term "race" was used interchangeably with "nationality" or "religion." When President Calvin Coolidge signed the Immigration Act in 1924, a measure supported by eugenicists that virtually cut off the flow of immigrants into the United States, he noted that "America must be kept American. Biological laws show . . . that Nordics deteriorate when mixed with other races." By "other races," he meant not only people of color, but Jews, southern Europeans, and other non-Nordic people.[14]

Coolidge's statement reflects the influence of decades of eugenic thinking. One of the most influential scientists to lend credibility to the American eugenic movement was biologist Charles Benedict Davenport, who became the leading eugenicist in the United States. A follower of Mendel's theories of heredity, Davenport became in 1904 the director of the Station for Experimental Evolution at Cold Spring Harbor, New York, a research facility where countless noted geneticists did research in the years between the world wars. Davenport was a biological determinist who did not believe that environmental factors made any substantial difference in human characteristics. Although the ideas of Sigmund Freud were gaining popularity, Davenport paid no attention to them. He believed that "Negroes" and new immigrants, including Poles, Irish, Italians, and "Hebrews," were racially inferior to the American-born Anglo-Saxon Protestant majority.

For eugenic theorists like Davenport, racial inferiority went hand in hand with sexual degeneracy. Davenport was particularly obsessed with sexual transgressions. His study of 350 "wayward girls" allegedly proved that prostitution resulted from bad genes. Davenport stated that all but one of his subjects entered prostitution because of "innate eroticism" caused by "an additional germinal determiner that less licentious persons do not have." He contended that immigrants and people of color were more likely to have this genetic predisposition and argued for immigration restriction, as well as compulsory sterilization. If the flood of foreigners into the country did not stop, he was certain that the American population would become "darker in pigmentation, smaller in stature, more mercurial, more attached to music and art, more given to crime and larceny, kidnapping, assault, murder, rape, and sex immorality."[15]

In the writings of eugenic reformers, race, class, sexuality, and ethnicity were all blurred. Nonmarital sexual activity was a code for class and a marker for hereditary inferiority. There is no evidence that middle-class or affluent women were ever labeled feebleminded or sterilized against their will. Most of the sterilized women in Indiana were poor and White, but their poverty and sexual behavior marked them as both racially and genetically inferior. A few of these women gave further evidence of their alleged depravity by consorting with Black men. One institution official described

a feeble-minded woman who herself is the illegitimate child of a feeble-minded mother. This woman, now in the asylum, has four feeble-minded children, all illegitimate. Of these four children, three are white and one black. One of the children, a 15-year-old girl, is away from the poor asylum going about the county as she pleases, and although but a child, has already started upon a life of immorality. There is little doubt that unless she is properly protected, she will in years to come assist in increasing the host of feeble-mindedness and illegitimacy in the state.

This official also cited the example of a feeble-minded woman who married, separated, and then married a "negro." It is implicit in these cases that sexual intercourse with a Black man was further evidence of the "feeblemindedness" and racial inferiority of these White women.[16]

Most eugenicists accepted the prevailing views of the inferiority of Black people, although they did not all agree about miscegenation. Some believed that White men impregnating Black women (though *never* Black men impregnating White women) would have a beneficial effect by lightening and improving the Black race. Others thought that any mixing of the races was bad and would destroy the purity of each race and lead to "mongrelization." The latter view was more prevalent and contributed to the passage of a number of antimiscegenation laws. The definition of a "Negro" was altered to include those who had one-sixteenth Black ancestry, or a single "drop" of Negro blood. The peculiar racial theories of the day found their way into these laws, including the "Pocahontas exception" that allowed a White person to marry a person with one-sixteenth or less Indian blood, that is, those who claimed to be descendants of Pocahontas. According to one contemporary physician, this provision was important to save "young women, perhaps, from being misled into marrying mulattos under the guise of Indians."[17] Antimiscegenation laws, grounded in prevailing theories of sex, race, and reproduction, set the stage for compulsory sterilization.

The Momentum of the Movement

In the early years, eugenic sterilization was performed on individuals whose antisocial behavior allegedly gave evidence of hereditary defects. But sterilization was also performed to punish criminals who were believed to be sexually dangerous. Given the racist assumptions of the day, it is not surprising that punitive eugenic policies were carried out with particular brutality toward Black men. In 1855, for example, Kansas enacted a law permitting the castration of any "negro or mulatto" convicted of rape, attempted rape, or kidnapping of a White woman. Later the law was amended to include rapists of any color. Only one legal castration is known to have taken place:

In 1864 a jury in Belton, Texas, convicted a Black man of rape, and recommended castration; the sentence was carried out.

Officials also used castration against people who were not convicted of crimes and without state sanction. In 1894, for example, Hoyt Pilcher, the physician and superintendent of the Asylum for Idiots and Feebleminded Youths in Winfield, Kansas, claimed that he had castrated fourteen girls and forty-four boys, adolescents he described as "chronic masturbators." Although Pilcher lost his job as a result, there were those who supported the practice. The brutality of castration had the peculiar effect of making sterilization without castration—vasectomy and tubal ligation—seem humane by comparison.[18]

The first vasectomy was performed in 1897 by A. J. Ochsner, a surgeon who wrote in the *Journal of the American Medical Association*, "If it were possible to eliminate all habitual criminals from the possibility of having children, there would soon be a very marked decrease in this class." By 1902, the surgeon for the Indiana Reformatory, Harry C. Sharp, advocated vasectomy for eugenic sterilization. He vasectomized forty-two prison inmates aged seventeen to twenty-five and claimed that the operation tamed their behavior. Sharp argued in favor of sterilizing every male inmate of prisons or asylums of any sort. He was apparently the first to perform mass sterilizations without consent or court approval. But his actions received little overt criticism. In fact, Sharp was instrumental in achieving the passage of Indiana's compulsory sterilization law in 1907.

Organized opposition to compulsory sterilization was minimal. A few eugenicists favored segregation over sterilization because they feared that sterilized women would be sexually promiscuous. The most powerful and consistent opposition came from the Catholic church. Nevertheless, American eugenicists were able to achieve their two major political goals: the restriction of immigration and compulsory sterilization. In the early years, owing to the zeal of a small but energetic group of advocates, most of whom were administrators of institutions for the feebleminded and their political allies, the greatest legislative successes were in the Midwest and Far West. Few compulsory sterilization laws were passed in the East coast or the South. Later, both the regional focus and the targeted population would change dramatically.[19]

The eugenics movement was not isolated to the United States; in fact, its founder, Francis Galton, was born in England, and the movement was strong there. But no eugenic laws were passed in England, while many were enacted in the United States.[20] British eugenicists were amazed at the legislative success of the American movement and believed that it was due, in part, to the

U.S. political structure: States could pass laws in the United States, whereas only Parliament could do so in England. But there were other reasons, including the widespread belief in the United States that scientific expertise would eradicate social problems. Moreover, the relatively homogeneous English population did not evoke the same racial and ethnic fears that surfaced in response to the increasing diversity of American cities.

The campaign for compulsory sterilization in the United States gained momentum in the early twentieth century. The *Readers' Guide to Periodical Literature* lists twenty-seven articles under the heading "eugenics" between 1905 and 1909, increasing to a total of 123 in the next five years. Although eugenics remained a movement of professional reformers with little mass appeal, the publicity campaign helped generate political support. At the same time, enthusiasm grew among some supporters in the medical community. Every article on the subject that appeared in the medical literature between 1899 and 1913 favored the practice; there were twenty-three such articles spanning 1909 and 1910 alone. Spearheaded largely by scientists in the emerging field of genetics and supported by reformers in various fields and across the political spectrum, the notion of weeding out the "bad stock" fit the Progressive-era faith in social progress and human betterment through scientific knowledge. Notable experts, such as the psychologist Edward A. Ross and the biologists Michael F. Guyer and Samuel Holmes, supported the movement. In 1911, *Scientific American* lent its support with an editorial in favor of eugenic sterilization.[21]

The 1907 Indiana law was the first to legalize compulsory sterilization. Within the next two decades, along with national laws restricting immigration, 23 states had compulsory sterilization laws on the books, 17 had active programs, and 6,244 people had been sterilized. In spite of these numbers, crusaders for eugenics were not satisfied. Not all the laws were equally utilized, and advocates of sterilization continued to push for enforcement and standardization. At the center of the movement was Harry Hamilton Laughlin, a zealous advocate of sterilization who joined Davenport at Cold Spring Harbor to head the Eugenic Record Office. According to Laughlin, the "socially unfit and their supply should if possible be eliminated from the human stock if we would maintain or raise the level of quality essential to the progress of the nation and our race." His long list of the "socially unfit" who should be sterilized included

the Feeble Minded: using the term generally . . . The Pauper Class: pauper feebleminded through successive generations . . . The Criminaloids: persons born with marked criminal tendencies . . . Epileptics . . . The Insane . . . The

Constitutionally Weak . . . Those predisposed to specific diseases . . . the Congenitally Deformed . . . Those having defective sense organs, such as the deaf-mutes, the deaf and the blind.

Laughlin concluded that "approximately 10 percent of our population . . . are an economic and moral burden on the 90 percent and a constant source of danger to the national and racial life."[22]

To give his work credibility, Laughlin went to Princeton University and received a Ph.D. in genetics; his doctoral project was the only rigorous experimental study he ever did. Nevertheless, he cultivated his image as a scientist, especially with the press, which gave him a measure of stature in the movement. Laughlin became known as the nation's eugenics expert and was influential in pushing for immigration-restriction legislation, as well as support for compulsory sterilization in the courts. The scope and stature of the eugenics movement was evident by 1921, when the Second International Congress of Eugenics convened at the Museum of Natural History in New York. The conference included 108 papers from the fields of genetics and medicine; 55 pedigree studies on humans; and 55 presentations on the consequences of marriage between different ethnic groups, especially across racial lines. In 1926, a group of professors at Yale University formed the American Eugenics Society. The support of experts and professionals contributed to the widespread acceptance of compulsory sterilization.[23]

Buck v. Bell

The campaign for legal sterilization culminated in the 1927 Supreme Court decision, *Buck v. Bell*. Advocates of eugenics manufactured the case to gain constitutional legitimacy for the practice. They selected the case of Carrie Buck to test the constitutionality of the Virginia compulsory sterilization law. At age seventeen, Buck became pregnant as the result of a rape and was sent to a state institution for the feebleminded. The daughter of an unmarried woman who was allegedly feebleminded, Buck was also described as feebleminded, as was her daughter, also born out of wedlock. No evidence was ever presented to "prove" that Buck, her birth mother, or her daughter were below normal intelligence. Laughlin was chosen to evaluate Buck as a candidate for sterilization. Although he never met her, he used sketchy information provided by the Virginia institution where she was incarcerated to determine that she was a sexually immoral "low grade moron" with a mental age of nine. Looking at her records, he described her as part of the "shiftless, ignorant and worthless class of anti-social whites of the South."

Buck was sterilized in 1927, allegedly because she was feebleminded, but actually because she was born out of wedlock and gave birth out of wedlock. The following year, her sister Doris, aged sixteen, was taken to the Virginia Colony for Epileptics and the Feebleminded and sterilized. She was told that she had an appendectomy. Later, Doris married Matthew Figgins and tried to get pregnant. None of the physicians she consulted gave her any reason why she could not conceive. She finally learned the truth in 1979. "I broke down and cried. My husband and I wanted children desperately. We were crazy about them. I never knew what they'd done to me."[24]

Neither Carrie nor Doris Buck was mentally retarded. In the Supreme Court proceedings, no experts testified on Carrie's behalf. It was not until 1940 that a few sociologists began to question the fact that no counsel ever argued against the sterilization on the grounds that neither Buck, her birth mother, nor her child were ever proved to be mentally defective and that all that is known about Carrie's biological mother was that she bore a child out of wedlock. Carrie's daughter died as a child, but her teachers described her as bright. In approving the sterilization, Justice Oliver Wendell Holmes declared, in his famous written opinion on the case: "Three generations of imbeciles are enough." Within the next few years, the number of states with compulsory sterilization laws increased to thirty, and the number of operations rose dramatically.[25]

Observers have argued that the Nazi sterilization policies gave eugenics a bad name and that the movement in the United States declined when the German policies became known.[26] But according to a study by Philip Reilly, "Revulsion over Germany's racist politics did little to curtail American programs before or after World War II. Indeed, American advocates pointed to Germany to illustrate how an enlightened sterilization program might quickly reach its goals." Actually, the United States provided the model for eugenic programs in several European countries. England was the only major nation in which eugenic laws were unequivocally rejected because British scientists refused to accept the premise that the "number of defectives" would be reduced through sterilization. Even Germany in the 1920s rejected compulsory sterilization. It was not until 1933 that the Nazis instituted a eugenic sterilization law, modeled on the program in California. Hitler's statements on eugenic sterilization sound remarkably like those of Justice Oliver Wendell Holmes. In *Mein Kampf* Hitler wrote:

To prevent defective persons from reproducing equally defective offspring, is an act dictated by the clearest light of reason. Its carrying out is the most humane act of mankind. It would prevent the unmerited suffering of millions of persons, and, above all would, in the end, result in a steady increase in human welfare.

Eugenicists in the United States hailed the German policy. In fact, Laughlin, one of the leading American eugenicists, argued that Jews fleeing Nazi Germany should not be exempt from the immigration laws, on the grounds that the threat to the American racial stock was worse than the threat to the Jews in Germany.[27]

The Taxpayers and the Poor

The Buck decision, combined with the economic crisis of the 1930s, fueled a renewed campaign for compulsory sterilization during the depression. The cost to taxpayers of caring for the "feebleminded" had always been an issue in the sterilization debate, but it took on new urgency during hard times. The high level of unemployment and the increasing number of Americans on relief raised the cost to taxpayers of caring for the poor. Advocates of compulsory sterilization argued that the practice would reduce the number of "relief babies." As late as 1938, a respected expert, Dwight E. Minnich, chairman of the zoology department at the University of Minnesota, called for "developing a better race" in an address to the Minnesota Birth Control League. Minnich advocated "sterilization of the unfit and equalization of the birth rate among various ability levels of the population," which he claimed would save the state $50 million annually.[28] Sterilization seemed a simple solution to the complicated problem of poverty. Therefore, it is not surprising that the 1930s was the heyday of compulsory sterilization. As waiting lists for state hospitals grew, the number of sterilizations reached new heights.

Eugenic reformers who had once been noted for their idealistic feminism, like Charlotte Perkins Gilman and Margaret Sanger, became more concerned with social control. By 1929, Gilman had become a strident advocate of compulsory sterilization: "Those who are able to earn are taxed to support those who are not. The best is handicapped by the worst . . . as we learn new ways of keeping incompetents alive. It is true that in some places we are applying drastic methods of birth control by sterilizing the patently unfit, but even that is objected to by some tender hearts." Paul Popenoe, a eugenics hard-liner, argued that 10 million Americans ought to be sterilized. He based his estimates on intelligence tests—instruments that were ultimately determined to be unreliable because of their class and cultural biases.[29]

Throughout the 1930s, compulsory sterilization continued to gain legitimacy. In the decade following *Buck v. Bell*, medical journals published sixty articles about sterilization, most of them favorable. The Human Betterment Foundation of California, along with many physicians' organizations, breathed new life into the crusade for sterilization. The board of the foundation included distinguished scholars and educators, such as the president of the University of Southern California; the chancellor emeritus of Stanford University, David Starr Jordan; and the psychologist Lewis M. Terman, also of Stanford. The foundation claimed that "modern sterilization is not a mutilation. . . . It is the only reliable method of birth control which many defectives can use. . . . Such persons may not have the intelligence, the foresight, or the self-control, to handle contraception successfully, nor the ability to care for children intelligently." The weight of professional advocacy fostered public acceptance, particularly among the nation's elite. According to a 1937 poll in *Fortune* magazine, two-thirds of readers favored the sterilization of mental defectives and criminals, and only 15 percent opposed it.[30]

As the number of sterilizations went up, the locale where they were performed shifted as well, from the West to the South. California was responsible for nearly half of all sterilizations until the 1930s, largely as a result of zealous officials in state institutions. But by the end of the 1950s, the majority of sterilizations took place in the South. Most of these operations were still performed on White women and men because state institutions were racially segregated. It was not until sterilization moved outside residential institutions that people of color became the primary targets.

Initially, the shift to the South had more to do with poverty than with race. During the depression of the 1930s, officials became less concerned with sterilizing "defectives" and more concerned with preventing parenthood among those they considered unable to provide for their children. The goal was to reduce the costs to taxpayers. This goal generated a change in who was sterilized; the number of young women who were sterilized increased dramatically, presumably to prevent them from having children who would then be dependent on the state. The majority of institutional sterilizations in the

1920s were performed on men and boys; by the 1930s, two-thirds were performed on women and girls, despite the fact that more men than women were institutionalized. Young women were often institutionalized for the sole purpose of sterilization and were released after their operations.[31]

These policies continued throughout the 1930s even though before the laparoscope, female sterilization was major surgery compared to vasectomy. In some states, sterilization continued to include castration. For example, North Carolina sterilized nearly two thousand institutionalized women and men between 1929 and 1947; these operations included 349 vasectomies, 58 castrations, 1,477 salpingectomies, and 17 ovariectomies. At least five women are known to have died from these involuntary surgeries while they were incarcerated in institutions during the depression.[32]

After World War II, in spite of the fact that Nazi sterilization campaigns had given eugenics a bad name, compulsory sterilization continued in the United States. Capricious criteria continued to be used to incarcerate and sterilize individuals for petty offenses. In 1946, for example, a desperate woman (with a Spanish surname) wrote to Hjalmar Petersen, the former governor of Minnesota, begging him to help get her daughter and brother released from the Minnesota School for the Feebleminded, where they were ordered to be sterilized.

> I am writing this letter conserning the Minnesota School for Feeble-minded. I have a daughter there since 1944, we've been trying very hard to get her out of there. She was put there for stealing some money. I should think that their isn't a Law for people being sterilization just for stealing money. . . . Coud you please try to see if you could get her out? I also have a brother there too, He's there for not going to school, And they also want to have him take the sterilization. The judge that sentenced my daughter in 1944, said that she was never handled by any boys. And I don't understand why she should have a sterilization. I want to know if you could try and have her home for Christmas.

The outcome of this case is not evident, but it is clear that compulsory sterilization of the so-called feebleminded continued into the postwar years.[33]

"Voluntary" Sterilization

Advocates of sterilization eventually shifted their emphasis to "voluntary" sterilization. But the principle of "consent" remained grounded in eugenic ideas, rather than in the concept of individual reproductive choice. For example, one of the most powerful organizations founded in the 1930s, the Sterilization League of New Jersey, evolved into a national organization, Birthright, by 1943. In 1950 it changed its name to the Human Betterment Association of America, then again in 1962 to the Human Betterment Association for Voluntary Sterilization, and again in 1965 to the Association for Voluntary Sterilization. These name changes emphasized choice over compulsion and located the organization within the birth control movement. It was not until the 1960s that the association came out publicly against compulsory sterilization, but its tactics and goals did not change even then. In 1963, the association's leader, E. Curtis Wood, claimed that voluntary sterilization would reduce the welfare rolls and illegitimacy. Some physicians used a wide range of coercive measures to "promote" sterilization among the poor, such as refusing to perform deliveries, abortions, prenatal examinations, or other types of medical care unless the patients agreed to be sterilized. Many did not even bother with the pretense of consent.[34]

For inmates of institutions, the "choice" was clear: they could agree to sterilization and gain their freedom, or they could refuse it and remain incarcerated. This alleged choice led some officials to claim that the operations were voluntary. According to one study,

> Many mentally deficient persons by consenting to the operation are permitted to return, under supervision, to society where they become self-supporting social units and acceptable citizens. Those inmates unwilling to consent to the operation remain segregated for social protection as well as individual welfare.

Dr. Hill from Oregon "didn't discharge from the feebleminded school until sterilization had been done. The patients now often ask 'when am I going to have my operation?'" If sterilization was the only way out of incarceration, it is easy to understand why the inmates might "volunteer." The line between voluntary and coerced sterilization was a thin one. As one judge concluded concerning the case of a female inmate at an institution in Nebraska, "The order does not require her sterilization. It does provide . . . that she shall not be released unless she is sterilized. *The choice is hers.*"[35] One survey in Minnesota reported that most of the institutionalized women who were sterilized and released were "successful" at reentering the society. But the study did not address the possibility that there was no reason to institutionalize them in the first place.[36]

The practice of sterilizing inmates before their release continued in several states, at the rate of 83 percent to 96 percent, according to a 1950 report. Other states employed additional methods to prevent the propagation of the unfit. In South Dakota, mentally deficient persons were prohibited from marrying unless they were sterilized. In 1944, of the 262 married mentally deficient persons "who were believed to be exposed to the risk of parent-hood," all but twenty-four had been sterilized. An official in Connecticut claimed that the 103 sterilizations performed in his institution prevented the birth of "80 second-generation morons whose upkeep would have cost tax-payers $490,000." Yet he considered that number to be low. "Connecticut is very cautious about this operation. . . . In California it is routine, once a girl or boy is brought inside a feeble-minded institution. It's that state's idea of thrift. We do this very rarely. In most cases we like to have the consent of the girls' parents." When asked why only the girls were sterilized, he replied, "In the long range, the mother is more important, or more dangerous. A man may be a moron, but it's the moron mother who will take care of the baby."

Truly voluntary (elective) sterilization was, ironically, prohibited. In the middle of the twentieth century, the only people who could get steril-ized were those who did not ask for it. The "120 formula," recommended by the American College of Obstetricians and Gynecologists, governed sterilization policies in most hospitals. Under the guideline, if a woman's age multiplied by the number of children she had totaled 120, she was a candidate for sterilization. She then would need two physicians and a psy-chiatrist to recommend the surgery. A twenty-nine-year-old woman with four children would be ineligible, as would a thirty-nine-year-old woman with three. Of course, these restrictions applied only to women who *requested* the operation; those who did not might be sterilized against their will at any age, even if they had no children. As late as 1970, one middle-class woman who was trying to obtain the operation complained, "Just like women who are sterilized without consent, we're treated as objects of population policy." Janet Stein, a twenty-seven-year-old mother of three, sued a New York hospital for refusing to perform her elective sterilization. A number of suits followed, but elective sterilization was not guaranteed until 1973, when the Supreme Court ruled in *Roe v. Wade* that along with abortion, elective sterilization was covered under the con-cept of the right to privacy.[37]

Even after *Roe v. Wade*, it was difficult for childless individuals to per-suade physicians to perform the operation. For example, in 1976 Maureen Arnold requested a tubal ligation.

I fully intended to get an abortion if I became pregnant, and told my doctor so in plain English. After three months of arguing with the doc and sex without birth control pills, she finally agreed to the tubal. It was three months of arguments with her because I was "young" in her eyes and at age 26 I was mentally 45 and felt 90 years old and couldn't wait to be "fixed."

Sally Cort also had trouble convincing her doctor. "I had my tubes clipped, not cut, which is easily reversed—it's the only way my doctor would do it." Marian Costello was married at age twenty-one, and when she requested the operation, "I really had to fight to get it, since the doctors I talked to 1) disapproved and 2) didn't think I was old enough to make such a decision." She finally convinced a physician to tie her tubes when she was twenty-four. Corinne Mason and her husband had trouble when he tried to get a vasectomy. "The doctor felt we were too young, we would change our minds, we had not recovered from the death of our child. We had to sign a paper in front of a notary that we understood what we were doing—that it was a permanent operation."

Institutional policies like the 120 formula reflect the continuing power of eugenic theories well into the postwar years: The "unfit" were targeted for sterilization, while the "fit" were prohibited from obtaining the operation. Nowhere is this philosophy more evident than in the correspondence of the physician Clarence Gamble, the foremost proponent of eugenic sterilization in the postwar years. Gamble, heir to the Gamble soap fortune who taught at the Harvard and University of Pennsylvania medical schools, launched a one-man media blitz promoting "voluntary" sterilization around the country. In 1950 and 1951, he published dozens of letters, in journals as varied as the *Journal of the American Medical Association* and *Newsweek*, all of which carried the same message. First, Gamble pointed out how much the state stood to gain in savings to taxpayers. To the Iowa *Marshalltown Times*, for example, he wrote that Iowa spent $4.5 million per year to support the insane and feebleminded, money that could be saved by a program of voluntary sterilization. Second, he said that the operation was simple and that no organ was removed, so it was not to be confused with "the barnyard form of sterilization." Third, he stated that sterilization did not affect one's sexual ability, performance, or enjoyment, and he minimized the risks of the surgery. He even suggested that the operation was not permanent. Finally, he claimed that the "compulsory" provision, still in the statutes of many states, was rarely used.[38]

But Gamble did not really favor voluntary sterilization, as several of his readers discovered. In 1949, Sam M. from St. Petersburg, Florida, wrote:

> Dr. Gamble, I have read your article, "Why Fear Sterilization?" in *Hygeia*. My wife's physical condition is such that it would involve risk in having children. Her passage is small and she has been anemic and in a general rundown condition for the past 3 years. Rather than have a Cesarean we have decided it would be better for me to have a vasectomy performed. We have gone over this problem thoroughly for the past 2 years and decided in favor of this action. I am fully aware of the fact that once this operation is performed I can never have any children. Since I am in better physical condition than my wife I would rather have the operation performed for sterilization on me instead of her. I have seen 2 doctors. They both told me to wait a few years, that I might change my mind etc. Doctor, I am 38, sound of mind, and have a willing ear for sensible advice. But I don't see why I can't have something to say about the way I want to live. . . . My wife and I do not want children under our circumstances that is definite. I have a wonderful wife and I don't intend to lose her or shop around for another just because of children. There is always adoption of some unfortunate should we decide in that manner. I would appreciate your help on this problem very much. Is this operation illegal in Florida? What type of a doctor should I see? A prompt reply will be eagerly awaited. Truly yours, Sam M.

Gamble was less than helpful. He replied that although surgical sterilization is not illegal in any state, "whether a physician will perform the operation depends, of course, on his individual decision. The hesitation of those to whom you have talked is undoubtedly intended to be for your own good." This man responded to Gamble's enthusiastic support for voluntary sterilization; he and his wife wanted to remain childless. But they were not the right volunteers.[39]

Clearly, Gamble did not believe that voluntary sterilization was for use by the middle class.[40] In 1957, he received another letter, from Mrs. Mary B. in a suburb of Philadelphia. Mrs. B. wrote that she had been married 6 years since graduation from college and had "4 grand children." But she had no success with birth control after each baby.

> The last time I talked to him (my obstetrician) about having something done to me or to my husband—he said nothing could be done to me unless something was wrong with me, which there isn't—when talking about the operation done on a man, called vasectomy I believe, he said it wasn't done anymore unless we had a reason. None of our reasons seem good enough—and so I talked to my parents and various urologists we knew and Dr. Guthmann suggested I write to you, and that you might be able to help us.

She added that she had no success when she called Planned Parenthood. Again, Gamble's reply was not helpful: "While there is no law against voluntary sterilization for those who wish no further children, physicians hesitate to perform such an operation too readily lest the patient should later regret the action."[41]

Emerging Opposition

Compulsory sterilizations declined during World War II. Although they increased again after the war, the rate of officially sanctioned institutional sterilizations never returned to the prewar levels. Most physicians abandoned the movement, and geneticists struggled to dissociate themselves from their earlier ties to eugenics. Only a few continued to crusade on behalf of eugenic sterilization well into the postwar era. One such advocate was the gynecologist Robert Latou Dickinson, an early pioneer in infertility treatment, artificial insemination, and birth control. Another was Gamble.

The response to Gamble's advocacy of eugenic sterilization illustrates the increasing hostility to the practice in the wake of World War II. If eugenicists were initially heartened by the Nazi eugenics program, the general public was thoroughly outraged by the time the Nazi horrors came to light. In one of many vehement responses to Gamble, Sidney Smith of Massachusetts called Gamble's plan for voluntary sterilization an

> immoral proposal, misnamed "humane" and "progressive." . . . It is of course obvious that in the case of the feeble-minded, incapable of normal judgment, it would be only by a highly unethical and extraordinary abuse of their confidence that they would be persuaded to "avail themselves" of this violation of their physical integrity and this surrender of one of their fundamental human rights. By no stretch of the imagination would sterilization under moral duress be termed "voluntary." . . . What would the founding fathers of our country think if they could see today the attacks being made on our fundamental liberties and rights, which they fought so zealously to assure us forever? Euthanasia, sterilization—what next, O God?[42]

In the *Woman's Home Companion*, Edith M. Stern also delivered a stinging protest:

> 50,000 Americans have already been deprived of all possibility of parenthood. More will be sterilized tomorrow. Do you know who? Or why? Don't turn to

the law for an answer. . . . Our laws on this vital problem are dangerously muddled and sadly in need of thorough overhauling. . . . Smudging the statute books of more than half our states is a muddle of laws designed to improve the quality of the human race in general and of the American people in particular. This goal is to be reached by sterilizing the so-called unfit. . . . More or less qualified individuals play God [by deciding who] would make undesirable parents. . . . It is relatively simple to obtain consent from a helpless institutionalized individual or from an indifferent relative or a guardian.

Stern then described three "tragic examples." "Jack" was a "mischief maker" and "difficult to handle" in an Oklahoma orphans' home. Although he was never tested, he was sent to the state institution for the feebleminded, where he was sterilized as a "purely routine matter." Infuriated, he escaped, enlisted in the army, and became a master sergeant and mechanic. After the war, Jack "married a normal young woman who very much wanted a child." Later he told her what happened to him, and she got a divorce. "Grace" was another mistake. A "graduate" of a midwestern state training school where she had been sterilized before her release, she wrote to its superintendent, telling of her new job, her marriage, and her desire to have a child: "Is there any operation I could have now to fix me up so I could? . . . My husband and I are so anxious to have a baby and we would take good care of it." Noting that one-fourth of all state laws on eugenic sterilization covered "moral degenerates" and "sexual perverts," Stern asked:

> Who are these people? What do West Virginia and Oklahoma mean by "the crime against nature" or California by "sexual depravity"? The Kinsey report has indicated that considerable behavior formerly considered "depraved" is actually fairly normal. Should enforcement of sterilization fall into the hands of a zealot, there's no telling who'd be safe.[43]

Some journals also backed away from supporting such practices. *Scientific American* had favored compulsory sterilization in 1911, but rejected Gamble's article in 1949. The *Saturday Evening Post* also rejected the piece: "It could be that we are kidding ourselves, but we feel that the majority of our readers are relatively free of misconceptions about the effects of sterilization." Gamble and his associates interpreted these rejections as evidence of timidity in the face of controversy over what they considered to be a "progressive" social measure. Janet Baird, who worked closely with Gamble, wrote of the publisher of *Reader's Scope*: "I think he hesitates to stick his neck out on anything so controversial. That's the trouble with things like the 'UnAmerican Committee' [sic]—everyone with any liberal tendencies runs for cover to avoid being branded a Communist."[44] It is highly unlikely that even the most zealous anti-communist considered sterilization to be subversive, but Baird's comments reveal the moral righteousness that she and her eugenic comrades carried into the crusade.

In spite of the efforts of crusaders like Gamble, popular opinion was hostile to the idea of compulsory sterilization during the postwar years. An official in Ohio stated that "sterilization had been submitted to the legislature several times, and had been uniformly and heavily defeated." Nevertheless, the abuse of sterilization continued, often on children. Some physicians actually admitted that class, not alleged intelligence, was the criterion for sterilization. In a letter to Gamble in 1948, Dr. Christopher Tietze cited a study of the parents of 1,280 institutionalized mental defectives: "It should be noted, however, that in many instances the parents were not actually tested but their intelligence estimated on the basis of their educational and occupational history." In other words, a child who did poorly on culturally biased I.Q. tests and whose parents were deemed feebleminded on the basis of their occupational and educational history would be recommended for compulsory sterilization.[45]

Abuse of Sterilization since 1960

Eventually, the question of feeblemindedness became moot. Institutional sterilizations declined in the 1950s and 1960s, although they never completely ceased and remained legal in nineteen states as late as 1985. But abuse of sterilization continued on a large scale outside the walls of institutions. The earlier criteria, which targeted the feebleminded—a category based largely on class and sexual behavior—shifted to a focus on race and poverty. Race had always been an issue in eugenic sterilization, and it came back into focus when expanding welfare policies provided support for poor women of color and their children. Although the majority of welfare recipients were White women, people of color were targeted for sterilization. Concerns about the rising costs of welfare provided a rationale for attacks on the fertility of Black, Hispanic, and Native American women.[46]

After World War II, sterilizations were performed disproportionately on women of color. A 1970 National Fertility Study by the Office of Population

Research of Princeton University found that whereas 43 percent of the women who were sterilized in federally financed family planning programs were Black, Black women represented only one-third of the patients. A study of New York City hospitals in 1973 showed that Spanish-speaking women were sterilized at three times the rate of Black women and six times the rate of White women.[47]

Native American women were the most vulnerable to the abuse of sterilization. The General Accounting Office found that "in four Indian Health Service hospitals alone, 3,406 sterilizations were performed between 1973-1976," without informed consent. Representatives of the Mohawk Nation charged that the U.S. Public Health Service sterilized young Native American mothers without informing them of the nature of the surgeries. In the single year 1973, the Indian Health Service Hospital in Claremore, Oklahoma, sterilized 132 Indian women. Connie Uri, a physician who documented the abuse, estimated that more than 25 percent of Native American women were sterilized.

Sterilization was so prevalent that some tribal peoples were likely to be wiped out as a result. Uri observed, "All the pureblood women of the Kaw tribe of Oklahoma have now been sterilized. At the end of this generation the tribe will cease to exist." These operations were not necessarily the result of blatant coercion, but many of the women had not been informed about the permanence of the surgery or told of other contraceptive options. In 1974, Gerhard Gisell, a federal district court judge, estimated that 100,000 to 150,000 poor women had been sterilized under federally funded programs and noted that the "dividing line between family planning and eugenics is murky."[48]

Physicians became the gatekeepers of reproduction, with the authority to make decisions about their patients' future fertility. In the late 1950s, Gamble and Alan Guttmacher argued that physicians are better equipped to make these decisions than are the patients themselves: "Men of the highest standing are furnishing this safeguard for their patients, recording on their histories adequate physical and mental indications for the operation. The time should soon come when serious economic indications that promise to be permanent are recognized as justifying protection at government expense." Sterilizing poor women under duress "within an hour or a few days after labor" was not considered shameful or surreptitious:

It is tube closure after oft repeated or hazardous delivery which has received the most rapidly increasing endorsement outside the procedures in state mental hospitals. This impulse started chiefly in the southern states with their larger proportion of people of very low incomes associated with a high reproductive rate.[49]

The lack of safeguards meant that individual physicians had enormous latitude in treating poor women. Whereas many physicians undoubtedly respected the wishes of the women in their care, others clearly took advantage of their patients' vulnerability. The federal government fostered this abuse by covering the costs of sterilization but not of abortion or contraception. For many poor women, the line between voluntary and involuntary sterilization was thin. Once the restrictions on elective sterilizations eased, surgeries became readily available, especially to low-income women. In 1969, the American College of Obstetricians and Gynecologists dropped the 120 formula, and in 1970 it removed the requirement that two physicians and a psychiatrist must approve the surgery. Although these developments made elective surgery more readily available, they also paved the way for abuses. Physicians often forced poor women of color to "choose" sterilization while in labor or delivery or as a condition of prenatal, obstetric, or abortion services.[50]

Whether or not these women wanted more children, they were not necessarily "ready to give up their fertility," according to one study. In many communities, especially where resources were scarce and children were precious, "a woman's greatest gift is still thought to be her fertility." Some physicians, however, had no qualms about destroying women's reproductive potential. Clovis Pierce, the only physician in Aiken County, South Carolina, who was willing to deliver babies for women on welfare, was one. But Pierce did it on one condition: that mothers of three children on Medicaid agreed to be sterilized. Mrs. Marietta Williams, aged twenty, was sterilized after the birth of her third child. She said that Pierce threatened to take her to court if she did not sign the consent form. "I wouldn't marry again. Who would want me, knowing I cannot have any children?"

Pierce defended his policy as saving taxpayers' money. The records of Aiken County Hospital showed that 18 of the 34 deliveries paid by Medicaid included sterilization; 16 of the 18 were of Black women. All eighteen sterilizations were performed by Pierce, who earned $60,000 from Medicaid in eighteen months. When two of the women whom Pierce sterilized sued, the federal jury in South Carolina did not agree that their rights were violated. The jury awarded one woman five dollars in damages, but awarded nothing for the other. Pierce testified that his policy saved children from being raised in the worst possible conditions. His disdain for his patients was undisguised. He said that he saw patients with dirty bodies and clothes and "an odor on them you can smell coming across the room."[51]

In a similar situation in Baltimore, fourteen young Black women were sterilized without their knowledge. One Black physician said, "Hell, sterilization of black women, especially those who are young . . . is a fact of life in this city." Bernard Rosenfeld, a physician who did an investigation, blamed the "incredible arrogance of medical power which permits a doctor to cavalierly subject an indigent patient to the personal whim of the physician." Such arrogance was not confined to Baltimore. A physician from Texas boasted, "I used to make my pitch while sewing up the episiotomy, when the anesthesia started wearing off. . . . It was house staff (residents) policy. They used to wear buttons saying, 'Stop at 2, damn it.'" Sometimes doctors performed unnecessary hysterectomies on poor Black women, simply for the practice. The New York Times found that these "hyster-sterilizations" were "increasingly popular among surgeons, despite the risks," and "so common among some groups of indigent blacks that they are referred to as 'Mississippi appendectomies.'"[52]

Civil Rights Leader Fanny Lou Hamer was one of the Black women who was deemed "unfit" to be a parent. When she was sterilized in 1961, she and her husband had already raised two girls who had come to live with them, and they believed they could have easily cared for more. Two pregnancies had ended in stillbirths, but they still hoped to have their own children. When she was hospitalized for the removal of a small uterine tumor, she was given a hysterectomy without her knowledge or consent. She learned of it later when the physician's cousin told her cook, who then told Mrs. Hamer. But there was nothing she could do. She helped bring the issue to light as an activist for civil rights, but the movement against the abuse of sterilization was still many years away. Hamer explained why she had no legal recourse: "At that time? Me? Getting a white lawyer to go against a white doctor? I would have been taking my hands and screwing tacks in my own casket."[53]

In the 1970s, feminist activists, concerned about the abuse of poor women of color, fought to bring the abuse of sterilization to light. As the result of a sustained and effective political campaign, a number of cases reached the courts. One such case was that of Norma Jean Serena, a Shawnee woman who was sterilized in 1970 in Armstrong County, Pennsylvania, without her knowledge, during delivery. According to her medical chart, the operation was performed for "socio-economic factors." Another case that attracted a great deal of media attention was that of two Black sisters, Minnie Lee and Mary Alice Relf, aged twelve and fourteen. The girls were sterilized in the Montgomery Family Planning Clinic, a federally funded social agency. The clinic staff insisted that the girls and their parents had been informed. But the girls' father, Lonnie Relf, said, "Nobody understood. The girls had been getting birth control shots for some time, and the clinic's nurses come here and said they wanted to give them some more. But they just took 'em away instead and then taken the life right out of them." Relf said that the sterilizations would not have taken place if he had been there. "I didn't want it done, and I'm still upset," he said. Mrs. Relf agreed: "I was mad. I wouldn't have let them do that." The investigation of the Relf case revealed that the same clinic had sterilized eleven young girls, ten of them Black. The Eugenics Board of North Carolina admitted that it ordered the sterilization of 1,620 persons between 1960 and 1968. Almost all were Black women and girls; more than half were younger than twenty years of age.[54]

As a result of the efforts of feminists and their allies, in 1974 the federal government established regulations to be followed in the cases of federally funded sterilizations. These regulations included safeguards for informed consent and the prohibition of sterilizations of women under age twenty-one. But follow-up studies revealed that most federally funded hospitals and clinics did not enforce these policies. Pressure by feminist groups and highly publicized court actions continued.

In the 1970s and 1980s, a number of women's organizations pressured the American Civil Liberties Union (ACLU) to file several class-action suits. One such case was *Doe v. Lynchburg*, filed against the state of Virginia on behalf of 7,000 women who were sterilized under Virginia's law between 1924 and 1974. One of these women was "Judith Doe," who was admitted in 1948, at age thirteen, to the Lynchburg Training School, a state mental institution, shortly after giving birth to a son who was conceived when she was raped by her stepfather. Records at the hospital say she was "not basically defective" but was "in an emotional and intellectual loss" after the birth of her baby, who was put up for adoption and became "a successful businessman." Doe believed that she was sterilized because she was poor. "I don't think of myself as white trash. . . . They told me I had to go through with the operation or they wouldn't let me out. I didn't know what else to do." Later she married, but the marriage did not last. "We were hoping we would have children, but we didn't and we just split up." The class-action suit did not ask for restitution; it merely asked that everyone be notified and provided with medical and psychological assistance, since the state agencies had refused to notify those who were sterilized.[55]

The ACLU also filed a class-action suit on behalf of Nial Ruth Cox and "others similarly situated." Cox, a Black woman, was sterilized under state law at age eighteen. Neither she nor her mother understood the nature of the operation. "She is not, and never has been, mentally defective, despite an assertion by the doctor who performed the operation that she was an '18 year old mentally deficient Negro girl.'" Cox's mother "consented" to what she was told was a temporary tying of tubes, under threat of removal from the welfare rolls of her entire family. Cox said:

> I was living with my mother and eight sisters and brothers. My father, who was married to my mother until I was six, is dead. My family was on welfare, but payments had stopped for me because I was 18. We had no hot or cold running water, only pump water. No stove. No refrigerator, no electric lights. It got cold down there in the winter. I got pregnant when I was 17, I didn't know anything about birth control or abortion. When the welfare caseworker found out I was pregnant, she told my mother that if we wanted to keep getting welfare, I'd have to have my tubes tied—temporarily. Nobody explained anything to me before the operation. Later on, after the operation, I saw the doctor and I asked him if I could have another baby. He said that I had nothing to worry about, that, of course, I could have more kids. I know now that I was sterilized because I was from a welfare family.

At the time of the suit, Cox was a twenty-six-year-old nurse's aide living on Long Island.[56]

Not all the suits were successful. Ten poor Chicanas in Los Angeles, who spoke little English, filed a class-action suit against the hospital where they were sterilized, charging that they were coerced and deceived. Some were presented with consent forms written in English while they were in labor or under anesthesia, and others were told they would die if they did not submit to sterilization. They lost their suit; the judge cited a "breakdown in communication between the patients and the doctors." In spite of all the efforts of feminist activists, the abuse of sterilization continued. Even after the federal guidelines were strengthened in 1978, 70 percent of the hospitals did not comply with them. In 1981, the *Boston Globe* reported that states were still sterilizing poor Medicaid recipients, many of them minors, without properly obtaining their consent.[57]

Such abuses of sterilization eventually declined in the 1980s, but they have not entirely stopped. In the 1990s, several states have considered or enacted legislation that would cap welfare benefits for women who have additional children while receiving aid. Some lawmakers have proposed incentives, such as additional subsidies for women who accept Norplant, capsules that are implanted in a woman's upper arm that prevent pregnancy for up to five years. As Alexander Cockburn noted in the *Nation*, "Just as, at the turn of the century, vasectomy allowed eugenicists to abandon advocacy of castration, so today Norplant . . . substitutes for grosser attacks on women's fertility." These proposals allow politicians to avoid the real sources of poverty and social disarray. Contrary to popular myth, welfare recipients average fewer than two children per family, and their fertility rate is lower than that of the general population. Still, those who advocate cutting welfare benefits for poor women and their children, using thinly veiled eugenic arguments, continue to blame the poor for their own plight.[58]

Compulsory sterilization represented social engineering of the worst sort. By focusing on the reproductive behavior of the "unfit," authorities and public officials avoided tackling the real sources of poverty: racism and the maldistribution of wealth. Similar uses of reproductive control occurred in industry, where sterilization allowed employers to avoid the problem of health hazards in the workplace. Employers in certain industries prohibited fertile women from working with materials that allegedly posed a risk to a fetus. Like the physicians who offered a "choice" to women in labor—sterilization or no medical attention—these employers gave women an "option." Five women who were working for American Cyanamid succumbed to the surgery to keep their jobs. According to Judge Robert Bork, "This is not an anti-woman decision. . . . The company was offering women a choice. That's all it was about."

But the women did not feel that they had a choice. Betty Riggs, one of the women who was sterilized, said, "Only a judge who knows nothing about women" could call it a choice. "I was only twenty-six years old, but I had to work so I had no choice. This was the most awful thing that happened to me." Betty Moler, who was sterilized at age twenty-seven, said, "It makes me feel different, like a part of me is missing." These policies also discriminated against men, who worked in hazardous areas with risks to their health and reproductive capacities. There is considerable evidence that many men working with hazardous chemicals were rendered sterile. According to a study by the political scientist Sally Kenney, so-called protective policies allowed companies to avoid making their workplaces safer and rendered men as well as women sterile against their will.[59] Like eugenic sterilization, these exclusionary policies were put into place presumably to protect those who they actually harmed.

The eugenics movement set a precedent for regulating individual reproductive behavior as a means of social engineering. Although the advocates were a small number of middle-class professionals, these crusaders had the power to

affect institutional policies, laws, and medical practice for much of the twentieth century. The successes of negative eugenics show how powerfully ideas of
parental worthiness became woven into the social and cultural fabric. If "unworthy" parents were allegedly responsible for poverty, crime, a drain on public
funds, and a host of other social problems, then the opposite must have been
true: "Worthy" parents were good citizens. By the middle of the twentieth
century, parenthood among the "worthy"—married, middle-class heterosex-
uals—became a primary marker of respectability. As the baby boom finally
put fears of race suicide to rest, the childless faced an even more ferocious
stigma, one that called into question not just their behavior, but their character, as well.

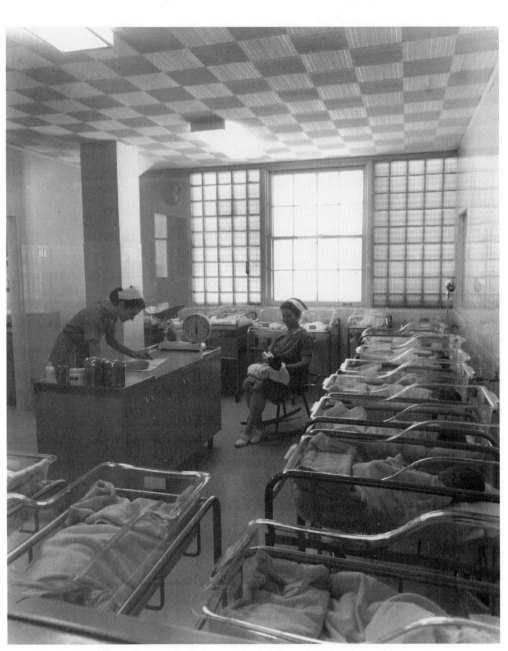

During the years of the baby boom in the 1940s and 1950s, hospital nurseries were filled to capacity. *(Courtesy of the Herb and Dorothy McLaughlin Collection, Archives and Manuscripts, University Libraries, Arizona State University, Tempe)*

CHAPTER 4

The Baby Craze: The Rise of Compulsory Parenthood

★☆

I was brought up by progressive parents who expected me to have a career as my mother and aunts had, even in the 1920s and 30s. Ironically, what I myself wanted was a home and several children.
    —Pamela Moore, born 1923, childless in the post–World War II years

Why, I suddenly find myself beating my breast and proclaiming my patriotism and exclaiming that I love my wife and kids, of which I have four with a fifth on the way. I'm all loused up. I'm scared to death, and nobody can tell me it isn't because I'm afraid of being investigated.
—Anonymous studio executive in the midst of the Hollywood red scare, quoted in Lillian Ross, "Onward and Upward with the Arts," *New Yorker*, February 1948

By the time Pamela Moore came of age in the post–World War II era, childlessness had declined precipitously, and the stigma surrounding it took on a psychological dimension. Now childlessness became a mark of social maladjustment. The focus shifted from "unfit" poor women to "neurotic" middle-class women who did not conform to prevailing gender roles. Childless adults no longer appeared merely unfortunate or selfish; they were vilified as downright un-American. The now-famous postwar suburban family placed children at its center. Polls indicated that virtually nobody considered the ideal family size to be no children, and only a tiny minority said that they did not want children themselves. As the number of childless adults plummeted, compulsory sterilization disappeared from view, and voluntary childlessness became virtually invisible. Researchers found that "nearly all American couples now in the childbearing ages have a strong aversion to childlessness."[1]

Gone were the days when a small cadre of professionals and experts felt they had to carry the burden of exhorting the middle class to procreate. Even before the war, crusaders for eugenics faded into the woodwork as Nazi breeding experiments became known. During the war, the stakes in having children intensified considerably, compared to the prewar years when the stigma attached to childlessness had eased somewhat. When demographic trends shifted dramatically and precipitously in the 1940s, the pronatalist message became ubiquitous. Suddenly, babies invaded the popular culture, from magazine covers to movie screens. And the baby boom exploded.

Although Pamela Moore, quoted at the opening of this chapter, was only about a decade younger than the women described in chapter 2 who were content to be childless, the demographic and cultural upheavals of the postwar years affected Pamela and her peers differently. The numbers themselves tell a dramatic story. Among ever-married women, 20 percent of those born between 1906 and 1910 remained childless. Yet the rate of childlessness for those born just a few years later, between 1913 and 1918, was only 14 percent—down by a third. Looking at the lifetime childlessness of all women, regardless of their marital status, fully 27 percent of those born in the three decades before 1915 never had children, compared to only 10 percent of those born between 1915 and 1930. This drastic decline in childlessness coincided with the dramatic rise in the marriage rate, as well as the birthrate, which gave rise to the baby boom.[2]

The Baby Boom

The baby boom affected everybody. Birthrates in America rose for every racial, ethnic, religious, occupational, and income group in the country. Scholars and observers generally explain the baby boom as the result of a transition from hard times to good times. The explanation is not so simple, however. The defensive nationalism that gave rise to the race suicide panic did not boost the birthrate, even in the relatively prosperous 1920s. But something in the quest for "national security" in the postwar years did.

Although the baby boom was fueled, in part, by the economic boom, it also resulted from a profound change in the national political culture: The nation's security suddenly became fused with a vision of the American home. The ideology of domesticity, focused on the nuclear family with children, came to embody the hope for the future of the nation and the ultimate achievement of happiness and personal fulfillment for its citizens. The dual functions of patriotism and personal happiness marked a change in the concept of parenthood and marginalized the childless in unprecedented ways.[3]

Childless women and men in the postwar era struggled to find their place in a society that wrapped happiness and meaning around having children. Some drew strength from faith and experience to help them deal with their disappointment and lived full and rewarding lives without children. Eliza James desperately wanted children. Like Pamela Moore, she grew up anticipating motherhood. But her experiences during the depression and the war prepared her to cope with the disappointment of infertility later in her life. As it turned out, her childlessness enabled her to pursue an exciting occupation. A farm-reared "depression-era teenager" from Texas, the youngest of eight children, she recalled the struggles of her family: "We were poor from a financial standpoint all my life but never felt the real pinch until the 1930s and the draught of those years." After her marriage in 1939, she "housewifed only for a couple of years" and then "started on a project of producing children."

That project was interrupted during the war when she went to work for Southern Bell Telephone, a job she continued after the war. She embarked upon infertility treatment and had surgery for blocked fallopian tubes. But the surgery was not successful. In spite of advances in infertility treatment, physicians still had a relatively limited repertoire. Decades later, reproductive technologies, such as in-vitro fertilization, would offer possible cures for women with blocked tubes. But in the 1940s, as her physician explained, the condition was probably incurable. Although the news was disappointing, it allowed Elizabeth and her husband to come to terms with their childlessness and move on with their lives.

> Of course, we went through years of people wanting to know why we had no children, we didn't know what we were missing . . . ad nauseam! . . . I had worked at containing my bitterness and my husband had accepted the situation even though it was a great disappointment to him. Having been reared in the Southern tradition of carrying on the family name, it hurt him.

Eliza finally came to accept her childlessness when her sister gave her a Bible in 1954, with a marker on the 54 chapter of Isaiah, "Sing, O Barren One, who did not bear." From that moment, "my bitterness left me. I have felt at peace with other people's children and have devoted my life to working with young people," two of whom she raised as her own.

Eliza was fortunate to have taken an exciting and challenging job during the war that laid the foundation for a lifelong career. Being childless was a misfortune, but it also enabled her to continue her work as an outside plant engineer for the Bell Telephone Company, "a job that I totally enjoyed. . . . I was the first woman the company put in the field in Tennessee." She retired in February 1979, to farm and raise cattle, but she also continued to work as a contract telephone engineer for several years. When a contractor called her in 1992 and asked the seventy-two-year-old retiree, "Are you ready to go back to stump jumping?" she returned to work full time, making construction draw- ings and helping "to bury 121 miles of fiber-optic cable." Eliza was part Rosie the Riveter and part Ann Bradstreet, the colonial poet who prayed for solace from God. Her interesting work, her faith, and her informally "adopted" chil- dren provided her with the means to escape the pain that many of her child- less contemporaries endured in the midst of the baby boom.

Unlike Eliza, Pamela never came to terms with being childless. Being a mother was much more important to her than it was to the older women in her family, "who expected me to have a career as my mother and aunts had." Pamela wanted "a home and several children," but her hopes were dashed. Like many others of her generation, she had an abortion as a young woman. In the postwar years, abortion had become more dangerous, more difficult to obtain, and more shameful.

> Regrettably, a few months following the end of World War II I discovered I was pregnant. There was no way I could get married and leave my family duties, but in those days, unwed motherhood was considered slightly less than murder in the moral code. I considered, and rejected, suicide and when my nerve-induced migraines threatened to give me away . . . I told my father and he agreed to find and pay for a doctor who would perform an abortion, on condition I give up my theatrical ambitions and get a regu- lar paying job.

She recalled the horror of the experience.

> Even now I can hardly bear to think of that Friday night. It was what was called a medically-induced miscarriage in that he used drugs rather than

surgery and I was sent home immediately since the doctor feared discovery and imprisonment. I was in sheer agony all night, cramping and vomiting, so weak I had to crawl on hands and knees to get to the bathroom. I remember a friend of my brother was home on leave and we said I had the flu and he sat by the bed telling me the plot of Gilda, the Rita Hayworth movie. By the next morning, I had lost the baby and though I didn't know it at the time, any chance of having another.

Years later she married a "fine man by whom I expected to have several children. I didn't dare tell my husband about this disgraceful episode of my youthful past." After pursuing infertility treatment, the physician "told me privately that my internal organs were irreparably scarred. . . . When I finally told my husband, he could not forgive me for not disclosing my 'past' and we subsequently divorced and he married again."

The abortion cast such a long shadow on her life that it destroyed not only her reproductive organs but her marriage. She never married again, and in spite of having "many friends, an interesting career and the opportunity to travel extensively," not having children "has been the greatest regret of my life." The openness of prewar society that made it possible for women to carve out respected and exciting lives without children had ended. After the war, according to the prevailing White middle-class ethos, only one worthy occupation remained for women: motherhood. Although Pamela's experience would have been heartbreaking in any era, the intensity of postwar pronatalism undoubtedly made it worse. "Being childless has been an ongoing cause of great sadness in my life—nothing else ever made up for that loss. To me children are the greatest source of happiness in life."[4]

Patriotic Parenthood

The passion for parenthood began during the war. The bearing and raising of children became a national obsession with powerful patriotic overtones. Fighting the Nazis with their infamous racism and eugenics policies made it unsavory to talk about having children as a duty to the "race," so the rhetoric shifted to child rearing as a contribution to the nation. Wartime propaganda continually reminded men that they were fighting for home and family and urged women to turn their postwar energies to marriage and child rearing. Radio programs broadcast the message that the war was about "love and gettin' hitched, and havin' a home and some kids, and breathin' fresh air out in the suburbs . . . like free people."[5] In the postwar vision, "the men would be secure in stable careers, the women in comfortable homes, and together they would raise perfect children. . . . It was the *Zeitgeist*, the spirit of the times," recalled a postwar psychologist.[6]

Even before the war ended, the declining marriage rates and birthrates of the depression years had turned around. Between 1940 and 1945, the birthrate climbed from 19.4 to 24.5 per one thousand population. The age at first marriage dropped, and the marriage rate accelerated, paving the way for the rush into marriage and parenthood that continued for two decades after the war ended.[7] Homemaker and mother became the most exalted identities for women, and fatherhood the measure of responsibility and respectability for men.

The patriotic meanings of parenthood expanded with the advent of the cold war. The explosion of the atomic bomb on Hiroshima in 1945 marked the beginning of the nuclear age. "On that day parenthood took on added responsibilities of deep and profound significance," warned a writer in *American Home*.

> Out of the smoke and smoldering ruins arose a great cry for leadership equipped to guide the stricken people of the world along the hazardous course toward peace. . . . Upon the shoulders of parents, everywhere, rests the tremendous responsibility of sending forth into the next generation men and women imbued with a high resolve to work together for everlasting peace.

Parenthood now became "an absorbing, creative profession—a career second to none." The writer in *American Home* directed her pronatalist arguments toward educated, middle-class women as the potential mothers of the nation's future leaders. As for those affluent women who were so preoccupied with "superficial culture, refinements and polish, luxury and ease" that they "failed to produce the quality of leadership needed," they were nothing more than "flabby, apathetic, indifferent, irresponsible members of society." She claimed that such "ignorant, lazy or selfish" individuals "have no place" in the postwar world.[8]

These exalted ideas about parenthood cast the old eugenic call for the "worthy" to procreate in new cold-war terms. Along with the scorn heaped on White middle-class women who shirked their reproductive duties, the pronatalist ethos of the postwar years both fed and reflected the demographic explosion. The huge increase in births that created the baby boom was not the result of couples suddenly having large families. The number of children per family actually went up only modestly, from an average of 2.4 in the 1930s to 3.2 in the 1950s. What made the baby boom happen was that everyone was doing it, and at the same time. The birthrate rose among all social, occupational, economic, and ethnic groups in a remarkable consensus of reproductive behavior.[9]

In the midst of this reproductive mania, childlessness appeared to be deviant, selfish, and pitiable. In spite of the increasing birthrate, many postwar observers feared that in the wake of new opportunities that opened for women during the war, women might be inclined to shirk their procreative responsibilities—to the nation's detriment, as well as their own. In one of many efforts to encourage women to direct their career aspirations to the home, J. Edgar Hoover, director of the Federal Bureau of Investigation, addressed American housewives as "'career' women. . . . I say 'career' women because I feel there are no careers so important as those of homemaker and mother." Linking domesticity to cold-war patriotism, he called upon "homemakers and mothers" to fight "the twin enemies of freedom—crime and communism."[10]

Many agreed with Hoover that women should focus their talents and expertise on motherhood. Harking back to turn-of-the-century suspicions of women's occupational and educational advancement, these alarmists dusted off and revived the old specter of race suicide. A 1946 study reported in the *American Journal of Sociology* concluded that the increase in women's employment "is related to the secular decline in the birth rate" and predicted (wrongly) that since the proportion of women in the paid labor force was likely to increase even more, the birthrate would continue to decline.[11]

Newsweek contributed to these postwar anxieties by reporting that education for women was equally detrimental to procreation: "For the American girl books and babies don't mix. Long ago scientists concluded that the American family's reproduction rate is in inverse ratio to the educational attainment of the parents. Now . . . they have discovered that it is the higher-educated wife, rather than the husband, who brings down the birth rate." A writer in the *American Mercury,* using classic eugenic terminology, argued that the "feeble-minded . . . are filling our asylums, juvenile courts and hospitals throughout the land." She claimed that "too many 'borderline' cases, are breeding too high a proportion of our infants," instead of "the sensitive and intelligent people who should have continued to dominate our land."[12]

Even as late as the peak of the baby boom in the mid-1950s, *U.S. News and World Report* echoed the same concern: "America's college women . . . are failing to keep up with the baby boom. It is the relatively uneducated women who keep the U.S. population on the rise." The report was inaccurate; the sharpest rise in the birthrate was among the most highly educated women. Nevertheless, distorted claims like these kept eugenic fears of race suicide alive and brought public shame upon women—particularly White educated women—who were childless.[13] The focus on the educated White middle class also ignored the plight of the poor and people of color, who had the highest rates of childlessness, owing to poverty and poor health care. According to one study, poor people were likely to be even more devastated by childlessness than were the affluent because they "experience proportionately more of their total [feelings of satisfaction] in the family than do the affluent."[14] They were also less likely to be able to afford infertility treatment or adoption.

For the poor, as well as the wealthy, having babies offered a major source of personal fulfillment. Unlike the early decades of the century, when American men and especially women were called to the duties and sacrifices of procreation as if called to war, postwar Americans approached patriotic parenthood as a major source of joy and satisfaction in life. Happy families became synonymous with the "American way of life." Fulfillment, rather than responsibility, became the ultimate reward. The "pursuit of happiness" took on a decidedly domestic cast in the cold-war era. According to a writer in the *Ladies Home Journal*, "Certainly the happiest women have never found the secret of their happiness in books or lectures. They do the right thing instinctively."[15]

Sexy Motherhood

The "maternal instinct" was the point at which ideas of happiness, patriotism, and reproduction fused, with an unprecedented focus on sexuality. In the past, motherhood had been explicitly identified with chastity, purity, virtue, and restraint. But in the postwar era, the glorification of motherhood reflected emerging ideas about eroticized marriage and the sexualized home. In their best-selling volume, *The Modern Woman: The Lost Sex*, Marynia Farnham and Ferdinand Lundberg insisted that the true fulfillment of female sexuality was motherhood.[16] The ideal of cold-war womanhood was the glamorous and sexy wife and mother.

Hollywood actively promoted this vision as early as the mid-1940s. In fan magazines and publicity photos, mothers became sex symbols and babies became romantic. If images of sexy sweethearts inspired World War II soldiers to fight for home and hearth, the promise of sexy mommies inspired men to don the "gray flannel suit" for the rewards that awaited them at home. "Hollywood's newest pin-up girl" was the infant daughter of Lana Turner, noted World War II "pin-up" herself. Joan Crawford, saucy and sexy star of the 1930s, became "another incredibly devoted and capable mother," according to writers in the 1940s. Everywhere the popular culture featured movie stars with their babies, in alluring and romantic poses. *Life* magazine ran a photo essay on professional models who were mothers, praising these "professional beauties who have found that having a baby is fine for their careers. . . . Motherhood, in fact, seems to help them. . . . Being a mother usually improves a girl's disposition, her attitude towards her work, her looks and even her figure."[17] Although most of these messages emphasized a newly glorified motherhood, fatherhood also took on heightened significance. It became the new badge of masculinity and meaning for postwar men, and Father's Day a holiday of major significance. In 1954, *Life* announced "the domestication of the American male." To those men who recoiled at the idea of tending to children, a male psychiatrist wrote in *Parents* magazine, "Being a real father is not 'sissy' business. It is an occupation . . . the most important occupation in the world." The historian Stephanie Coontz noted that in the postwar years, "For the first time, men as well as women were encouraged to root their identity and self-image in familial and parental roles."[18]

The shift also surfaced in the popular culture. According to *Photoplay* magazine, when film star Maureen O'Hara told her husband she was pregnant: "He walked more briskly, like all prospective fathers. His eyes sparkled. His voice had a new ring of authority." Male movie stars who played heroic tough-guy loners in the 1930s and 1940s appeared deranged and dangerous in postwar films; the new heroes were domestic sorts who spent their time with their families.[19] Carl Corning's young adulthood spanned the years when these images of manhood changed. He recalled that in the 1930s, "all I wanted was to make myself financially independent. . . . I had to work to go to school, I had to go to school in order to do what I wanted to do . . . and I liked the independence." That spirit was rewarded before the war, but not in the postwar era. "I changed my ideas," he explained, and began to think about having children.

Fatherhood

Fatherhood was a major marker of middle-class manhood in the years after World War II. According to the historian Robert Griswold, the new prosperity, mass consumerism, and routinized jobs blurred the distinctions between working-class and middle-class men.

> If consumption was declining as an effective barometer of class standing, child rearing could become a new index of middle-class sensibility. And where better to realize the key assumptions of masculine domesticity than in the burgeoning middle-class suburbs of the postwar era? Here middle-class men had the job security, financial wherewithal, education, and leisure to practice a style of child rearing that underscored private rather than public life and solidified the social standing of middle-class men imbued with status anxieties.[20]

Fatherhood was not just a matter of pride, however. It, too, was an important responsibility and evidence of maturity, patriotism, and citizenship. In *Penny Serenade*, one of the most popular films of the 1940s, the hero, played by Cary Grant, gives up his adventurous, reckless ways for a settled job, a steady income, and a child. In the film, the child is the reward for the drabness of postwar white-collar work for men. Pleading with the judge to let him keep his adopted daughter, he claims that he has been transformed and is now worthy of parenthood:

> I'd always been, well, kinda careless and irresponsible, I wanted to be a big shot. I couldn't work for anybody; I had to be my own boss—that sort of thing. . . . Look I'm not a big shot now. I'll do anything—I'll work for anybody—I'll beg, I'll borrow—Please, Judge . . . she'll never go hungry and she'll never be without clothes not as long as I've got two good hands to help me.

The happy father triumphs as the judge agrees to let him keep the child.[21]

At a time when social observers, such as David Reisman and William Whyte, lamented the monotonous, routine, unsatisfying work of middle-class postwar men, there appeared to be few opportunities for robust, virile, masculine productivity. Even for industrial laborers, much of the work was now done by machines. Thus, few opportunities remained for men to be productive with their bodies. Procreation offered that possibility. As one man remarked in 1955, "I'd like six kids. . . . It just seems like a minimum production goal."[22] Along with virile procreation, manly child rearing was also a vigorous endeavor. To avoid raising "sissies," men had to be physically active with their children, playing sports with them, building things with them, and taking them on rugged adventures. Without such masculine influence, children, especially boys, might become weak and dependent from "overfeminization."[23]

Men also understood that fatherhood was a mark of good citizenship and that the absence of children was a sign of possible subversion of the American way. Parenthood also provided proof of virile heterosexuality at a time when "homos," like "pinkos," were targets of rabid homophobic anti-communism. The studio executive quoted at the beginning of this chapter remarked in the midst of the Hollywood red scare, that in order to prove his patriotism he had to proclaim "that I love my wife and kids, of which I have four with a fifth on the way." He was "scared to death . . . and afraid of being investigated," so he promoted himself as a good husband and father.[24] Kate Foley recalled that when she and her husband finally had a baby, "People's attitude toward us really changed. We were now a 'real family.' We were now *adults*—childless adults are only quasi-adults, I guess. My husband's employer saw him as more 'permanent' and worthy of company investment."

Procreation reflected optimism and abundance, a sign of faith in a better future. But the emphatic, almost desperate, pronatalism of the era suggests that anxieties and fears about the future remained. The same sort of defensive nationalism that fueled the race-suicide panic now spurred the postwar baby craze. Governmental policies and major social institutions did everything possible to keep the baby boom booming. Countless incentives, from federally financed mortgages to tax deductions, supported the establishment of nuclear families with children. Contrary to the myth of the self-sufficient nuclear family of the 1950s, often held up as a model to disparage the single-parent families of the 1990s who receive "government handouts," the postwar suburban family was far from independent. In fact, in the years following World War II, virtually the entire White middle class was subsidized by the government. As Coontz pointed out, "the 1950s suburban family . . . was far more dependent on government handouts than any so-called 'underclass' in recent U.S. history."[25]

Federally subsidized housing was located not in the inner cities, but in the suburbs. Governmental spending spurred much of the upward mobility of the middle classes, which rested largely on home ownership. Federal Housing Authority and Veterans' Administration loans made home ownership available to millions of blue- and white-collar families. Redlining policies that marked off neighborhoods for home loans were based on racial residential barriers. As a result, most suburbs were integrated by class, but segregated by race. For White Americans, nuclear families gained tremendous benefits from governmental support; it paid to have children and settle in the suburbs.[26]

These policies were not meant to support children directly, however. They were intended to support families—particularly families with male breadwinners and full-time mothers at home. Even Aid to Families with Dependent Children (AFDC) supported full-time motherhood instead of child care centers and jobs. Except for a brief period during World War II, federally funded child care centers were never put into place. Rather, the incentives for women to stay home and care for their children, along with the disincentives to pursue careers, gave the government's pronatalist policies a decidedly gendered cast. With the help of generous subsidies from the government, developers and architects carved out huge suburban tracts across the country that were designed specifically for women to remain at home and rear children. Architects assumed that men would be away at work during the day and houses would be occupied by women and children. In Levittown, New York, the giant 17,400-unit suburban development, the interior walls of houses were flexible and could be expanded if families increased. Kitchens were near the front entrance, so mothers could keep an eye on their children playing in the yards. Formal living rooms and parlors gave way to "family rooms," where parents and children could enjoy their leisure time together. It is no wonder that Levittown earned the nicknames "Fertility Valley" and "The Rabbit Hutch."[27]

Children and the Good Life

Postwar abundance was nowhere more evident than in the child-centered, gadget-filled suburban home, symbol of the American way of life. Americans spent their money on themselves as *families*, not as individuals. In the five years following World War II, consumer spending increased 60 percent, but the amount spent on household furnishings and appliances rose 240 percent.

Increased expenditures for household operation, recreation, appliances, and automobiles far outdistanced those for food, clothing, personal care, and education. From the housing market to the supermarket, everything seemed geared to families with children. Grocery-store bargains came in "family-size" packages, automobiles were big "family sedans" and station wagons, television sets sat in family rooms and featured family sitcoms, "family restaurants" cropped up everywhere, and new theme parks like Disneyland beckoned families to travel and play together. In this atmosphere, it was rare to find anyone complaining about the cost of raising children. Children were not perceived as competing with adults for family resources, but as the opportunity for collective enjoyment. The good life appeared to be "cheaper by the dozen."[28]

During these years, marked by an overwhelming celebration of parenthood, childless adults were marginalized and disadvantaged more than ever before. Judging from the popular culture, everyone was either having children or desperately trying to have them. Intentional childlessness during these years was so stigmatized that it virtually went into the closet. Writer Letty Pogrebin recalled that voluntary childlessness was one of the family secrets hidden from her as a child, something as shameful in the cold-war era as marital discord or communism. When she was old enough, her mother let her listen to the women speak in Yiddish.

> That's how I learned that the aunt and uncle who wore glamorous clothes and won tango contests were actually miserable in their marriage; that another aunt was a card-carrying Communist throughout the McCarthy period; that still another aunt, a childless woman who'd been the subject of collective pity, was actually quite fertile. She used contraception and had once had an abortion but had chosen to call herself barren rather than admit she didn't *want* any children.[29]

Demographers assumed that childlessness by choice was practically extinct, even though later research showed that among some upwardly mobile segments of the population, voluntary childlessness was not uncommon. Even then, researchers assumed that childlessness was not an end in itself but a sacrifice to pursue a strategy for socioeconomic advancement: "Couples with the greatest disadvantages must make the greatest sacrifices of child-centered behavior."[30] Presumably, anyone who was childless was unhappy about the situation. But not everyone bought into the baby craze. Hugh Hefner tapped into fantasies of resistance and capitalized on a backlash against compulsory domesticity. His magazine, *Playboy*, unapologetically promoted individualistic over family-centered consumerism, nonmarital over marital sex, and self-indulgent masculinity over responsible fatherhood.[31] But the *Playboy* lifestyle remained largely a fantasy—men were flocking to become dutiful dads, just as women were eager for the crown of wife and motherhood.

Infertility and Adoption

It was during this era of compulsory parenthood that infertility first entered the public imagination in a major way and captured the attention of the media. The plot of popular films like *Penny Serenade* revolved around not only parental worthiness but infertility. In that film, the hero's pregnant wife miscarried and became sterile in an earthquake injury, making her so despondent that she was virtually suicidal until the possibility of adoption occurred. In *Close to My Heart*, an infertile woman and her husband tried to adopt, and again the man had to prove that he would be a responsible and caring father. Childlessness entered the popular culture not as a dangerous situation caused by selfish adults shirking their duty to posterity, but as a monumental personal tragedy.

Readers of almost any mass-circulation magazine could follow the story, week by week, of Janet Leigh and Tony Curtis's struggle to have a baby. When they finally had their long-awaited child, *Look* magazine did a huge photo essay, and the proud father announced, "She's the star of the family." Elizabeth Taylor, another screen goddess, finally became "A Woman At Last" when her baby was born. And virtually everyone knew of Marilyn Monroe's deep disappointment when the nation's number one sex symbol was unable to reach that ultimate expression of female sexuality: motherhood. Even though the actress refused to discuss her childlessness with the media, that did not stop contemporary observers from commenting on it endlessly.[32]

With babies everywhere and many of the nation's institutions encouraging, supporting, and celebrating procreation, infertility became increasingly difficult to accept. According to most estimates, infertility affected one out of ten married couples, or approximately 10 million people in the United States. Childless couples had two choices if they wished to pursue parenthood. They could seek infertility treatment, or they could try to adopt. Neither route necessarily guaranteed that they would end up with a child, but the medical profession, as well as the adoption establishment, increasingly catered to childless couples. Because only about half the infertility cases could be accurately diagnosed and only a third could be successfully treated, many infertile couples sought to adopt.

In the postwar years, adoption became primarily a service for infertile couples. One article, for example, written by a social worker, urged physicians specializing in infertility to encourage their patients to consider adoption as a route to "substitute parenthood." The article reported on a survey of adoptive parents in the late 1950s, on the assumption that all adoptive parents were infertile. When asked to describe their feelings about their infertility before they had adopted, the men gave responses like "deep disappointment," "inadequate," "resigned to the fact," "feeling I had failed my wife," and "disappointment but largely because of wife's feelings." Typical of women's responses were "absolutely heartsick"; "frustrated, depressed"; "a terrific desire for children and a desolate fear that we might not have any"; "despair"; "bitterness"; "longing"; "feeling a flop as a wife and woman"; "misery"; "self-pity"; and "desperate feeling of hopelessness and inferiority." The author concluded that "unwanted childlessness is a deeply depriving experience, principally for wives." He urged physicians to take on the role of counselor: "Although he may be unable to help the couple fulfil [sic] their desire for fecundity, he can help restore their flagging self-respect. The physician's role as manipulator of nature gives way to the educator's role of coming to grips with the inevitables of nature."[33]

Largely abandoning their mission as a service for children who needed homes, adoption agencies turned their efforts to serving couples who wanted babies. The new philosophy also favored the creation of nuclear families over the preservation of biological kinship, unlike previous strategies that included support for birth mothers and their extended families. The doctrine of the "best interest of the child" was redefined in the postwar years to mean a home in a nuclear family, rather than support for a biological mother.[34]

Like infertility treatment, legal adoption was a relatively recent phenomenon. First developed to protect orphaned children from exploitation and to secure a legal inheritance for them, it emerged in the late nineteenth and early twentieth centuries as a system geared to finding suitable homes for children who needed care, owing to the misfortune or death of their biological parents. In the early years of the twentieth century, the majority of all children who were relinquished for adoption were born to married parents and lived with one or both parents for several years. The average age of children placed for adoption was four and a half years. Because poverty, divorce, and desertion were the most common reasons that biological mothers relinquished their children and because close emotional bonds had already been established, caseworkers often endeavored to keep channels of communication open. Confidentiality and secrecy were rarely enforced, and both biological and adoptive kinship networks were frequently maintained. Couples who were hoping to adopt children gave a range of motivations. The most common one was the desire for children or the love of children, but other reasons were altruism, companionship for a sibling, desire for a boy or girl, replacement for a child who died, childlessness, "to further our own happiness," a wish to pass on their inheritance, or even a need for someone to do chores. All these motivations were considered legitimate. Infertility was rarely mentioned; the term itself was not even used before 1940.

The relatively flexible and open prewar process, focused on the needs of children and sympathy for the plight of biological parents, changed drastically in 1946. Suddenly, children's need for parents became secondary to childless couples' desire for children. According to a Washington State study by the historian E. Wayne Carp, after World War II only one reason was given and accepted for adopting a child: infertility. Helen Louise West remembered the policy. She and her husband adopted four children before giving birth to a daughter. She felt fortunate that the last child did not arrive sooner. "No, we should not have had Annette sooner because if we could have had a family of our own, we would not have been permitted to adopt children." The Wests' experience reflected a new priority in adoption policy: the creation of nuclear families. At the same time, the demographics of adoption changed radically in the postwar years: The percentage of adopted children born to married women dropped from 65 percent to none; virtually all were now born to unwed mothers. And the average age of relinquished children dropped from four and a half years to a few days.[35]

With the striking exception of unwed Black mothers, agencies no longer endeavored to keep biological families together or to encourage birth mothers to raise their children. The new goal was to create intact nuclear families by taking White infants from "unworthy" birth parents and giving them to "worthy" White infertile couples. At this point, in an effort to create pseudo-biological relationships, agencies became much more rigid and secretive, refusing to reveal information to any part of the adoptive triad—adoptive parents, adopted children, or birth parents—even if that information would not identify the parties involved. The idea was to construct an entirely new family—not an overtly adoptive family, but a fictive genetic family in which everyone "matched" as closely as possible. Adoption seemed to be the "perfect solution" for both infertility and illegitimacy. That is, while it protected the parents from the stigma of infertility and the children from the stigma of illegitimacy, this system also erased the visible reminders of illicit sex as the reproductive agent and created the appearance of "normative" marital procreation.[36]

In addition to this shift in adoption policy, the idealization of the postwar nuclear family stigmatized unwed mothers in new ways. These women's undomesticated sexual behavior marked them not only as "fallen women," but as "neurotic" and a threat to the familial order. Social workers convinced many young single women that they were not worthy to be the mothers of their children. As the historian Rickie Solinger demonstrated, after World War II only unwed Black girls and women were encouraged to keep their children; White teenagers and single women were virtually forced to relinquish their babies. No longer treated with compassion, these women were now vilified as "neurotic at best, psychotic at worst." Both Solinger and Carp noted that psychoanalytic theories came to dominate casework, supporting the idea that unwed mothers were incapable of raising their children. In the words of the Freudian psychoanalyst Helene Deutch, unwed pregnancies represented "infantile narcissism" and "parthenogenic, puberal fantasy."[37]

Since these unwed women were considered unfit to become mothers and so many infertile couples were desperate for children, adoption agencies became brokerage houses for childless couples, rather than service centers for children in need of homes. In the process, unwed White women who gave birth became the supply side of the adoption industry. Agencies became preoccupied with finding healthy "desirable" infants for adoption, at the expense of other children who may have been in desperate need of homes. According to an article in the *Saturday Evening Post*, about half the postwar adoption agencies rejected children whose mothers had histories of mental illness, suggesting that the children who were most in need of care were those the agencies refused to serve. Even though unwed White women continued to produce babies for adoption, the demand quickly outdistanced the supply. Ironically, the Children's Home Society of Washington, which had been placing children in adoptive homes since the late nineteenth century, all but ceased placing children in 1973 because of the shortage of White infants, although there was no shortage of children in need of good homes.[38]

Given the desire to "match" children and adoptive parents, screening of potential parents through intrusive home studies, and the shortage of suitable infants, it was not easy to adopt children. Florence Barkley, who married in 1939, adopted two children during the baby-boom years. She recalled, "It was hard to adopt. It took 7 years to get first son and three years for second one—and I did go through a lot of painful infertility treatment—I'd do it again, I'm not sorry—and I get very angry when people say, 'Oh you got yours the easy way.'" While agencies tried to mask adoption by matching children and parents as closely as possible, some infertile couples hoped that adoption would provide what their biology denied: a child who resembled them. Prospective parents who wished for children similar to themselves in appearance were reluctant to adopt a child from a different background. Pamela Moore recalled, "I wanted to adopt but I was nearly 40 by then and in those days the only children available to older couples were Asian children which my husband would not consider."

Janice Stiles eventually adopted two children in the 1950s, but only when she found children who matched her and her husband. At first she did not have strong feelings about physical resemblance, but soon she became "obsessed with likeness." Infertility had a profound impact on her life and her marital history. Her first husband had impaired fertility and became an alcoholic, and she believed that "the childlessness may have started his downward slide because he felt that it was his 'fault.' I tried to spare his feelings, but the whole situation was not something I could hide." Her own feelings drove her to

cross the street, sometimes, to avoid walking past a pregnant woman; I'd go to baby showers (and this was during the baby boom—there were *lots* of showers) and come home and cry in the bathtub while the water poured in; I even used to daydream while we went on long drives that I'd see a baby in a blanket by the side of the road and take it home. . . . I had always wanted to adopt from childhood, wanting to take home every pale, thin little Depression-era girl I saw. . . . But I became obsessed with likenesses—how much the children looked like the parents. I didn't want to adopt children who looked too different from us.

When a lawyer friend approached her about a pregnant young woman who was looking for a couple to adopt her baby, Janice "considered it but knew the child wouldn't fit our home. Both parents were Polish working class people who didn't resemble us in the least." (She described herself as of Dutch, German, Swedish, English, and French-Swiss descent.) Even though class did not affect appearance, she mentioned it in those terms.

Although there were more healthy newborns available for adoption in the postwar years than there are today, there were not enough to fill the demand. Agencies established elaborate screening procedures to determine parental worthiness, and hopeful couples competed for the available children. Dorine and Bob Donald recalled their 1940s adoption ordeal:

> At that time there were 30 applications for every child that was available, from the 30 there were 10 couples that were approved and then the 10 were narrowed to 3 couples. We had asked for an infant baby girl but when the Case Worker called and said there was a two and a half year old boy that would be needing a home we forgot all about an infant baby girl. We were selected to have the honor of adopting our little boy. The thrill of seeing him for the first time, well, it really cannot be put into words. We so enjoyed our Son that about a year later we applied again, this time a girl to complete our family. Sure enough again we were the fortunate ones to be selected. We brought home a beautiful 8 week old baby girl.

Many couples, like the agencies that served them, considered adoption to be primarily a service for childless couples; they, not the children they adopted, were the beneficiaries. Looking back as proud grandparents and great-grandparents, the Donalds recalled the remarks that offended them as adoptive parents: "'How can you feel toward them as you WOULD YOUR OWN?'" and "'How fortunate those poor little children are for you to give them a home.' Our response to that remark was 'We are the fortunate ones to have been allowed the honor to have our son and daughter grace our home.'"

Some postwar adoptive parents were indifferent to concerns about physical resemblance or similar backgrounds, but they were likely to find themselves out of synch with the policies of adoption agencies. It took a year of bureaucratic hassles before Raymond Tressle and his wife were able to adopt their daughter. After their marriage in 1959, his wife had several miscarriages. When Raymond was called to Korea, they agreed that he would try to adopt a Korean child while he was there.

> After arriving in Korea, my chaplain put me in touch with an orphanage in Inchon which was operated by a French religious order. Several thousand children were housed there under conditions of absolute poverty. The staff was pitifully small and barely able to cope with the constant influx of desperately sick and starving infants. At this orphanage I fell in love with a tiny girl, about six months old at the time. A Korean policeman had found her in a trash pile where she had been abandoned shortly after birth. Rats had attacked her before her rescue.

Finally, after endless wrangling with the U.S. State Department, the Korean government, and the U.S. Army, he was able to adopt her. "Lisa was a delightful daughter and young woman, and is now married and the mother of three children of her own." He added at the end of his letter, "Interestingly, nearly fifteen years ago, after many years of being unable to bear a child, my wife gave birth to our son, one week after our daughter's seventeenth birthday." Here was a couple who never even tried to adopt a healthy newborn who would resemble them. She was as much "theirs" as the biological child they ultimately had.

For many postwar adoptive parents, like Raymond and his wife, the biological tie of the child made virtually no difference at all. Barbara Worthen was another who devoted her entire life to acquiring and raising her biological, adopted, and foster children. No sacrifice was too great in her effort to build her family. "I have experienced 8-10 miscarriages, fertility (obviously!), childbirth, temporary sterility, adoption, foster parenting and having guardianship." As a child during the depression, she recalled that most families she knew were small. "I wanted to have six children when I grew up. . . . My mother, tidy, responsible, 30's homemaker, told me that one child was enough, and that I'd change my mind when I grew up." But Barbara never did. Married in 1950, she and her husband wanted "lots of kids." She was so impatient that after only one month of marriage, "I cried from disappointment and wondered if there was something wrong with me!" Her reproductive history did not go smoothly. After two babies and three miscarriages, one during the Korean War "under the 'tender' (not!) care of the U.S. Navy. . . . I remember feeling . . . a great emptiness. . . . such a failure and wanting another baby so much." Even though she stayed in bed for seven months to avoid a miscarriage with her second pregnancy, Barbara wanted still more children.

"For a while, I was too busy to feel that yearning again, but, by the time [our daughter] was 18 months old, I started looking with longing at the corner where we had kept the bassinet. About that time, my husband came DOWN, literally, with the mumps and was apparently left sterile (though he was never checked) but I certainly wasn't getting pregnant." In 1959, they adopted a baby boy, and in six months she was pregnant again. "The doctor said that mumps can cause *temporary* sterility. So, now we needed a bigger house." But she miscarried again, in her seventh month, after three months in the hospital. Barbara was so keen on having more children that she was willing to risk her life. "This time, the doctor said that he hadn't been sure that I was going to survive, and he suggested sterilization. Los-

ing the baby was bad enough, without losing hope forever, so I refused."
They adopted a girl the next year, in 1961.

Barbara was on the extreme end of the scale in her indifference to biology
and background. There were some, however, who felt differently toward
adopted children because they were not their biological progeny. One
woman, signing her letter Anonymous, married when the war ended. She
continued to teach while her husband finished his law degree. After fourteen years and "numerous tests," they had no children, but finally adopted a
newborn boy they learned about from their physician. Four years later they
adopted a three-month-old boy from an agency. "Then a year later the social
agency asked us if we would take a five year old neglected girl. We accepted
her. But her language and filthy songs were so bad, we didn't send her to
kindergarten. . . . She has been a real challenge from the beginning!" This
woman and her husband are now seventy and seventy-one, and her husband
has been a successful banker and attorney and "owns several large cattle
farms. . . . [We] wish any of our three were capable to take over. However,
that is not the case. I don't want to sound arrogant but I do believe genes
play a very important part in your make-up and the old saying 'You can't run
water uphill' is certainly true."

Anonymous was surely not the only postwar parent whose children,
whether biological or not, did not turn out as they had hoped. But she
blamed genetics. Given the persistence of eugenic ideas, along with the
notion that adoption was "second best," it is not surprising that some parents would express such thoughts. Even for couples who were thrilled to
become adoptive parents and never had any regrets, a stigma still surrounded those who "failed" to have "their own" children. Many infertile
couples pursued medical treatment before turning to adoption. Medical
research made great strides in treating infertility during these years, improving the odds of successful diagnosis and treatment. Although medical intervention by no means guaranteed a cure, postwar optimism and faith in
scientific expertise prompted many couples to see the bottle of "miracle
cures" as half full rather than half empty.

Infertile couples who were contemplating medical treatment in the postwar era did not need to look far for encouragement; they saw photographs of
beaming, cherubic "miracle babies" everywhere they turned. In huge headlines, words like "help" and "hope" jumped off the pages of popular magazines. *Hygeia* presented a two-part series, "More Help for Childless
Couples"; *Today's Health* gave "Hope for the Childless"; *Science Digest*
offered "New Hope for Childless Couples"; and *Ladies Home Journal*

chimed in with "New Hope for Childless Women." *Look* promised that "In one out of three cases, CHILDLESS COUPLES CAN HAVE BABIES." *The American Weekly* gave better odds, telling readers, "Maybe You CAN Have a Baby. . . . Doctors are able to help up to half of all sterile couples to have children." These articles described new medical treatments for infertility. Often they were written by physicians and scientists who were leaders in the field of infertility research and practice, or they included interviews with these experts, or they reported the findings of medical research initially published in scientific journals. There were also personal testimonies, like the saga of one formerly infertile woman in *Cosmopolitan* magazine, "I Was Sure I Was Sterile." *Parents* magazine explained "Childlessness and what can be done about it" in one issue and "How To Combat Sterility" in another.[39] With so much medical information available to lay readers about advances in treatment, it is no wonder that infertile couples flocked to clinics hoping that they would be among the fortunate ones who could be helped.

There were several reasons for the increased interest in infertility treatment by both physicians and couples. Researchers were indeed making major strides in the rapidly expanding field of reproductive medicine, improving on earlier therapeutic strategies. In part, clinicians and scientists were responding to the demand for treatment. In the heightened pronatalist atmosphere of the baby-boom era, more and more childless couples sought medical intervention to enable them to become parents. Considering the powerful negative stigma that surrounded childlessness during these years and the pain of living on the margins of a family-centered culture, it is no wonder that childless couples turned to physicians for help as the odds for treatment improved.

At the same time, the postwar infatuation with experts in every field contributed to the exalted stature of physicians and the willingness of many childless couples to put their faith in medical science. Every article in the popular literature carried the same message: Do not resign yourself to a life without children; trust the experts to help you achieve parenthood. Postwar physicians were much better equipped to treat infertility than they had been in the past. I. C. Rubin, the physician who developed the Rubin test for diagnosing blocked fallopian tubes, told the readers of *Parents* magazine that science had made great strides in recent decades. "It isn't too long ago that any honest doctor would have been forced to say, 'I'm sorry—there's nothing I can do.' . . . But today, the doctor can honestly say, 'There may be a chance.

We'll see.'"[40] But science could only work if people put their entire faith in it. When infertile couples turned to the medical profession in the postwar years, they put their faith, bodies, and bank accounts into the hands of the experts. Sometimes they ended up with their hearts' desire; at other times they ended up with heartache.

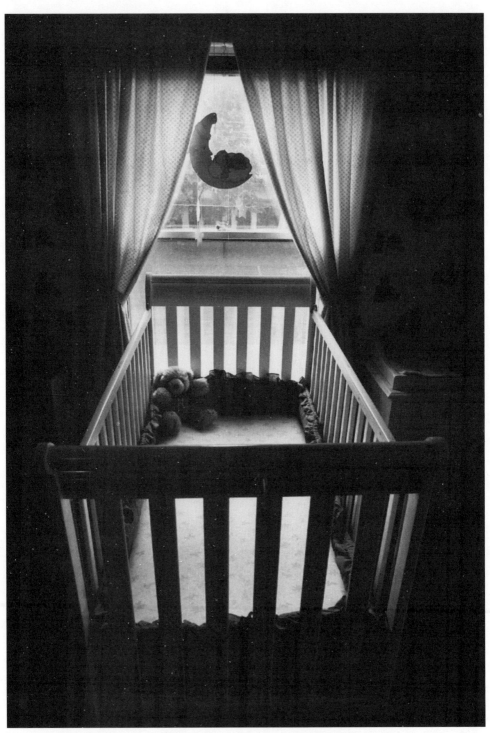

(Courtesy of Jeff, Susan, and Rose Gottleib; photo by Mary Lou Nemanic)

CHAPTER 5

Infertility: Freud in the Bedroom, Sex at the Clinic

★☆

Medical writers have sometimes observed that sterility groups contain a larger than average number of persons who are self-centered and show a lack of warmth in their social and personal relations. People of this kind frequently are the victims of frigidity and an abnormal reaction to the family relationship.
  —Albert Horlings, "Can They Have Children?" *Harper's*, January 1942

One of the greatest difficulties in treating childless couples is not medical but just stubborn male pride. Many men refuse to believe that they may be to blame and will not submit to examination or treatment.
  —"Advice to the Childless," *Time*, May 1, 1950

In 1950, the *Ladies Home Journal*, in its regular feature, "Tell Me, Doctor," ran a two-part series on infertility. The first of the two fictional stories, written by a physician, featured the good patient, a docile and obedient woman. As the physician gently and politely explained the course of treatment, she replied, "I'll be glad to co-operate in any way I can." But when the woman requested information about the most controversial midcentury treatment, donor insemination, the physician avoided the issue.[1] Instead of answering the question, he replied after a long pause: "If you mean artificial insemination by means of the husband's semen, I have tried it a number of times with some success."

Rather than pursue the matter in an effort to obtain more complete information, the good patient replied, "Thank you, Doctor, you've given me an awful lot of your time."

The next installment described the bad patient, who not only managed to contract gonorrhea, but abandoned the treatment prescribed by her previous physician. This woman's worst offense was clearly her disobedience. "Do you mean to say, that knowing you had such an infection, you stopped treatment?" asked the angry physician.

"I told you—I got tired of going there every day and being smeared with little balls of cotton on sticks. The doctor was in a huff about it, but I never went back to him," she replied.

The physician scolded her harshly: "You were a foolish woman not to have done as you were advised—criminally foolish!" Although the invented dialogue said nothing about her economic situation, his reply suggested that the fictitious patient was an outlaw from the poorer classes: "If you couldn't afford private medical attention, there are clinics. You never would have got away with it in this town!" But now there was nothing left to do but a complete hysterectomy.

"Remove all my organs!" she exclaimed. "Why?"

The physician's gentleness and tact, evident in his dialogue with the good patient, was gone.

> Your tubes are closed, enlarged to the size and shape of a frankfurter sausage, doubtless filled with pus, and so tightly adherent to what is left of the ovaries that it is impossible to distinguish where one leaves off and the other begins. Your uterus is of no use, for it is unlikely you could ever become pregnant; and if you did, you could never carry the pregnancy.

The woman had not only destroyed her body, she became a social outcast, of no use to society. "In my opinion—and God knows I don't want to operate upon you, for it will be a tough job under any circumstances—you will never get to the point where you will become a useful member of society again until you are rid of that mass of disease that fills your entire pelvis."

Chastened, she became meek and submissive: "What do you suggest, Doctor, for me to do?" He urged her to enter the hospital, cure the infection, and have the surgery. "The woman tugged silently at the corner of her handkerchief as she weighed the doctor's words. 'Well,' she finally said, 'I guess I had to learn the hard way. And now that I've learned, it's too late.'"[2]

The "bad patient" was probably a figment of the writer's imagination, but the worshipful, cooperative "good patient" was less likely to be. During the years of the baby boom, when couples without children felt the sting of exclusion from the parent-centered culture, their extreme social isolation heightened the private anguish of infertility. For women, childlessness was particularly painful in the midst of the renewed glorification of motherhood that emerged after World War II. Infertile women, more often than men, actively sought medical help and cooperated fully in their treatment. They put their faith in physicians to help them conceive the children they desperately wanted. Most embarked willingly, even eagerly, upon a process that invaded their bodies, bank accounts, bedrooms, sex lives, and psyches. Nowhere are the high stakes in procreation and the cultural meaning of childlessness more evident than in the infertility industry.

Infertility in the Cold-War Era

As the cold war unfolded, reproduction remained a highly politicized concern, but the politics of reproduction took a new form. With the onset of the baby boom, exhortations to the middle class to procreate seemed unnecessary. The alleged threats to the nation's future no longer appeared to be the degenerate offspring of the "feeble," the poor, or the "inferior" races. Now there were new internal enemies, bred within the middle class itself, who posed a danger to the nation's security because they were "soft." Anticommunist crusaders, such as J. Edgar Hoover, director of the Federal Bureau of Investigation, and Senator Joseph McCarthy, claimed that many so-called subversives, pinkos, and homos were the children of "neurotic" women. Patriotic women, according to these cold warriors, embraced the role of submissive wife and devoted themselves wholeheartedly to motherhood. In the cold-war era, any woman who consciously or subconsciously avoided the "natural" female role of wife and mother was likely to be labeled neurotic and unfit for parenthood.

Few physicians shared the rabid anticommunism and extreme sexism of the most fanatic anticommunist crusaders. But the gender assumptions the anticommunists articulated permeated the culture and were widely accepted by both professionals and the general public. In 1950, for example, Abraham Stone, medical director of the Margaret Sanger Research Foundation and a major researcher in the areas of contraception and infertility, explained the postwar version of a woman's "natural" role:

For conception to take place a woman must be a woman. Not only must she have the physical structure and hormones of a woman but she must feel she is a woman and accept it. A girl child becomes and feels herself a developing woman if she has made a proper identification with her own mother and has also learned to accept her femininity and also masculinity as represented by her father and later, by her husband. Being a woman means acceptance of her primary role, that of conceiving and bearing a child. Every woman has a basic urge and need to produce a child. Being a woman means a complete readiness to look forward to the delivery of that child when it is sufficiently nourished by her to take its place as an infant in the outside world. Being a woman means her feeling of her own readiness and capability to rear that child and aid in its physical, emotional and mental development.[3]

Few experts at the time questioned the definition of womanhood articulated by Stone, and many based their treatment on such beliefs. Margaret Valen encountered this theory when she consulted a physician in 1945 to discover why she was not getting pregnant. She was twenty-five and her husband was twenty-seven, and they had been married only a year, but since they married "late" by 1945 standards, most of her friends no doubt had children already. Medical experts encouraged childless couples to seek help early, warning that "the longer sterility has existed, the harder it is to correct. Only a qualified physician can answer for each man and wife the question of when they should undergo examination." Margaret went through the usual infertility workup and tried "everything kookie," but nothing worked. The physicians could find no physiological cause for the Valens' childlessness.

The Valens were among the 50 percent of infertile couples at the time who could not be diagnosed.[4] But that did not prevent her physician from suggesting treatment. When no physiological cause could be found, some physicians looked for psychological explanations. As a working woman in the postwar era, Margaret was not behaving in an appropriately feminine way. Perhaps, the theory went, she was inhibiting her own fertility because she held a job—an unwomanly thing to do and evidence that maybe she did not *really* want a child. Particular warnings were directed toward employed women, who allegedly put their fertility at risk: "The pressures of modern living and the strains of occupations in which women have been engaging are ... significant causes" of infertility, cautioned a leading expert. "The same can be said of men, but to a lesser extent."[5] In keeping with such theories, Margaret's physician told her she should quit her job, so she did. Like most infertile women who sought medical advice, she did whatever her physician told her to do, even if she thought it was "kookie." But Margaret never got pregnant. Quitting her job did not do the trick.

Advising a woman to quit her job was not a standard treatment for infertility, but it was one approach to a problem that was still difficult to diagnose and treat. Researchers had found that stress could be a factor in infertility, by causing fallopian tubes to contract or by affecting the motility of sperm. If employment was a cause of stress, it was not entirely "kookie" for physicians to suggest quitting a job to relieve stress. The problem, however, is that there was no way to be certain that job-related stress caused a woman's tubes to contract. It was just as likely that stress at work affected a man's fertility. But it was unthinkable to suggest that a male breadwinner should quit his job. The woman's job during these years appeared to be expendable. Moreover, in most cases it was the woman, not the man, who sought treatment.

Lois M. was one such woman. She read an article in a popular magazine about artificial insemination and wrote to the California physician who was quoted in the story. She was desperate for a child, but her husband was infertile and refused to seek treatment. "When my husband was 8 he had an operation," she explained.

> His testes didn't come down properly and they had to pull them down. . . .
> They told him at that time he might or might not be able to have children.
> . . . I have tried to get him to have himself checked but that is a very touchy subject. He said it has something to do with his ego and I can understand it. He said if he doesn't know then he can always have hope. He loves children very much and if he could have one it would mean alot to him. We have talked about artificial insemination and he said he wouldn't mind. The only thing is he said he'd rather I went ahead and did it without him knowing and then he could feel like it was his. . . . I know this letter sounds sort of crazy but it is true. I promise I have talked to him but I just think it would do more for his ego if I could have this done. We both love children very much and it seems so terrible that if we want children so bad we can't have any and some people who don't want them can have children. Is there anyway I can do this without him knowing. Is it a state law that he has to sign a paper? Believe me I'm not just trying to do anything behind his back, he just feels so bad because he can't have children.

The physician replied that although there was no law, virtually no medical practitioner was willing to proceed with artificial insemination without the husband's informed consent.[6]

The responses of Margaret Valen and Lois M. were not unusual. Although the cause of infertility involved the husband about as often as it did the wife, women were more likely to seek medical intervention and were more willing than men to submit to treatment.[7] Why were men so reluctant and women so eager to seek treatment? The answer is not as simple as "stubborn male pride," as *Time* magazine suggested, or female docility, like the case of the fictional "good patient" implied. In fact, both men and women helped to shape as well as responded to the medical approach to infertility, which focused on the female patient and often ignored the man.

As the result of new research on ovulation, hormonal contributions to fertility, the role of secretions, the production and viability of sperm, and other functions of the male and female reproductive system, physicians could offer their patients new diagnostic tools and treatments in the baby-boom era. Infertile couples might seek help from their family physicians or from the growing number of specialists in reproductive medicine. Among the treatments now available were hormonal therapies to stimulate ovulation or improve the quality of semen, new surgical techniques for opening blocked passages in the woman or the man, artificial insemination with either the husband's or a donor's semen at the appropriate moment in the woman's cycle, and a number of nonsurgical interventions to increase the likelihood of conception and to reduce the chances of miscarriage. These therapeutic strategies represented major advances in the field in just a few decades.

At the same time, new medical societies, dedicated to the treatment of infertility, emerged and grew rapidly. The American Society for the Study of Sterility, for example, which was founded in 1944 by 30 members, had 425 members by 1954, 2,095 by 1964, and 4,885 by 1973. The society held meetings at which research findings were presented, and published guidelines for thorough diagnostic evaluations of both husbands and wives, to be used by specialists and general practitioners alike. With this rapid expansion of expertise in the field, childless couples found increasing opportunities and encouragement to seek medical treatment.[8]

Reflecting this trend, the Birth Control Federation changed its name to the Planned Parenthood Federation of America in 1942. At the same time, the Margaret Sanger Research Foundation, which had been dedicated to the development and dissemination of contraceptive services, shifted its focus to infertility. Abraham Stone, the clinic's medical director, described infertility as "a tragic waste of potential parenthood [that] causes an inestimable amount of heartbreak and human suffering." At the annual meeting of the

Planned Parenthood Federation of America in 1945, he told his colleagues, "In a democratic society parents should have easy access to the best available knowledge for preventing conception, but social and medical measures should also be promoted which would make it possible for responsible parents to have children when they desire them."[9]

Stone believed that encouraging childbearing was as important as providing contraception:

> Planned Parenthood organizations . . . have a two-fold program. Their primary objective is to make available scientific knowledge and measures for the control of conception, so that children may be born by choice rather than chance, and the health, welfare and stability of the family be preserved. At the same time, however, they also aim to encourage childbearing whenever this appears to be medically and socially indicated and to make available to couples denied children because of some disturbance in their reproductive powers, scientific information and aid to help them overcome this lack of fertility. [According to the] birth control philosophy . . . Control does not necessarily mean limitation. It implies the power to regulate, to exercise choice and direction.

Stone also lamented the frequent neglect of the male partner. Although specialists since the nineteenth century had been exhorting their colleagues to examine the husband as well as the wife, the problem persisted. In 1945, he wrote:

> One of the most significant recent advances in the study of childlessness has been the realization that the fruitlessness of a couple depends upon the physical condition of both partners and that the responsibility for a barren marriage must be shared by both husband and wife. Formerly it was the woman that was nearly always considered to be responsible for a sterile mating and it was she alone who was subjected to various examinations and tests; today we recognize that the male, too, may be an important factor in the infertility of a marriage, and that in perhaps some forty percent of barren marriages the cause of the childlessness may be due largely to some deficiency in the reproductive powers of the husband.

He urged clinics to have on staff "a gynecologist and a urologist, or at least someone trained in both of these fields."[10]

Yet six years after Stone's statement, another specialist noted the continued neglect of the male partner and cautioned his medical colleagues against assuming that infertility was a female problem: "These misconceptions . . .

may be due to the fact that much greater effort and research has been devoted to the female sterility problem than to the male." He noted the "persistent casual attitude on the part of many of us toward the husband as an etiologic factor."

> Possibly one of the most persistent errors in the management of infertility, despite the growing emphasis on male sterility, is the readiness of some physicians to employ fairly radical diagnostic, or even therapeutic, procedures on the wife, without first obtaining a careful evaluation of the husband's fertility status. It cannot be too strongly emphasized that, under ordinary circumstances, no woman should be subjected to tubal studies, endometrial biopsies, etc., unless it has been demonstrated that the primary cause of infertility does not rest with the husband. The fact that in most sterility problems the wife is the one to seek medical aid makes it relatively convenient to start the investigation with her. This is even more often an approach of least resistance when the husband is one the who is reluctant to come in for examination.

In spite of researchers' and clinicians' continued efforts to improve the diagnosis and treatment of male infertility, these exhortations went largely unheeded, and the neglect of men continued.[11]

Most infertility practitioners were specialists in female reproductive medicine. The vast majority of the members of the American Society for the Study of Sterility, for example, were in the field of obstetrics and gynecology, followed by urology, with a few in related fields, such as internal medicine, endocrinology, general practice, and pathology.[12] At its annual meeting in 1963, Herbert H. Thomas, the president of the society, justified the continued focus on the female patient: "This does not indicate that we are unaware of the responsibility of the male in the problem of infertility, but the incidence of primary male infertility is variable but relatively low and, in our culture, it is usually the women who initiate the request for assistance." Surely, the president of the society knew the widely published statistics by its own members indicating that approximately half the infertility cases involved a problem with the man. Yet he remained focused on the woman as the patient:

> In seeking counsel with us, she . . . admits to frustration and failure . . . as we endeavor to probe and explore the innermost secrets of her life in order to alleviate her barrenness. As she bares her personal life before us and submits to many indignities and both painful and somewhat hazardous diagnostic procedures . . . we must not betray this trust. . . . The responsibility to our frustrated patient and her husband is a great one.[13]

The definition of the patient as female extended into medical language itself, which cast the female body as inherently flawed. Medical texts, as well as physicians and their patients, routinely described infertility in terms of "failure," "blame," and "fault." One woman, for example, who wrote to a noted specialist about her repeated miscarriages, wondered whether he agreed with her local physician that surgery might correct her "defective cervix." The specialist agreed that surgery might solve the difficulty, but referred to the condition not as a "defective cervix," as the woman's letter had, but as an "incompetent cervix."[14] Medical terminology was filled with metaphors of the "incompetent" female body, while presenting the male reproductive system as robust. This cultural casting of biological phenomena not only described women's physiology as weak and flawed, it also disadvantaged men, whose reproductive systems might need attention and repair.

The anthropologist Emily Martin analyzed the language of reproduction in standard twentieth-century medical textbooks that have been used routinely in medical schools. She found such statements as these: Ovaries "shed" eggs but testicles "produce" sperm, unfertilized eggs "degenerate" and are "wasted," and "menstruation is the uterus crying for lack of a baby." In contrast, although millions of sperm that do not fertilize eggs die within a few hours, the textbooks never called them "wasted," "failed," or "degenerating"; rather, they described the male reproductive physiology as a "remarkable cellular transformation . . . amazing characteristic of spermatogenesis is its sheer magnitude." Descriptions of fertilization in these textbooks reflect cultural ideas about male aggressiveness and female passivity. Although research documented the active role of the egg in traveling through the tube and showed that the process of fertilization involves mechanisms in both the sperm and the egg that make them "mutually active partners," the loaded language persisted. As if cast as a villain in a film noir, the advancing egg "captures and tethers" the sperm and "clasps" the sperm to its nucleus. The egg has became the femme fatale or the overbearing Mom, devouring its male victim.[15]

Infertility, His and Hers

While depicting female reproductive physiology in a negative light, this language also subtly connected male fertility to virility, inadvertently perpetuating an unfortunate myth. In spite of all the scientific evidence that infertility did not signal a lack of virility, the close association between procreation and potency remained powerful, sometimes discouraging men from seeking treatment. One infertile husband "equated fertility with virility and was both depressed and angered to have the whole issue questioned."[16] An article in the *American Mercury* reported the case of a woman who refused to bring in her husband for an examination: "Tears filled her eyes. 'He couldn't take it . . . it might break up our marriage. Rather than risk that I'll reconcile myself to going without a family.'"[17] An infertility specialist explained:

> Unfortunately, the average patient closely relates his ability to reproduce with his ability to perform coitus. As a corollary to this, most men feel that any question of their ability to reproduce casts reflections upon their virility. . . . If the various physiological concepts are explained tactfully at the initial visit, much can be done to win over the husband's subsequent cooperation.[18]

Childless men frequently endured cruel taunts about their sexual prowess. Norma McKinley, who was married in 1958, remembers a reception at a midwestern university at which a noted physician asked her husband, upon learning that they had no children, "What's the matter young feller? Are ya shootin' blanks?" Doreen Hall, a young military wife, was furious at her husband "when he wouldn't give semen samples because he was too embarrassed to have the corpsman on base know that he might be 'shooting blanks.'" Dorothy Norwich recalls the humiliation when her husband's friends taunted him, "Do you want me to show you how to get her pregnant?"

Few other medical conditions evoked such snickers. Considering the myths that surrounded male infertility and the powerful pronatalism directed primarily toward women, it is no wonder that women were more likely to seek help and that some physicians would try to avoid reluctant husbands, if possible. Women themselves often contributed to the neglect of male partners by trying to protect their husbands from the humiliations of infertility treatment or from the disgrace of acknowledging a male problem. Betty Shinder was fertile, but her husband was not. "I never told the families because I knew it would hurt his pride. Everybody just concluded it was my fault. I didn't really care because what happened to him happened to both of us." In this charged atmosphere, some physicians undoubtedly thought that it was in their patients' best interests to examine and even treat women first. After all, female infertility was more likely to be treated successfully because it was better understood.

Norma's physician examined her first because, he explained, "the cause of

infertility was most often found in the female whose apparatus was more complex and more often the cause of disfunction than the male and that in any
case males were reluctant to consider any questioning of their reproductive
functioning until the female component had been thoroughly investigated."
Because her physician did not abide by the standard medical guidelines that
emphasized the importance of examining the man first, Norma went through
a painful ordeal before her husband was evaluated. This ordeal included the
Rubin test, described by one leading physician as a "simple . . . introduction of
a gas . . . into the uterus under a certain degree of pressure. . . . [It is] quite a
painless procedure and takes only a few minutes."[19] But Norma recalled,
"I believe they must have used an air compressor on a par with Rapid Oil
Change." After all that, "it was finally determined that all of my essential parts
were in working order and my husband was dispatched to a urologist. . . . I was
bamboozled by the physician's finding me unflawed. I assumed that I was to
blame." As it turned out, there was a problem with her husband's semen that
was easily corrected, and the couple eventually had two children.

Women themselves sometimes contributed to the squeamishness surrounding the treatment of male infertility. Dorothy was another wife who went
through an excruciating ordeal before her husband was examined. After her
tubes were tested, "I was in severe pain for 3 days . . . but was told that everything looked fine and all of the tests came back that there was nothing wrong
with me." In spite of her pain, she described the semen analysis, which required
ejaculation into a glass jar, as a much greater ordeal: "This has to be the most
humiliating test that a man has to do. But they were kind enough to let us do
this at home. I then had 30 minutes to race 30 miles to the clinic to get it
tested and [was] told that I could find the results out in 3 days." It was *his*
semen, but *she* was the one racing to the clinic. In spite of the fact that she
went through unnecessary tests and that she was fertile, she continued to be
the one to visit the clinic. The results of the semen analysis were given to her—
not to her husband. "The nurse came on the line and said, 'Your husband's
result came back there was *no* sperm seen.' I asked 'Could this be possible?' She
said 'All I can say is no sperm was seen.' I was broken hearted to say the least."

Women who would willingly subject their reproductive organs to surgery
were sometimes as nervous as their husbands about surgery to male sex
organs. One woman wrote to the noted specialist John Rock after medica-
tion failed and the local physician told her and her husband that "the only
thing left would be an operation. Dr. Rock please help is there anything you
can do for us[?] I don't want my husband to have an operation. My husband
and I make novena after novena. . . . [Give] us an answer to our prayerful

novenas." Rock's associate replied, "I think you are much too worried about the seriousness of the operation. . . . A varicocelectomy is not a serious operation at all, and it has resulted in marked increase in fertility in some men. I really feel that you are much too concerned about it."[20]

A major stumbling block to treating male infertility was some women's eagerness to deflect the problem away from their husbands. One woman learned about male infertility from an article in a popular magazine and wrote to the physician for advice. Although she suspected that her husband might be infertile, she wrote as though the problem was entirely hers:

> I came across something you said or wrote about Subfertile husban's + it interested me very much because I have wanted to have two more children, but have been unable to get pregnant. I have gone to so many doctors + they have all told me there is nothing wrong with me but then, "Why Doctor can't I get pregnant?" . . . I will tell you a little of myself Doctor + I hope you can help me.

She described getting married at age seventeen and having three children and two miscarriages. "Then Doctor I got married for the second time but that didn't last very long because I caught a Venereal Disease from him it was pretty bad but the Doctor who took care of me said he cured it on time, before it was worst." Finally she

> found the right man. . . . [We] have been married 6 yrs + I have had lots of test done on me + even an operation but so far Doctor Im still praying to have a child. Could it be punishment from our Lord or is there an explanation. I'll pray that you can help me Doctor + answer my letter. . . . Sincerely, Mrs. Frank L.[21]

It is obvious from Mrs. L.'s letter that she was not infertile, since she had gotten pregnant at least five times and had given birth to three children. Mrs. L. did mention the possibility that venereal disease had affected her fertility, but claimed that the physician who treated her had cured it in time. She did not mention any examinations or treatment of her husband, although she had already undergone considerable medical intervention herself, including surgery. Reminiscent of Ann Bradstreet three hundred years earlier, Mrs. L. wondered whether her lack of children with her present husband was punishment from God for her past mistakes, even though the only mistakes she related in her letter had to do with poor choices of husbands.

Another stumbling block to the treatment of male infertility was that it required men to engage in one of the most stigmatized sexual acts: masturbation. For centuries, both medical experts and social reformers warned men of the dangers of masturbation, claiming that at the least, it would sap their energy and make them useless and lazy and at the worst, would cause a wide range of serious symptoms and illnesses, from warts to insanity and even death. Masturbation was even said to cause infertility. And now physicians were telling their male patients to engage in the one act that, from childhood onward, they had been warned never to do.

Masturbation phobia was alive and well in mid-twentieth-century America—and, of course, so was masturbation.[22] One unfortunate man had a powerful dose of both, so much so that he believed he was unfit to father children. Although his reaction was undoubtedly extreme, his concerns reflected the cultural taboos against masturbation and its threat to the "virility" of the nation. In a 1964 letter to Rock, a Catholic physician and birth control researcher who had appeared on television discussing the benefits of the oral contraceptive pill, Thomas R. connected his own "self-pollution" to reproductive damage, the cold war, and nuclear destruction. He worried that the loss of healthy offspring—resulting from practices like his own, which he believed would "alter or foreclose the generative processes," and might leave the nation underpopulated. "This could be our downfall. Russia could triumph." Rock responded promptly, recommending readings on overpopulation in the United States and adding, "I think like the rest of us you have a lot to learn. Let us do our best to find out the facts. They are much more dependable than theories."[23]

With ideas about the evils of masturbation still culturally powerful, some men may have found masturbation abhorrent and the test itself literally impossible to accomplish. The collection of the specimen could be psychologically and physically awkward or religiously unacceptable. Semen analysis required that the man bring in a sample "obtained by coitus interruptus or masturbation into a clean glass container." The preferable method was masturbation in the physician's office. The second best method was masturbation at home, if the specimen was brought in within an hour. Use of a condom to collect semen during intercourse was not considered reliable because of certain ingredients in the condom that were damaging to the sperm. If it was impossible to collect a semen sample, an estimate of male fertility could be made by examining the wife within twenty-four hours of intercourse.[24] This option, developed by Max Huhner in 1913, avoided the problem of examining the man at all. "One cannot help but surmise that in the beginning this was a sly way to evaluate the fertility of a sensitive and often uncooperative man," noted the president of the American Society for the Study of Sterility.[25]

Even when husbands were eager to do whatever was necessary to conceive a child, they were disadvantaged in the treatment of infertility because of the persistent assumption that women were the primary patients. All kinds of medical and surgical therapies seemed to be available for women, but men with low sperm counts had few options, and physicians were often discouraging. In 1964, for example, Donald W. of Pensacola, Florida, wrote to Rock after the physician appeared on television. He said:

> We have been to the Dr., and he says my wife is normal in every respect, but I am not. He says that due to my testicles being abnormally small, we will never have any of our *own* children. What I'd like to know is, is there anyway in the World I can build up my sperm count so as to give my wife pregnancy? If this would involve an operation or what, I would do it for a child. . . . We have talked over adoption, but feel that there is still some chance for pregnancy to happen. If there's anything I can do or you can advise us on, we will honor it.

Here was a man eager and unafraid to do whatever was necessary, but the response to his letter was discouraging: "In general, the treatment of infertility in men is very inadequate, but we have had some small measure of success in a few patients. We could better answer your question after we receive the actual doctor's report." Although researchers were developing a variety of methods to improve the production and function of sperm, from hormonal therapies to surgery, success rates remained low.[26]

Larry L. was also eager to do whatever was necessary to conceive a child, but was not certain that his rural physician was doing everything possible. Mr. L., a self-employed farmer, and his wife, a nurse at the county hospital, had been married seven years "and have had no children, which we would like very much." He noted that his wife "has been checked and is OK," but he had a low sperm count.

> Dr. Rock can you help us in any way as we would like very much to have 1 or if possible 2 children by natures way with my sperm. We don't care for artificial way, only if it can be with my on (sic) sperm. We have been doctoring for 5 years now with no luck. At the present I'm taking shots every week to try and increase the sperm. Dr. Rock, I would like if you would . . . tell us of anything we can do, of anything available to us.

Rock's secretary replied in his absence, with referral to a physician in Mr. L.'s area who was a "certified obstetrician and gynecologist. . . . I am sure that he will be able to help you." She referred Mr. L. to a gynecologist, not a urologist, because infertility cases were routinely referred to specialists in female reproductive medicine.[27]

Although treatment opportunities for men with infertility problems were limited, many men tried desperately to get help. A thirty-year-old army private wrote to the Margaret Sanger Bureau after reading an article in *Newsweek* in 1945. After seven years of marriage, he and his wife were childless

> because I am sterile, altho I believe my case is not hopeless. I have been to doctors with my condition but the Army interrupted my treatment. I love children and desire more than anything in the world to raise a family. Any way you can help me now or later would be appreciated.

Stone, medical director of the bureau, replied with a sympathetic but not optimistic note, explaining that the young man could not expect much help from the army:

> I very well understand your situation and I should like to help in whatever way I can. . . . It seems to me that under the circumstances you can hardly expect adequate care. If you will communicate with me after you have been released from the Service, I shall be glad to direct you to a hospital or physician in your community where you will be able to obtain the necessary care and treatment.[28]

Some men were eager for treatment, not in spite of, but perhaps because of concerns about their masculinity. One man wrote to Stone: "I can't help feeling like a eunuch, psychologically, if not completely physically. I don't mean to sound pathetic. I don't want to go through life with that kind of damnation." He had discontinued infertility treatment because, as a writer, it was interfering with his work. But now he wanted to return to the clinic: "My manliness is now much more important to me [than] any silly writing."[29]

There was, of course, one sexual malfunction that was positively linked to infertility: male impotence. *Look* magazine reassured readers that out of a study of 1,000 subfertile men, "85 percent had fine physiques and enjoyed a normal sex life." The other 15 percent, however, did not.[30] Stone acknowledged that there were psychological factors involved in male impotence. "Some men are unable adequately to penetrate into a woman, or they avoid sexual relations at the most fertile time and yet seem anxious to have a child. . . . Unconsciously, this may be due to fear and anxiety resulting from experiences, ideas, or attitudes in early childhood which had never been resolved." But impotence was difficult to treat. Rock described the state of the art as "still very unpromising and unsatisfactory, and though successes are sometimes obtained with very little therapy, failures often follow a variety of prolonged treatment and psychiatric analysis."

The most effective treatment for infertility caused by impotence was artificial insemination with the husband's semen, which, of course, did not cure either the impotence or the infertility. "This procedure should be undertaken only after a careful evaluation of the situation and of the future stability of the marriage, and carried out only when it is felt that the chances of the marriage enduring are sufficiently promising." Rock gave one example of a successful insemination that achieved not only conception but potency. When the impotent man's wife was inseminated with his semen, she became pregnant and subsequently delivered a healthy baby boy. "Incidentally, the husband's potency improved greatly, and he has since been able to have normal relations." The case suggests that the husband may have felt—and become—impotent partly because he was not able to father a child. Once he did so, even with the help of a syringe, his impotence was cured.[31]

A few infertile couples, recognizing that infertility treatment, especially for men, was imperfect, attempted to participate actively in their own treatment. One couple tried to gain the knowledge and skills to figure out their problem themselves. With a treatment success rate of less than 50 percent and relative inattention to male infertility, this couple may have surmised that with enough information, they could do as good a job as a physician. As was often the case, the wife, Mrs. H., wrote to Rock on behalf of the couple, even though the problem was with her husband. She explained that after seven years, they had no children. Three semen analyses revealed that Mr. H. had a low sperm count. Their doctor "gave little hope, because thus far very little has been accomplished to improve sperm mobility and count. We have limited means and can't readily afford the numerous sperm tests needed for an accurate evaluation." So after considerable research, they decided to pursue a do-it-yourself diagnosis:

[We] purchased a microscope to try our own sperm tests. ... We have stained a drop of the ejaculate with Gentian violet, without results. ... The books that are available to us do not give instructions for preparing a slide on sperm count. We are very concerned, that is why we have gone to the extent of trying our own tests. Of course this is not a subject readily discussed. We would be laughed at for attempting such a thing. Could you help us and explain the procedure for preparing a slide. If you feel our microscope isn't powerful enough we will stop trying.

Rock did not provide the information requested, but his response was generous. He suggested that Mr. H. make an appointment to see him in his office and assured him that he need not worry about the cost: "You can pay what you can."[32]

Few infertile couples were as ambitious as Mr. and Mrs. H., but many did complain about the lack of attention to male reproductive needs. When Rock appeared on television in 1964 discussing the birth control pill, he also mentioned infertility. Among the hundreds of letters he received after the broadcast were several commenting on the lack of attention to male reproductive concerns. Some called for male contraceptives. "Grandma of 9— Mother of 3" asked, "How about developing a pill or ?? for the men? The women more than do their share, the men are the most passionett so why not control them for a change. . . . So please let us women have a rest from pills and put the cure where it belongs—on men!" Rock replied:

> You are not the first to propose a change in target. You are somewhat gentler in approach than a correspondent from Kansas who suggested that clamps might be applied to appropriate places such as cattlemen use on bulls. Have no fear, we are working hard on the male end of things. The difficulty with medical approaches so far has been that if the medicine works the way we want it to, it very soon takes away all sexual desire and ability. That would not be very gratifying. However, it will not be long now when you can feel that you are getting even.[33]

Others had different reasons for wanting a reliable male contraceptive. Mr. A. wrote:

> I think you have been working on the wrong side of the ledger. If you want a real challenge, perfect a pill that will render a man sterile for 1 day, one week, one month, without serious side effects and the world's [population] problem is over. With a man you can reason but not a woman. In this business, after a certain time she passes into remote control, while a man always retains his power to reason.

Rock replied:

You may be sure that biochemists are working on the very difficult physiological problem of rendering a man temporarily sterile. The matter is much
more complicated than the one concerning ovulation. Even that, however, is
still not completely solved, I think, but there is reason to expect steady
improvement.[34]

Despite the optimism Rock expressed in his responses to these letters, the
promise of an effective contraceptive for men never materialized, and several of the advances in infertility treatment, such as donor insemination
with frozen sperm, represented progress in bypassing, rather than curing,
male infertility.

Given the odds against achieving a cure, along with the cost and the ordeal,
the fact that so many couples pursued treatment reflects the intense desire for
children, the faith in expertise, and the profound optimism of the era. Infertility treatment often disrupted everyday routines from work to sex.[35] Treatment
itself could become a full-time occupation. Some couples persisted for
months and even years with the grueling routine of clinic visits and sex-on-a-
schedule. But others burned out. Records at a clinic in California, for example,
show that many gave up treatment and decided to adopt. One couple tried to
conceive for nearly two years. The wife's medical chart noted that "patient
seems to be rather tense individual. . . . I suspect they are having a coital problem because . . . they're trying actively on a schedule and it has become quite
mechanical." After twenty-eight visits to the physician with no diagnosis, the
chart stated that the "patient is somewhat discouraged . . . everything appears
to be normal." The couple discontinued treatment and proceeded with adoption. Another couple was instructed to "concentrate on trying to conceive"
and to "concentrate intercourse [on] alternate days," but after fifty visits to
the clinic without results, they, too, filed adoption papers. After four years and
forty-four clinic visits, another couple gave up. Because the husband had low
sperm motility, the treatment included artificial insemination with his semen.
Thus as part of the treatment, they had to abstain from sex. His sperm and her
egg were to join in the clinic, rather than the bedroom. According to the
physician's tactful notes, eventually Mr. Barnett "got a little tired of producing
specimens" for the inseminations and discontinued treatment.[36]

Marilyn Dillon remembers being so

desperate to conceive, I remember once even having intercourse in our car,
parked in a secluded spot, between the end of my work day at the University
of Minnesota and the start of my evening class there. Two or three times arti-

ficial insemination was attempted. To my recollection, every possible infertility procedure known at the time was done. And though the suggestion was made that my husband might have some abnormality contributing to my inability to conceive, "our" infertility was generally considered to be due to something amiss with me.

Although she suspected that her husband was infertile, she continued to pursue treatment herself because "infertility was deeply painful, humiliating, and frustrating; there also were shame and stigma. I felt, 'why me'?"

Specialists understood that sex on a schedule, often required as part of infertility treatment, might cause sexual malfunction in both men and women and might end up being counterproductive to the procreative effort. According to Stone,

a woman who normally has little difficulty in achieving a satisfactory orgasm, may be unable to do so under the rather artificial conditions [and] a man may have great difficulty in having sex relations if these have to be carried out on medical instructions. If the wife follows a temperature chart and watches closely for the propitious days, the husband may become impotent at that very time. Sensitive people find it difficult to have intercourse "to order," and they may be reduced to temporary impotence by such pressures.

One counselor in a postwar infertility clinic suggested that female patients keep the ovulation chart to themselves. Rather than tell their husbands when the "right" moment arrived, they should simply seduce them.[37]

Studies in the 1940s and 1950s of thousands of patients admitted to the Infertility Services of the Margaret Sanger Research Bureau revealed a high drop-out rate. Only one-fourth to one-third of the couples achieved pregnancies. In 16 percent "conception was found impossible or inadvisable on the basis of male factors," and 10 percent were "failures," defined as "those cases completely or almost completely worked up and treated but with unexplained failure to conceive." With such dismal results, it is not surprising that nearly half (47.4 percent) of the admitted couples discontinued treatment. The researcher noted that "the high rate of abandonment before our investigation and treatment could be completed seems most interesting. . . . [It] reflects a basic human characteristic. (If we could eliminate almost 50 percent of our cases as deserters, our 'success' rate would be gratifyingly high!)"[38]

Psychological Diagnoses

Infertility treatment was frequently unsuccessful because half the cases eluded diagnosis. Clinical research continued to focus on the development of more precise diagnostic methods and more effective treatments. Practitioners did not all agree about the basic underlying causes of infertility. Some staunchly believed that if a physiological cause could not be identified, it simply had not been discovered yet. Most, however, agreed that emotional factors could be involved. Researchers had already established that stress could affect hormonal secretions, tubal contractions, and even sperm motility. But the causes of the emotional stresses that led to these physiological outcomes, as well as the prescriptions for reducing these stresses, were a subject of considerable debate. Some leading physicians downplayed the psychological factor. "It is easy to overestimate its importance," said the medical director of the Planned Parenthood Center of Los Angeles. "Admittedly, emotional disturbances can play a part in infertility, but physical conditions are a more frequent cause."[39] Others, however, emphasized psychological causes.

At the extreme end of this debate in the 1940s and 1950s were the psychoanalytically oriented practitioners. If they could find no physiological cause for a couple's childlessness, they often looked for evidence of their patients' unconscious desires to avoid parenthood. This psychological scrutiny was generally directed toward women. Although men were more likely than women to resist treatment, physicians rarely considered the possibility that reluctant men had a psychological difficulty that contributed to their impaired fertility or that they "subconsciously" did not really want children. Stress caused by pressure at work was the only psychological factor mentioned in the medical literature on the evaluation of male patients. Experts in the field never suggested that men thwarted their own potential for parenthood by "unconscious wishes" or "a rejection of their masculinity." On the contrary, specialists frequently reassured men that infertility did not mean they were lacking in masculinity. Clearly, most physicians believed that masculinity was not something that men were likely to avoid. But psychoanalytically oriented physicians claimed that some women contributed to their own infertility by their reluctance, consciously or unconsciously, to "accept their femininity." According to these practitioners, even the most eager and cooperative female patient might "subconsciously" wish to avoid motherhood.

As infertility continued to gain attention from the popular media, as well as the scientific community, these psychoanalytic perspectives began to infuse the discussion of childlessness. The postwar years witnessed a romance with all forms of psychology, especially Freudian and neo-Freudian theories. Psychoanalytic jargon appeared everywhere, from scientific journals to popular articles, and even in casual conversations. Some neo-Freudian theorists breathed new life into prescriptions that were first voiced by their Victorian forebears about the importance of women attending to their proper role. Old notions that education and careers hindered women's reproductive potential resurfaced, as did exhortations about women's sexual behavior. Although many infertility experts were skeptical of psychoanalytic explanations, neo-Freudian practitioners received a remarkable amount of attention in both the medical and popular literature.[40]

One example of this approach was a 1951 article by a sociologist, a psychologist, and a gynecologist that was published in the *Journal of the American Medical Association*. The authors began with the premise that normal, healthy adults naturally desire children. "Most people who do not truly want them probably have personality defects—for example, infantilism. . . . Women totally lacking the desire for children are so rare that they may be considered as deviants from the normal." Infertile women, they reasoned, might subconsciously thwart their own fertility by rejecting their femininity. They described three "types" of such women:

> The masculine-aggressive woman insists on having a child of her own body, cost what it may. She is a ready, though rarely ideal, candidate for donor insemination, sometimes obtaining her husband's reluctant consent by a species of emotional blackmail. Second, there is the wife who accepts childlessness and lives on good terms with her sterile husband but demands from him constant proofs of his masculinity in the way of achievement and material success. And, third, the truly motherly woman compensates for her lack of children by directing her motherliness toward other persons or objects, real or symbolic.

The three male authors asserted that whatever intrusive procedures were required to enable a woman to get pregnant, including artificial insemination with the sperm of an anonymous donor, the women did not mind. In fact, they argued, the women may even enjoy it.

> The patients are seldom troubled by any notion of violation of their bodies; indeed, some of them derive a peculiar satisfaction from the coldly scientific nature of the operation. Successful results create a feeling of superiority and triumph over the male, as well as a sense of fulfillment.

These writers expressed almost as much disdain for male patients. Claiming that the reproductive drive "is less powerful in men than in women," men were nevertheless more upset by infertility: "The traditionally proud lord of creation, finding himself unable to create a baby, is likely to develop a strong sense of personal devaluation."[41] Filled with unsubstantiated assertions, gross gender stereotypes, and virtually no data, this article in the nation's premier medical journal illustrates the weight of psychological theories in the postwar era.

Some specialists who agreed with these psychological theories warned other practitioners not to treat "neurotic" women for infertility. One advised: "The wise physician will be able to ascertain the psychic health of his patients. He will then be in an enviable position to determine whether or not attempts should be made to relieve sterility." It was important to do so, he argued, for "allowing an emotional [sic] immature woman to become fertile may open up the proverbial hornet's nest. The repercussions may result in neurotic children, broken homes, and divorce."[42] Some gynecologists, as well as psychologists and psychiatrists, pointed to "personality" factors in infertility. "The emotional maturity of the patient, that is, her ability adequately to meet the demands of pregnancy as well as motherhood, should always be considered in the treatment of sterility," argued W. S. Kroger, director of Psychosomatic Gynecology at Mount Sinai Hospital in Chicago and one of the leading voices in the application of psychoanalytic theories to infertility treatment. Kroger urged his fellow practitioners to take note of "those unhealthy attitudes and personality factors likely to complicate or contraindicate pregnancy." To determine if a woman should be treated for infertility, the physician should "seek answers to the following questions:"

1) Is the patient a cold, selfish, demanding person, or is she a warm, giving woman?
2) What is her motivation for becoming pregnant?
3) Could the absence of so-called "motherliness" be due to environmental factors, permanent or temporary, and does this account for her sterility?
4) How much does her emotional past . . . influence her attitudes toward motherhood?
5) What are the deeper meanings underlying her surface attitudes toward pregnancy, motherhood, and sterility?

Those who should be rejected for treatment included "the aggressive and masculine women who are competitive, strong, ambitious, and dominating. They 'wear the pants in the family' and are usually successful career women, possessing considerable executive ability." The greatest exemplar of the maladjusted female was the career woman. "We have all seen a long-desired pregnancy follow the renunciation of a career. This may be the result of the development of 'motherliness' and the consequent hormonal changes." Kroger concluded that "it should not be necessary for every physician to have training in psychoanalysis" to understand these basic principles. In other words, physicians who were not trained in psychology should make a psychological diagnosis that would determine whether the personality of the patient disqualified her for motherhood, in which case the physician should refuse treatment.[43] Kroger ended with a word of caution to the physician who might unwittingly treat a woman who was emotionally unqualified to become a mother: "If such a woman finally does conceive, the same psychological difficulties which once prevented conception, may adversely affect the child's psychic development, and . . . another individual is added to an endless procession of neurotics."[44]

Sexuality and Infertility

The "endless procession of neurotics" is reminiscent of Justice Oliver Wendell Holmes's proclamation that "three generations of imbeciles are enough." Although one was a eugenic argument and the other a psychoanalytic one, they had in common an assumption about fitness for motherhood based on a woman's sexual behavior and conformity to the prescribed gender role. For the eugenicist, a woman was unfit for motherhood if she was "promiscuous," meaning that she engaged in sex outside marriage and therefore should be sterilized. For the neo-Freudian, a wife was unfit for motherhood if she was "frigid," meaning not appropriately passive and submissive and therefore she should not be treated for infertility. In both cases, the gatekeepers of parenthood used their ideas about appropriate female gender behavior and sexuality to determine women's fitness for motherhood and to block some women from their opportunity to become parents.

Theories about the relationship between sexuality and procreation were nothing new. But whereas Victorian codes of the nineteenth century warned that women might become sterile if they were *too* sexual, neo-Freudians claimed that women might remain childless if they were not sexual *enough* or not "sexually correct." Frigidity was a major concern among these psychoanalytic theorists in the postwar years, and many associated frigidity with sterility. Some claimed that the vast majority of all women in Western countries were frigid, using as their definition "the incapacity of woman to achieve a vaginal orgasm during intercourse." These practitioners disagreed with the zoologist Kinsey, who identified vaginal as well as clitoral orgasm as equally "valid." Dismissing Kinsey's "statistical and non-medical approach," they relied on a psychoanalytic explanation of female sexuality:

> In the child, the clitoris gives sexual satisfaction, while in the emotionally mature woman the vagina is supposed to be the principal sexual organ. In frigid women, the shift of sexual satisfaction and excitement from the clitoris to the vagina, which usually occurs with emotional maturation, does not take place. ... The active emotional overvaluation of the clitoris must be relinquished, and a passive-receptive attitude toward the vagina is instituted. Many women fail in this task—hence the spectacle of a 70 to 90 per cent vaginal frigidity![45]

Another study argued that women who were "tomboys" as children became frigid and sterile as adults. The researchers described one allegedly frigid infertile woman in their sample as having been a "Boisterous Tomboy" and an "ill-adjusted child." The woman provided the evidence for their judgment in her description of her childhood:

> I was very bright and full of beans, fidgety, and quick-tempered. ... I was called a tomboy, a scatterbrain, and a Bolshevik. ... I imagined myself having exciting adventures and had an ambition to be on the stage and a great actress. ... I was a brilliant scholar and a good organizer. I was always captain of the forum and of the hockey team.[46]

Researchers and practitioners who labeled such women abnormal believed that women who did not conform to prevailing gender norms were unfit for motherhood. They included in this category women who they considered sexually maladjusted—aggressive or "frigid" instead of "passive-receptive"—and whose infertility was presumably the result of their psychosexual deviance. Curiously, the same diagnosis was used in "treating" another group of reproductive misfits: single White teenagers who became pregnant. As the historian Rickie Solinger has shown, Black and White teenage mothers faced different institutional responses to their situations. Social workers assumed that Black teenagers were sexually mature and potentially "maternal" and sent them home to have their babies. In contrast, they diagnosed White teenagers as mentally ill and asexual, which made them unfit for motherhood. These teenagers were whisked off to maternity homes, where their "mistakes" were "erased" and their children were placed for adoption. Psychoanalytic theorists at the time defined both unwed teenage mothers and "frigid" infertile wives as unfit for parenthood because of their alleged deviance from the marital heterosexual norm.

According to Solinger, "Females who violated gender-determined sexual norms were routinely designated as formally ill. One observer found so much frigidity that it was not even worth cataloging." Apparently, frigidity could cause unwed pregnancy as well as wedded infertility. The logic of this contradiction was never examined by the experts who so quickly labeled women frigid if they did not have babies in the expected marital mode. Sounding like the neo-Freudian physicians who described infertile women and expressing the virulent homophobia of the era, professionals who worked with White unwed teenage girls characterized them as exhibiting "marked rebelliousness . . . a lot of latent homosexuality . . . coupled with contempt for men." One social worker described a young client as "boyish in appearance and seemed to have adopted behavior which was symbolic of her unconscious conflicts. In all her activities . . . she was aggressive, almost as if she denied her femininity by redirecting her sexual energy."[47] Professionals in the postwar years redefined single pregnant girls and women. No longer described as "feebleminded," these women, like their infertile sisters, were diagnosed as psychologically disturbed, mentally ill, and sexually maladjusted.

Psychoanalytic ideas moved easily from the medical journals to the popular press. An article in *Coronet* magazine in 1953, entitled "Sterility Can Be a State of Mind," asserted that emotional states—hatred, fear, anxiety, poor adjustment to marriage—could inhibit fertility in from one-fourth to one-third of all cases of involuntary childlessness. According to the author, infertility often resulted from "high-strung women"; "strong parental prohibitions against sex"; and other psychological inhibitions, such as unresolved Oedipal conflicts. "Some specialists point out that to many persons, the doctor has become the highest authority in the conduct of their personal lives. . . . [He] has taken the place of the father of their childhood." Sometimes a visit to such a physician "may be reassuring to the wife and lead to a relaxation of her Fallopian tubes." The author also argued for the importance of sexual adjustment. "'The act of love' must, in truth, *be* an act of love, rather than just an act of sex, if fruitful union is to ensue." Repeating a common refrain, the article concluded, "If the wife is working, perhaps she can take a leave of absence for a while, or quit her job and stay at home. Rest and relax, and just forget all about doctors for a while. And see what happens."[48]

Some experts claimed that mere association with children would bring out a woman's "maternal instinct" which could stimulate fertility. *American Magazine* suggested a "plan that sometimes does wonders for childless couples. This is to go out babysitting. . . . [A] woman's maternal instincts are tremendously stimulated when there are children around." This was also the argument frequently given for the alleged "cure" of infertility by adoption. "Sometimes the adoption of a child is the secret," wrote an observer. "In the sunlight of a new happiness, the adoptive mother bears a child of her own." In one case, a psychoanalyst argued that the reason pregnancy followed adoption was because the wife quit her job after adopting a baby.

> Her conflict . . . resolved (sic) around the fact that if she became pregnant, she would have to stop working outside the home and abandon the masculine role. The decision to adopt a baby solved this unconscious conflict by making it absolutely necessary for her to give up her job. This, in some strange way, added to her femininity, and allowed her to conceive. Cases in which pregnancy follows the adoption of a baby are by no means rare. Everyone knows of similar instances.[49]

Some physicians were skeptical of these explanations. One cautioned those who believed that adoption often leads to biological parenting. "This popular belief has no justification. Some couples adopt a child, then subsequently have children of their own, and when this occurs, there's a lot of comment. But we don't hear about the many more couples who do not have children subsequent to adoption." This physician was also cautious about placing too much emphasis on emotional factors in infertility. He noted that emotional tension was as likely to be a *result* of infertility as a cause, since trying to conceive a child and seeking medical help in the effort were stressful activities in themselves: "Many childless couples are emotionally upset because of their failure to have children, but often the tensions have been built up as a result of years of frustration and hence may be an effect rather than a cause of the problem."[50]

This physician had a point. Infertile couples in the postwar years faced tremendous stresses. First, there was the stigma of childlessness at a time when having many children, at a young age, was the norm. Next was the suggestion, reinforced by psychoanalytic theories and echoed in the popular press, that infertile women were to blame for their own condition. Women were labeled abnormal if they were ambivalent about having children, they were suspected of not *really* wanting children even if they truly believed that they did, they were accused of unconscious wishes to remain childless, they were chastised for holding jobs or aspiring to careers, and they were admonished if they were not adequately passive and submissive. They were made to feel guilty if they had an abortion, held a job or pursued a career, or found sexual satisfaction in any way other than through a vaginal orgasm resulting from male penetration.

Since researchers had determined that stress might affect fertility, some of these pressures may have had the ironic effect of contributing to infertility. Women who were accused of being "abnormal," "selfish," "neurotic," or "immature" as a result of normal and healthy ambivalence toward or resistance to the accepted female role of full-time wife and mother may indeed have suffered enough stress to cause their fallopian tubes to contract. Meanwhile, in spite of the efforts of many specialists to improve the treatment of male infertility and the recognition that most infertility cases involved some problem with the male partner, infertility remained defined as a female complaint.

There is plenty of evidence to suggest that the profoundly gendered understandings of infertility and patterns of treatment influenced the way individual couples experienced and responded to their own childlessness. An extreme example is the long struggle of Lorna and Henry Anderson, who married in 1965, thinking that "everyone could have children whenever they wanted." When it did not happen to them, they began to discuss their options.

> Henry seemed reluctant to commit to any plan of action. He felt that if we were supposed to have children, we would just have them. I began to be so troubled by my childlessness that I went to the doctor on my own without Henry's knowledge. I was probed and prodded and the doctor said everything looked normal and before he did more tests, Henry should come for a sperm count. He refused to go.

Finding herself at a dead end with infertility treatment, Lorna "decided that it really didn't matter where I got the baby, my arms just ached for one, and it would be OK if we adopted." But Henry refused.

Lorna then turned to religion, where the advice she received from church authorities was virtually identical to that of the neo-Freudian experts who wrote in medical journals. She attended Bible study and

> found faith in God. With that, though, came teaching about women's roles and how they relate to men and God. At first I was totally awestruck and

believed that women were to be subservient to men and that Henry was to rule over me and I was to do as he said. I was taught that his will should be mine and that I must keep the peace in the family by not putting pressure on him to do anything he did not want to do. I began to pray. (That's what they taught. If I just was a better wife, God would reward me by giving me my heart's desire.)

So while thousands of her peers became caught up in the reemergence of the feminist movement, challenging the very precepts she now embraced, Lorna became a modern-day Ann Bradstreet, bending her will into submission while praying for a child. "So began a 20 year journey in making a wonderful home, cooking, canning, taking care of a large house and yard. . . . I was so submissive. . . . And the years rolled by." Not only did her prayers remain unanswered, but submissiveness took a huge toll on Lorna.

Needless to say, resentment began to build until I was on the verge of a nervous breakdown. No matter how hard I prayed, Henry would not open up, nor did I get pregnant. All I wanted was a child! Was that such a big deal[?] Everyone else had them. Some people had too many, abused them, aborted them. Why not me?

Lorna blamed herself—not her body, but her character. "What had I done wrong? Was I being punished for something? I wasn't a bad person. Why, why, why! The Bible says that nothing satisfies the barren womb. Certainly that was true."

Although she described a full life, including her work for a university, and Henry's good job as a construction supervisor, "I am filled with a sense of hopelessness. I don't have the strength or desire to end the marriage—he's all I have—my only connectedness to the past. . . . And what would be the point—I'm too old to be a mother now, anyway." Lorna's desire for a child motivated her to embark on a twenty-year effort to live a life of submissive domesticity. Few went to such extreme measures, but her obsession to become a mother reflected the heightened stakes in parenthood that had emerged in the postwar years. The medical profession responded to the pronatalist pressures by carving out and expanding a new field of infertility research and practice; however, as an imperfect science, it also absorbed and acted upon the prevailing gender assumptions of the day.

Perhaps inadvertently, the increased attention to infertility during the baby-boom era contributed to the heightened stakes in parenthood. More than at any time in the past, parenthood became a marker of full adulthood and normality. The childless became objects of curiosity, pity, scorn, and suspicion. Single men and women, as well as married childless couples, no longer found a cultural space that afforded them respect. And with the popular press filled with stories of miracle babies and new infertility treatments, those who found themselves childless were increasingly willing to seek a cure for their condition, rather than accept their childlessness and carve out their lives in ways that did not include parenthood. It is perhaps no surprise that childlessness declined to an all-time low during these years, with virtually everyone marrying and having children, and with increasing pressures as well as opportunities to seek treatment for infertility. In the postwar era, ideas of happiness, security, maturity, and good citizenship all revolved around the nuclear family with children. Those who did not marry and procreate were left out in the cold.

The patterns established in the midcentury decades continued to influence the treatment and the perception of infertility in later years, even though the tight ideological connections that linked marriage, reproduction, and respectability began to weaken. As the cold war began to wane, along with the unique ideology of domesticity that accompanied it, more and more young adults began to question and resist the powerful prescriptions to marry and multiply. The second wave of feminism made the kinds of gender claims articulated by midcentury Freudians unutterable, if not unthinkable. Still, the stakes in having children kept getting higher, and the lure of treatment—with its endless possibilities for a technological "fix"—propelled infertile men and women who were in pursuit of happiness on an ever-lengthening medical path. Ironically, the same high stakes that made some people so desperate for children made others equally eager to avoid parenthood like the plague.

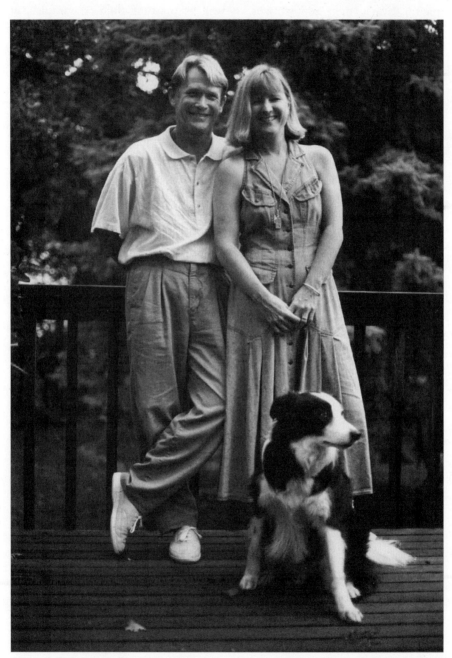

Political theorists and citizen activists James Farr and Mary Dietz, happily married for ten years without children, pictured here with their border collie, Willie, who reads at a second-grade level. (*Courtesy of Mary Dietz and James Farr; photo by Mary Lou Nemanic*)

CHAPTER 6

Childfree: The Revolt Against the Baby Boom

★☆

A Minnesota lawyer I know, married for ten years with no children, "dates" his wife; they live together in a fun-fun lifestyle that is close to that typified in Playboy *magazine.*

—Ellen Peck, *The Baby Trap*, 1971

MAKE LOVE, NOT BABIES

—Zero Population Growth Bumper Sticker, 1972

I'm constantly hearing about my biological clock, blah, blah, blah. I've had it up to my ears. . . . I don't want to share my life with anyone other than the man I choose to live with.

— A childfree rock musician, 1993

Me, I'm partial to romance.

—A childfree feminist professor, 1993

Belle Sander, a "casino change girl,"[1] lives in Las Vegas with her retired husband. Having chosen to be childfree, "I felt that we should stand up and be counted." They are "poor people," she wrote. "However, to be honest I must admit that our having chosen a childfree lifestyle had nothing to do with finances. We like the freedom." She calls herself "childfree" because it suggests the absence of something undesirable, "as a food without choles-terol is 'cholesterol free'." Janet Dewey, who has a Ph.D. in epidemiology, also prefers the term "childfree" because the term "childless" "implies that one's natural state is to have children, and I'm not at all convinced that mine is."

Such sentiments would barely have been whispered, if admitted, dur-ing the baby-boom years. Researchers in 1966 concluded that "fecundity impairments" caused nearly all cases of childlessness and that voluntary childlessness was "nearly extinct." But the next generation would prove those predictions wrong. In 1993, *Health* magazine described a "quintes-sential contented baby boomer:" happily married, affluent, a good job—a nineties woman who "has it all." But the one thing she does not have and does not want is children. Totally rejecting the ethos of the baby boom, she remarked, "Kids are fine. It's just that taking care of another human being is not what I want to be doing with my life for the next twenty years."[2]

Since the peak of the baby boom, along with the declining birthrate there has been a dramatic increase in childlessness, and most studies agree that the increase is largely due to a rise in voluntary childlessness. In 1990, for example, 25 percent of all women aged thirty to thirty-four were childless, compared to only 16 percent in 1976. Demographers predicted that fully 22 percent of all women born between 1956 and 1972 will never have any children, and most of them will be childless by choice. Many of these baby boomers are fed up with what they consider to be "a tyranny of parentism," according to Leslie Lafayette, founder of the 2,500-member Childfree Network, one of several groups formed since the 1960s to sup-port the choice to be childless. Voluntary childlessness increased so rapidly that fifteen years after it was declared "nearly extinct" another writer declared pronatalism "laughable and passé" and proclaimed that "the childless are finally in the mainstream of American life."[3]

Both statements were exaggerations. Voluntary childlessness increased after the 1960s, but it was not a new phenomenon, nor did the stigma sur-rounding the childless entirely disappear. What changed in the 1970s was the visibility and the stridency of the voluntarily childless. For the first time, advocates for the childfree began to argue that voluntary childless-ness represented not simply a legitimate alternative to parenthood, but a better lifestyle—better for individuals, better for couples, better for the planet.

The childfree movement emerged in a particular historical moment, in part as a reaction to the intense pronatalism of the baby-boom years and in part as a function of feminism, environmentalism, and the increasing tolerance for alternatives to the nuclear family. Although the movement gave voice to the voluntarily childless, it neither erased the stigma nor fully articulated the various motives for opting against parenthood. It may have widened the cultural space for the childless in American society, but that space remained on the margin. In spite of the efforts of childfree activists, researchers in the 1970s found a "high level of consensus that nonparenthood is not an advantaged status."[4]

Even the most satisfied of the childfree chafed at the persistent stigma. Louise Hanson, a happily married baby-boomer feminist college professor, wondered, "Why do people who are not in favor of limitless breeding always feel they have to prove they're not monsters? Even me?" Janet Dewey and her husband resented being labeled "eccentric" at best and "selfish hedonists" at worst. "Child-less-ness makes one a freak," echoed Sandra George. "It's [easier] to sympathize with the woman who spends a fortune on fertility treatments that ruin her health and destroy her marriage than it is to understand a woman who says, 'I'm doing other things with my life.'" Susan Conroy complained, "I am tired of being looked at as an oddity. . . . I don't walk around asking people why they have children." But she is constantly asked why she does not. As late as 1993, an article in the *Los Angeles Times* noted that the voluntarily childless are "treated like traitors to the American Way."[5]

One reason that the voluntarily childless sought each other out and began to form organizations like the Childfree Network was the intense isolation they felt. Stella Sims and her husband felt "left out" like "aliens from another planet because we don't have children of our own at home." Emma Stein McCoy was "impatient with the cult of parenthood among baby-boomers." Yet, she wrote, "a tiny part of me, tired of being a perennial outsider, wants to be a parent because I would immediately have something in common with a gazillion peers." Martin North felt "isolated and 'different' as a result of our choice. We have virtually no friends and very few acquaintances with whom we can relate in this regard." These comments indicate that even after the baby boom turned into the "baby bust," parenthood remained a powerful cultural norm. Nevertheless, the stigma surrounding voluntary childlessness eased somewhat, and an increasing number of American adults chose to be "childfree."

The Childfree Movement of the 1970s

The childfree movement emerged in the wake of the baby boom because a growing number of young adults rebelled against the powerful postwar ideology of domesticity. Hoping to avoid what many saw as a life sentence to the suburban nuclear family, many baby boomers decided not to have children. Although no single cause explains the trend, the rise in childlessness reflects a number of cultural developments that took place during the waning years of the cold war.

Improvements in contraception do not in themselves explain the rising rate of childlessness. If that were the case, childlessness would have increased steadily throughout the twentieth century. The availability and effectiveness of contraception correlates neither with the fertility rate nor with the rate of childlessness. It certainly cannot explain the high birthrate and the low rate of childlessness during the baby-boom era, when contraception was widely available. Nor can the mere availability of contraception and reproductive technologies explain the dramatic differences in childbearing behavior among different ethnic groups. Other factors—cultural, economic, political, and personal—all contributed to reproductive decisions.

For decades, social scientists have puzzled over the growth of childlessness. Even though the rate of childlessness since the 1960s has not reached pre–World War II levels, the increase has attracted a great deal of attention. The rise in the marriage age may help explain the declining birthrate, but since the vast majority of Americans continue to marry at ages young enough to have children, late marriage does not explain increased childlessness. Most studies attribute the rise to voluntary childlessness.[6] It is logical to connect the increasing number of childfree persons to the political movements of the 1960s and 1970s. Voluntary childlessness may well have increased because it was consistent with and supported by a number of political philosophies, including feminism, environmentalism, zero population growth, gay and lesbian rights, the movement for reproductive choice, and the New Left's rejection of the domestic ideology and compulsory pronatalism of the early years of the cold war.

The politics of the era no doubt supported those who made the choice and helped to create a more tolerant cultural environment for the voluntarily childless. Many rejected parenthood because of a greater commitment to careers or public life. Like their predecessors in earlier decades, they believed that without children to raise, they could contribute to society by devoting their energies to other endeavors. The couple pictured at the opening of this chapter represent the voluntarily childless of today who chose to devote their energies to public life and civic activism, rather than to child rearing. But a far greater number of the voluntarily childless who responded to the author's query for this study explained their decision in terms of personal pleasures. According to a summary of twenty-nine studies of the voluntarily childless conducted during the 1970s and 1980s, 79 percent of all respondents gave "freedom" and "self-fulfillment" as the reasons for their choice.[7] Most chose private life *without* children over private life *with* children. In all likelihood, these childfree baby boomers shared the same dreams of their parents for a secure and comfortable private life free from hardship. They did not reject the idea of marital romance and domestic bliss. Togetherness still reigned, as it had in the 1950s, but now children had dropped out of the romantic picture and only the couple remained.

At first glance, the childfree movement of the 1970s appears to have been a dramatic rejection of the postwar ideology of domesticity. During the baby-boom years, it was rare to find any public affirmation of life without children.[8] But a closer look reveals a profound continuity: the preoccupation with private life fueled both the nuclear family ideal and the reaction against it. Even at the height of the baby boom, there were glimmers that not everyone found parenthood to be the surest route to the good life. Whereas most messages in the popular culture equated having children with fun, leisure, and happiness, a 1958 article in the *American Mercury* argued just the opposite. The tongue-in-cheek piece, entitled "Pity the Childless Couple," began this way:

> There's nothing sadder than the childless couple. It breaks you up to see them stretched out relaxing around swimming pools . . . all suntanned and miserable . . . or going off to Europe like lonesome fools. It's an empty life. There's nothing but more money to spend, more time to enjoy, and a whole lot less to worry about.

The piece did not advocate childlessness; it was merely the "musings of a good mother—on a bad day."[9] Nevertheless, it was a preview of things to come.

By 1963, the unmentionable became mentionable. The same year that Betty Friedan's *The Feminine Mystique* appeared to wide acclaim, Gael

Greene cast "A Vote Against Motherhood" in the *Saturday Evening Post*, pro-claiming, "I don't want to have any children. Motherhood is only a part of marriage, and I am unwilling to sacrifice the other equally important femi-nine roles upon the over-exalted alter of parenthood." In many ways, Friedan's statement was a much more radical call to middle-class wives: Get out of the house and escape the trap of domesticity. Greene's message was that domesticity was bliss—without children:

> I champion the wondrously satisfying love of a woman and her husband, two adults enjoying the knowledge and mystery of each other. . . . Femininity is the acceptance, appreciation and enjoyment of being a woman. Motherhood is only part of it. The complete woman is also devoted wife, lover, playmate, buffer, a man's stimulant and tranquilizer, a creator (in the kitchen if not at the easel or typewriter).

Although her far-from-feminist motives were completely consistent with the togetherness ideal of romantic marriage and blissful domesticity, Greene obviously recognized the political stigma that surrounded the decision to avoid one's most patriotic duty during the cold-war years. When she told friends that she and her husband were not planning to have children, "the shock and disbelief could not be greater if my hus-band announced he had just accepted a job spying for the Russians and I was busy running a Communist Party cell in the basement boiler room." Apparently, her readers felt the same: Friedan—feminist and mother—was admired, while Greene was vilified: Three thousand letters came to the *Saturday Evening Post*, most of which attacked her for her heretical ideas about motherhood.[10]

Several writers have noted that the rise of voluntary childlessness ran parallel to the rise of the second wave of feminism, and there are indeed some obvious intersections. In the early 1970s, some of the radical partic-ipants in the women's liberation movement attacked the entire idea of motherhood. But few "mainstream" feminists advocated childlessness, and not all advocates of voluntary childlessness or childfree women con-sidered themselves to be feminists. Researchers in the 1970s found that most of the voluntarily childless they studied were not aware of the women's movement until after they had decided not to have children. Although many childfree women thought that feminism supported their choice, others were cool toward the movement because of its historical connection to motherhood. While radical feminists argued against motherhood, mainstream feminists called for child care centers, flexible work hours, and other supports so that women need not choose between careers and children.[11]

Nevertheless, feminists were frequently stereotyped as man haters and child haters, and voluntary childlessness seemed to feed the stereotype. As late as the 1990s, Louise Hanson, a self-proclaimed feminist, felt that she had to defend herself against such stereotypes. She and her husband were not "child-hating curmudgeons," she said. And she was anything but a man hater. She simply did not want her marriage to suffer the fate of those of her friends who became parents: "The intimacy of the relationship, not to mention romance, is long gone in the struggle for survival." Sounding a theme that echoed throughout the sentiments of childfree baby boomers, she wrote, "Me, I'm partial to romance."

In several widely read books and articles, childfree advocates called upon women to reject motherhood in favor of romance, claiming that the two were mutually incompatible. Betty Rollin's provocative piece in *Look* magazine in 1970 proclaimed, "Motherhood cleaned up sex!" Rejecting the baby-boom era's fusion of sexuality and motherhood, she warned, "When the stork flies in, a woman's sexuality may fly out."[12] Most of these tracts were written by and for women, with the explicit goal of countering the powerful postwar message that motherhood was the true fulfillment of womanhood. But these works were more powerfully influenced by the "sexual revolution" of the 1960s than by feminism. The first and most strident of these tracts, Ellen Peck's *The Baby Trap*, published in 1971, turned the message of the 1950s on its head but kept the goal the same. *The Baby Trap* was simply a new version of "How To Catch Your Man and Keep Him."

Peck advocated a life of excitement and sex. She argued against the cultural mandate of the baby-boom era that motherhood was the fulfillment of a woman's sexuality and the surest route to marital intimacy and bliss. She argued instead that children were a hindrance to those goals:

For many women, the birth of children marks the end of adventure, of growth, of sexuality, of life itself. A woman caught in the Baby Trap has less time to spend with the man she married and is less free to share his world. And a man, harassed by mounting bills and the awesome two-decade obligations of fatherhood . . . caught between the demands of family and his own needs as a man—that man may look elsewhere for the joy and excitement his marriage has lost.

Peck argued that parents were sold a false bill of goods and that the best way to achieve a satisfying and erotically charged marriage was to avoid having children. To make her point, she taunted, "The men I meet who don't have children talk about their wives. The men who have kids ask me out." The formula had switched from "become the mother of his child and keep romance alive" to "never have a baby and keep romance alive." Peck's book was a lengthy warning to women that if they had babies, their husbands might stray. Proponents of motherhood

> never tell you that many men find themselves less attracted to their wives after the physical changes of pregnancy and birth. They never tell you that there may be a correlation between fatherhood and infidelity. They never tell you that, rather than keeping a marriage together, children can often very quickly drive it apart.

Childlessness was the married woman's answer to the *Playboy* promise to men of endless consumerism and sex. If you do not have a baby, Peck told her female readers, you and your husband can both live the *Playboy* lifestyle together:

> Marriage should not signal a "settling down," but a waking up. . . . Take your pick. One or the other. Housework and children—or the glamour, involvement and excitement of a free life. . . . The girls I've talked to who don't have children are, almost without exception, prettier, more conversational, more aware, more alive, more exciting, more satisfied. They have . . . better marriages and happier husbands than those wives who do have children.

Peck also advocated jobs for women, but not for personal fulfillment, as Friedan suggested. Rather, wives should work because a husband

> has to know his wife is still attractive to other men. . . . If she works, she'll stay attractive, and stay interesting. . . . Men want women that *other* men want. And if you're working, your husband knows that other men are seeing and appreciating you. Result: he appreciates you more, too.

A job need not detract from a woman's role as a wife. As an example, Peck described the home life of Helen Gurley Brown, editor of *Cosmopolitan* and author of the 1962 best-seller *Sex and the Single Girl*, who cooked gourmet meals for her husband and decorated their home with a sensual touch. Peck quoted Brown: "Everything is comfortable and sexy: there's a lot of fake leopard. . . . I fix him a drink and settle him down, like a geisha . . . then I serve dinner. The atmosphere is intimate. There is no one else around." Nearly a decade after Friedan's book called for an end to the "feminine mystique," Peck called on women to be "like a geisha." Speaking for herself and her husband who lived in childless bliss, Peck asserted, "Barren we are definitely not."[13]

The Baby Trap was enormously popular and influential. The first printing of 10,000 copies sold out in ten days, and the book went through several additional printings.[14] After Peck's book came a number of other tracts that promoted similar ideas.[15] In 1972, advocates on behalf of the childfree formed the National Organization for Non-Parents (NON). Like Zero Population Growth, NON had an environmental rationale, but it also focused on lifestyle issues. Among its founders were Ellen Peck, author of *The Baby Trap*, and Shirley Radl, who wrote *Mother's Day is Over*. The organization attracted hundreds of members by the mid-1970s, two-thirds of whom were women, mostly White married urbanites under age thirty-five in the higher-income and educational brackets, generally not committed to religion. Most of the members believed that children got in the way of personal independence, required too much responsibility, and interfered with the marital relationship.[16] By 1978, the organization had softened its message somewhat to emphasize choice and had changed its name to the National Alliance for Optional Parenthood (NAOP).[17]

Optional parenthood began to gain legitimacy. One study found a noticeable change in attitudes in the late 1960s: College students in 1970 expressed much more tolerance of childless marriages than a similar group polled in 1965.[18] Books like *The Baby Trap* both reflected the trend and contributed to it. For those who were uncertain about having children, advocates like Peck helped them make up their minds. Faith Bayard was uncertain about parenthood when she first married, but after reading Peck's book she decided against it. Corinne Mason was devastated when her only child died at the age of seven weeks. "I was totally torn apart and wanted to adopt," she said, feeling that she could not go through another pregnancy. Then she read *The Baby Trap* and decided that life without children would be OK.

By the mid-1980s, voluntary childlessness was no longer considered pathological. A Roper poll found that while 94 percent of American women favored marriage, 82 percent did not feel that children were an essential ingredient for a happy marriage. Most women still planned to become parents, however.

A survey of college women in New England in 1985 found that most respondents expected to have nontraditional occupations and planned to delay marriage and childbearing until they were established in their careers. But again, few expected to remain childless.[19]

According to Kate Harper, who wrote *The Childfree Alternative* in 1980, "the key word . . . is choice." Her message was much less strident than Peck's, but she nevertheless encouraged her readers to think carefully before having children, and her book made a strong case for childlessness. She suggested that those who contemplate parenthood should ask themselves, as she asked herself:

> Can I be giving on demand, for as long as I am needed? Will I resent those demands so much that I hurt my child? Will I lose the very things I most value about myself—my peace and radiance and joy? Will I go crazy with the unending responsibility? . . . Will I still be able to enjoy a full and intimate life with the man I love, or will motherhood replace being a lover and friend?

For Harper, the decision was clear: "I fear spending years of my life too tired to enjoy myself, my child, or my mate." Work life was not an appealing alternative: "I fear getting myself into the trap of needing to provide for my child and having to work at something I despise." And she found the ideal of the nuclear family intimidating: "I fear most of all that I simply don't know how a healthy family works and that I will collapse under the strain of trying to achieve one."[20]

As Harper's anxiety suggests, the childfree choice did not necessarily reflect a rejection of the baby-boom ideology of full-time motherhood. In 1979, Carole Baker, director of NAOP, scoffed at the idea of "quality time," claiming that parenting required a woman's full attention: "The super woman image is a myth. You can't program tender loving care between 7 and 8 at night when you're at home. I think it's an injustice. You can't replace quantity with quality."[21] Many of the childless believed that parenting was a full-time occupation that demanded expertise and dedication and that if it could not be done successfully and correctly, it should not be done at all.

This message had a particularly powerful impact on women. The equation of good motherhood with full-time motherhood made it difficult to imagine pursuing a career while trying to raise children properly. Many of the childless career women believed that child rearing was a full-time commitment and would not consider holding a job and raising children at the same time. In surveys of the voluntarily childless, the women listed careers as a reason for childlessness almost as frequently as freedom and self-fulfillment; 74 percent of the women mentioned careers compared to only 29 percent of the men.[22]

Annette Andrews, for example, a single, childless librarian, expressed disdain for both teenage mothers on welfare and "well off wives working to the last minute in pregnancy, leaving young children from infancy while they pursue careers." In her condemnation of welfare and yuppie mothers alike, she argued that unless women planned to be full-time mothers and to devote adequate resources to the task, they should not have children. Shelly Gordon agreed. She was critical of "half-hearted attempts at parenting using leftover love and energy from the grueling pace of just surviving in today's break-neck paced world. That's not enough and it shouldn't be enough."

These responses reflect not only an assumption about the proper way to raise children, but an awareness that the job fell to mothers alone, with little participation from fathers and no assistance from the larger community. No respondents suggested that men should quit their jobs or take time off from work. But several suggested that women do so. The economic downturn in the 1970s and 1980s, combined with the expectation of child-centered consumerism, made full-time child rearing an even more difficult prospect. Janet Dewey complained, "I feel that for all the lip service about 'family values' (that term makes me nauseous now the way it's been used), there is almost a societal contempt for people with children, unless they are wealthy enough to do the Ozzie and Harriet routine." She said that her friends struggle to

> do right by their children, and all they get by way of societal support is inadequate public schools, unaffordable housing, and a perpetual guilt trip for having to rely on what little child care is available. Of course, if one chooses to stay home with the children it's going to be hard enough trying to pay for their health care, let alone a decent education.

Race, Class, and Voluntary Childlessness

This burden on parents may be one reason why voluntary childlessness has been more common among those who live in highly privatized communities and less prevalent where child rearing is shared. Voluntary childlessness has been lower among Black Americans than other groups. Hispanic women have had the lowest rate of childlessness, often explained as being a result of cultural and religious beliefs. Social scientists have not yet been able to explain why some groups are more inclined toward voluntary childlessness than are others. But one possibility may be that among the poorer communities of color, some of the communal patterns of child rearing still operate.[23]

Rates of childlessness for different groups have fluctuated throughout the twentieth century. The percentage of childless for all groups dropped dramatically in the decade following World War II, but in the 1960s the rate for Whites began to rise steadily and steeply until 1980, and the rates for people of color dropped just as steadily and steeply over the same years. Black women, who had the highest rates of childlessness of any group throughout the first half of the twentieth century, suddenly had a lower rate than White women.[24] Although the causes are not evident in the aggregate statistics, most studies agree that childlessness among urban people of color decreased as better health care and treatment for venereal diseases became more readily available after the 1940s and that voluntary childlessness accounts for much of the increase in childlessness among Whites.

If groups are compared according to class, however, the racial differences fade. Black women who had a college education or were married to professional men had the same rates of fertility and childlessness as did White women in similar circumstances.[25] Nevertheless, the rhetoric of the childfree movement never seemed to catch on among Black women, even among the affluent and highly educated who had high rates of voluntary childlessness. They were more likely to point to economic and cultural factors in their decision.

One forty-year-old Black executive, for example, married and voluntarily childless, said that she could not imagine taking on the full burden of raising children while her husband struggled in his career: "The black male is under such tension today just to survive, just to make it, to accomplish something in life, that it requires all of his energies." Another Black professional, Barbara Daniel Cox, executive director of the Women's Resource Network in Philadelphia, noted in the early 1980s that within the Black community, "there certainly is peer pressure in the direction of parenthood. . . . Family is a very important value to most black people, and I think we buy into the traditional concept that woman is here to procreate." As a childless woman in midlife, she was not sure whether she should have a baby: "Can I, Should I? Will I? Must I?" She pointed to the politics of the 1960s as giving a different message to Blacks than to Whites. Never subject to the Feminine Mystique that affected affluent, educated White women, Black women were less likely to see domesticity and children as a trap. "I think a lot of traditionalism came out with the black power movement, and blacks became more focused upon their roots and keeping family life together. . . . Black women want to hook up with black men emotionally more than white women do with white men."[26]

For some, that secure connection was a necessary precondition for parenthood. Arvonne Newton, a thirty-five-year-old divorced Black attorney who had grown up in a "secure two-parent family," wanted to have children as part of a committed relationship with "two on-site, full-time loving parents." She had two abortions because the men involved "weren't ready for the responsibility of fatherhood," and she did not want to be a single mother. She counts herself "lucky that I can exercise control over my own life."

In a 1994 column for *USA Weekend*, journalist Janet Singleton discussed the issue of childlessness among young professional Black women like herself and complained about the ubiquitous image of the Black welfare mother. "In the land of poisonous stereotypes," she wrote, "black women always have lots of (often state supported) kids. The truth is different. Almost none of my thirtysomething friends is a parent." Noting that childlessness is almost as common among college-educated Black women as among White women, she observed that

> the rough realities of race could provide formidable complications. Black women I know who entered adulthood hoping to follow a path to motherhood stumbled into barbed wire. They discovered that dating meant entering the eligible-black-male lottery: lots of deserving ticket holders, but only so many can win.

Although she has considered adopting as a single woman, she is "uneasy about money. Thrusting a black child into America without the insulation of financial security is like exposing a vein to Count Dracula." As a child of blue-collar parents, she knows "how draining it is to try to break into the middle class." Although she enjoys the freedom she has as a childless woman, "In my dreams I will continue to see motherhood as a possible destination."[27] For Black women like Janet Singleton and Arvonne Newton, childlessness resulted more from circumstance than from choice. Unlike their White peers, they did not explain their childlessness in terms of a "lifestyle."

The Childfree Lifestyle

In 1936, when childlessness was even more common than it is today, the noted eugenic advocate Paul Popenoe wrote about the unhealthy "refusal" to bear children and concluded that most cases were "motivated by individualism, competitive consumption economically, and an infantile, self-indulgent, frequently neurotic attitude toward life." Later researchers abandoned these harsh judgments and considered childlessness an "alternate lifestyle." One of the first sociologists to examine voluntary childlessness from a sympathetic perspective was Jean E. Veevers, who in the early 1970s studied a group of voluntarily childless urban middle-class wives in Canada. These relatively affluent women viewed children as "interfering with their lifestyle." They emphasized "new experiences," "spontaneity," and the large amount of leisure time childless women have, compared to mothers.[28]

Other researchers in the 1970s also examined the political and career commitments of the childfree people they studied, in an effort to find out if their subjects' choices reflected a commitment to public, professional, or community involvement over domesticity. The researchers found that most childfree people worked full time in jobs they said they enjoyed and that their philosophical beliefs tended toward liberal and feminist politics as well as religious skepticism. But their careers and beliefs seemed to support rather than determine their decisions to remain childless. More important was the lifestyle they wanted to enjoy together. It was almost as though the "togetherness" ethic of the postwar nuclear family had a new incarnation among the childfree baby boomers, geared more toward the "couple" than the "family" and focused on a different style of leisure and consumerism.

Although the early 1970s was a time of relatively high levels of political consciousness and grassroots activism of all kinds, the voluntarily childless were not predisposed to high levels of engagement in public life. Rather, they were likely to be loners, preferring to spend their leisure time with each other. According to one study, they "did not tend to join organizations."[29] They used their combined incomes for "leisure and luxury" more than did couples with children, well aware of the need for two salaries to support their standard of living. Many remarked that if they had a child, they would not be able to count on the income from two full-time jobs, and even if they could, the child would require a large share of it.

In one study of thirty childfree couples in the 1970s, all but two of the wives had full-time jobs and intended to continue working in their chosen careers. But they were clear about the fact that they had not chosen careers over children. They worked because they "would be bored staying at home" and indicated that they would continue working even if they had a child. Only 20 percent said that they would quit their jobs if they had a child. Most said that "having a child would make little difference in their basic orientation toward their employment situations." These researchers found, along with others, that "a career and career satisfaction is not a sufficient cause for choosing a childfree life—but it may be a necessary one," to provide the income required for the private lifestyle they desired.[30]

The trend continued into the 1990s. Like the voluntarily childless couples studied in the 1970s, few of the childfree respondents to this study wrote that they chose careers over children, or public life over private life. Evidence of 1960s sensibilities permeated many of the letters, but direct expressions of political, public, or career motivations for childlessness were rare. The impact of the women's movement was either implicit or explicit in letters from men as well as from women. Many women said that feminism gave legitimacy to their choice to pursue a career rather than parenthood. Stacey Downey stated unequivocally, "My energies, admittedly have been (and continue to be) focused on my career." But more typical was the response of Christine Newberry, who said: "I didn't really pick a career over the kids, but that does give me a somewhat convenient, noble excuse for not having them." Describing herself and her husband as "yuppies," she wrote, "I like going where I want, doing what I want, having light-colored carpets and art in the living room. I hate drinking out of Tupperware." Sally Cort echoed these sentiments:

> I think I would strongly resent the baby for ruining my life. My husband and I would not be able to afford a child without selling our land and probably our house. (We have 45 acres in the country.) We are both fiercely independent and basically do what we want to do when we want to do it. . . . I realize that this sounds extremely selfish, but what better reason for not having children?

Many of the childfree who wrote emphasized their desires for a close intimate relationship with their partners that they could enjoy in ample leisure
time with enough resources for consumer goods; travel; "spontaneity"; and,
above all, "freedom." Recognizing that "selfish" is the adjective most
frequently attached to voluntary childlessness, they variously admitted,
embraced, or rejected the term. Jason Domquist confronted the question of
selfishness directly. "Is the desire to be child-free selfish? Yes and no. 'Yes' if
commitment to a child means the sacrifice of concerts, opera, travel, and
other personal pleasures. I chose not to make that sacrifice. 'No' if having a
child can itself be construed as a selfish act."

Randy Almont fully admitted that his motive for childlessness was self-
indulgence. He is forty-six and had a vasectomy as a single man at the age of
twenty-three, for the sole purpose of sexual freedom.

> I simply did not want the troubles and commitment associated with raising
> children. . . . It took some convincing on my part, as the doctor really grilled
> me about it. I'd been raised to be extremely careful about pregnancy, and
> remained a virgin until I was about 22 years old. The vasectomy was like the
> cutting of a chain bonding me to a wall. . . . I married shortly after my vasec-
> tomy, shamefully not telling my wife of it.

The marriage lasted only a few months.

> I've been fortunate to have been able to experiment extensively sexually with
> loving friends, and others. I enjoyed that a lot, but I must say, this damn
> AIDS epidemic sure has messed up being a sexually active single man! Cur-
> rently, I've been celibate for several years, but happy in the knowledge that I
> was able to enjoy complete sexual freedom for a time.

Unlike Randy, Carolyn Macey is married. But she, too, acknowledged
"selfish" motives: "We were selfish in that we really did not care to have
others (children) interfere in our relationship, i.e., have to *share* ourselves
with them." Unlike the ethic of shared consumerism that marked family
life during the baby-boom era, Carolyn, like many of her childfree peers,
believed that children would compete with their parents over family
resources. With children,

> our standard of living would be significantly different. . . . We have a nice
> home with fragile glass sculptures and light carpets—very different from our

family homes of tough wood tables, Herculon upholstery and dark, stain-guard carpet! As we see our friend's teens total dad's car, we quietly enjoy our new car. As they drag off to Disneyland with 3 whining little ones, we hop a plane to the Caribbean for snorkeling. As they struggle with the din of cranky kids at the dinner hour, I'm returning from a ride on my horse to come home to peace and quiet and a relaxing night with my husband.

Perhaps the most extreme example of a woman who decided against having children in favor of a consumer-oriented private life with her husband was Valerie Moira, a thirty-five-year-old engineer, whose husband was also an engineer. Valerie quit her engineering job three years ago "to become a full-time housewife," but not to become a mother. She always made sure that her bosses knew that she and her husband had a permanent form of birth control "because a lot of them looked at me and wondered, 'When is this little engineer going to get pregnant and toddle off home and we'll never see her again?'" She did, of course, "toddle off home," but became a full-time housewife, not a mother, and they never saw her again. However, she assumed that her employers would never suspect that she would abandon her career for the home if she had decided against motherhood. Valerie tells people she is childless "because I don't want to share my toys." Her comment gets a laugh, she says, "but there's a measure of truth to it. We have a three-bedroom house, and the two spare bedrooms are *mine* . . . the house is *mine*, and my time is mine." Unlike the parents of the baby boom, whose consumer desires were family oriented and included items and leisure pursuits that parents and children would enjoy together, the childfree described children as competing consumers, who would draw resources away from parental pleasures. As Candace Rosovic explained, "I do not know how I could stand it if a child began demanding of me $100 sneakers and $400 Nintendos."

Several of the childfree respondents embraced the term "selfish" without apology. Some even delighted in their "immaturity." In a society that worships youth, many took pride in their youthful looks and lifestyles and hoped to avoid "maturity." Frank Seller, a fifty-four-year-old twice-divorced professor of health and physical education, mused on maturity in a dictation while driving to work:

I think my not having children has had a significant effect on how I view myself, how I view my maturity. I see myself as, mentally . . . probably thirty-ish. I think self-image to a great degree is learned. . . . I think people when they have children allow themselves to assume a different role in the world than when they were single and had other kinds and levels of responsibility. So I think people teach themselves to act differently, i.e., older, as a parent. . . . I don't need to act like a parent 'cause I'm not one, and I won't be associated with the behaviors that go along with that role. . . . I've got so much working on myself and nurturing myself and taking responsibility for myself and getting on with my life, it's a full time job for me.

Youthful Bodies and the Child Within

Combining the language of the therapeutic culture with that of the youth culture, a surprising number of respondents said that they did not want children because, as Doreen Cassedy wrote, "Goodness, I've got my hands full nurturing the child with-in me!" Dawn Gilroy said of herself and her current husband, "We are both believers in 'an inner child' and feel, together and separately, that our time is better spent nurturing *those* 'kids' than bringing a new form into being." Sandra Este is thirty-four, but "I am still growing up, and I don't think anyone should parent a child until she can successfully parent her own 'child within.'" Only a small minority of the voluntarily childless shared these sentiments, but the extent to which nearly identical statements surfaced in these letters suggests a culture that not only condones but encourages a preoccupation with one's private life, inner self, and physical body.

The body itself was a major concern for a number of women who wrote. Women in earlier times feared that childbirth could leave them disabled or even cost them their lives. Late-twentieth-century women also worried about the physical dangers of pregnancy and birth, but they were more likely to mention pain and disfigurement than illness and death. Alicia Coseti wrote, "I want to keep my hour-glass figure instead of sacrificing it for someone who probably won't appreciate me anyway!!!" The birth process seemed primitive and barbaric to some childfree women. Katherine Migan has

been terrified all my life of the agony and pain of pregnancy. Even as a little girl I used to pray and beg God to never let me have a baby. . . . Also, the agony and torture of childbirth; being in extreme pain for 18 or more hours and screaming from the pain also made me never want to have a baby. . . . I could never endure a pregnancy.

Tammy Bolen wrote that she is

> very queasy about stuff about the body and hospitals and medical proce-
> dures. I don't like pain. . . . I don't want to be pregnant. I see pregnant
> women and think, "Ugh! Glad it's not me." I don't want to give birth—it
> freaks me out . . . the "miracle" of birth freaks me out. It's so—barbaric!
> Some little live creature emerging from an orifice of my body! Like Alien!
> And then breast-feeding! Like some cow! I know it's all supposed to be all
> beautiful and everything, but it grosses me out.

Sally Cort also worried about sacrificing her body:

> I guess the main reason I never wanted kids is the birth process. It
> absolutely disgusts me and seems *unbearably* painful. I don't see how any-
> one would want to go through that hell. The nine months of sickness and
> getting fat would be horrendous, not to mention after the birth—sleepless
> nights, being stuck at home with a screaming baby, having to give up
> things I enjoy.

Andrea Moray echoed, "Sometimes I blame vanity. . . . I'm slim and don't
ever want to look fat or have stretch marks, or (God forbid) C-section scars. I
absolutely cannot see myself experiencing the pain of labor, which I can list as
my #1 fear regarding pregnancy." This body consciousness was not the exclusive preserve of the childfree. Many of their peers were equally preoccupied
with the physicality of the birth process, rejecting the anesthetics and bottle
feeding that were popular in the early postwar years in favor of "natural childbirth" and breast-feeding. Their impulses were diametrically opposed, but
their preoccupation with the physicality of childbirth represented two diver-
gent but related aspects of the body consciousness of late-twentieth-century
Americans.

The Population Bomb

Another trend providing support for the voluntarily childless was the
emerging concern about overpopulation and the environment in the postwar
years. Initially, experts hailed the "population boom," saying that it would
create prosperity. But gradually, the optimism surrounding the population

boom shifted to fears of the "population bomb." A national poll showed that support for population control jumped from 17 percent in 1966 to 44 percent in 1972. Concern about the population explosion initially focused on the developing world and incorporated the language and ideology of the cold war. In 1965, Philip Appleman argued in *The Silent Explosion* that the Soviets and Chinese opposed population control in underdeveloped countries to promise impoverished nations that communism would solve their problems.[31]

In his 1968 book, *Population and People*, Edward Stockwell used the rhetoric of the threat of nuclear war:

> Regardless of whether or not the "population bomb" represents a greater threat to the peace and security of mankind than the hydrogen bomb (and more and more writers and scholars are beginning to regard this assertion as valid), the inescapable fact is that the rapid and accelerating rate of population growth in recent years has created an extremely dangerous situation in many parts of the world.

Although his book focused largely on the threat of communism in overcrowded and impoverished countries, Stockwell also expressed concern about the danger to the American lifestyle if the population continued to grow. Like earlier eugenics advocates, he was concerned that the "wrong" people would be on the increase: "Many groups in the society do not have access to [contraception]. . . . Year after year these people continue to have many more children than they want to have or are capable of supporting at a decent level of living."[32]

The most influential of these tracts was Paul Ehrlich's *The Population Bomb*, published in 1968. Ehrlich's message was a powerful environmental argument for limiting population at home as well as abroad: "We must have population control at home, hopefully through a system of incentives and penalties, but by compulsion if voluntary methods fail. . . . Population control is the only answer." As one of the most visible leaders of the environmental population-control movement, Ehrlich had a huge impact. He followed his original book with *The Population Explosion*, coauthored with Anne H. Ehrlich in 1990, explaining, "In 1968, *The Population Bomb* warned of impending disaster if the population explosion was not brought under control. Then the fuse was burning; now the population bomb has detonated." He pointed to environmental, economic, and health problems, such as traffic gridlock, homeless people, drug abuse and crime, AIDS, global warming, holes in the ozone layer, and acid rain.[33]

Ehrlich was among the founders of Zero Population Growth (ZPG), which had 3,000 members by 1969. The organization called upon Americans to have no more than two children and advocated the distribution of free birth control pills, legalized abortion, voluntary vasectomy, and tax exemptions for those who had no more than two children. So powerful was the movement for population control that it became an important political rallying cry. In a message to Congress in 1969, President Richard Nixon claimed that population growth presents "serious challenges for our society." ZPG also gave impetus to the childfree movement.

Perhaps the most extreme expression of the commitment to childlessness on environmental grounds was the policy of childlessness in the Synanon community from 1976 to 1989. Synanon, founded by Charles E. Dederich in 1958, was originally established as a rehabilitation program for alcoholics and drug addicts. By the 1960s, it began to attract young people who had no history of drugs or alcohol, but who were drawn to its idealism, communalism, and alternative lifestyle. Like most of the utopian communities of the nineteenth century, Synanon functioned as a commune and offered an alternative to the nuclear family and traditional child rearing. Initially, the group was committed to communal child rearing. But in 1976, Dederich established a policy of childlessness, citing overpopulation as the main reason. He required all members to undergo sterilization operations or leave the community. Women who were pregnant at the time were required to have abortions if they wished to stay in Synanon. Most members complied with the policy.[34]

Synanon represented an extreme position. But it also reflected the power of the environmental rationale for childlessness. Of the voluntarily childless people studied in the 1970s and 1980s, 32 percent of the women and 14 percent of the men included population growth as a reason for their decision, making it the fourth most frequently mentioned factor.[35] In this study, 41 percent of the men, but only 12 percent of the women who wrote, included population control as a factor. Those under age thirty-five were nearly twice as likely as were those over thirty-five to express environmental concerns. Mandy Crowell-Downey was just a teenager when she decided not to have children and claimed to be motivated almost entirely by population concerns. "My parents provided the perfect environment for love, trust, respect, and friendship. . . . So after discovering how intensely important family life is, my decision to have a tubal ligation did not seem to follow. It was not a popular one." Her husband agreed with her, but it took

> a long time for Mom and Dad to get over [it]. . . . My decision came from what I can only call research. . . . My parents had, after all, taught me to be responsible! The trends and statistics were depressing at best and fearful at their worst. Age 14 is perhaps a bit young to be reading stuff from the Guttmacher Institute, WHO [World Health Organization], and others, but if that seems a bit strange, consider the doctor's reaction to a 16-year-old who asks for a laparoscopy! Imagine his reaction when he finds out I don't even have a boyfriend yet! He refused to perform the surgery; I would wait almost a decade before another doctor would take me seriously.

Mandy was one of the few women who felt this strongly about the issue. Most respondents who mentioned population concerns did so at the end of their letters, after explaining their choice in more personal terms. A typical comment was that of twenty-seven-year-old Circi, who used only her first name. Circi wrote that there are "enough people in the world" and deplored "the tragic spawning of people who are cursed with poverty." But her main reasons for being childfree were personal. "I'll admit I'm selfish! I don't want to share my life with anyone other than the man I choose to live with. . . . You'd think that in this day and age people would understand, but they don't!" Vanity was also a consideration: "I'm constantly hearing about my biological clock, blah, blah, blah. . . . Geez, not to mention the irreversible changes my body would have to withstand. . . . It's just out of the question and not up for discussion." Like many other childfree people, she rejected organized religion, although she "believes in karma." Circi lives happily in Portland, Oregon, where she and her husband perform in rock bands, and she also makes costumes and jewelry. "Birth control earrings are my specialty and most popular design!"

Some of the environmentally conscious childfree wondered why they did not get some credit or appreciation for doing their part. Marian Costello noted that "there are, quite simply, far too many people in the world, and support for those who choose not to add to the planet's burden is sorely lacking." Janice Nester considered her childlessness "my gift to Planet Earth, and to all the other living beings, human and animal, who are finding it more and more difficult to compete for dwindling resources." Louise Hanson was childless because she "looked around and decided that there were a lot more interesting things to do with one's life than 'momhood'." Nevertheless, she, too, wanted some credit for not bringing more

> polluting, resource-wasting middle class Americans into the world. . . . I don't want the Medal of Honor for it. I just want 30 or so years of responsible birth control, continued throughout two marriages, and at times, through risks to my health, to be acknowledged as something other than fiendish selfishness.

The strongest statement in support of population control came from Les U. Knight, editor of *These Exit Times*, a publication of the Voluntary Human Extinction Movement. "May we live long and die out," is the motto on the masthead. The group advocated the extinction of the human race on the grounds of saving the environment. In the first issue of the newsletter, Les wrote a column "Man to Man," advocating vasectomy and exhorting men to "take our fair share of the responsibility for contraception." His argument was not about the environment, however. It was about the good life, good sex, and liberation from possible child-support payments: "A vasectomy could pay for itself the first time you use it." Best of all, "when fear of pregnancy is banished from your sex life, a whole exciting world of enjoyment will move in to take its place. I can't tell you what it's done for mine. But don't take my word for it, find out for yourself just how appreciative your partner can be." He ended not with an environmental pitch, but rather, "I gotta go now, something just came up."[36]

Children: Pro or Con?

Knight's message was not antichild: "One of the main reasons I've chosen not to breed is because I like children. Until we can take good care of the ones we have, we shouldn't make any more." But other respondents were more hostile to children. Following environmental and population concerns, next on the list of reasons given for voluntary childlessness was a dislike of children. Earlier studies reported that 43 percent of the men but only 26 percent of the women said that they did not like children.[37] Relatively few of the childfree respondents for this study actively disliked children, but those who did were vehement. Like Camille Goshen, who called herself a "die-hard child hater," these militantly childfree women and men considered children to be an unpleasant intrusion into their personal space and had no tolerance for their presence. Circi wrote, "I do not like children and do not find them amusing." Janice Nester found infants "ugly, noisy, and altogether too much work and responsibility . . . but I absolutely cannot resist a puppy." Murray Parson "just never liked kids. Even when I was a young child, the cries of babies would make me nuts. I still can't stand that noise. I do not like dealing with children at all." Sherry Alasi had no use for "ten pounds of screaming, demanding and diaper-messing baby . . . I do not like babies." Lorena Cash "confessed" that she is not fond of children. "I say 'confess' since one is led to believe that such a sentiment is unnatural and quite abnormal." But she could not tolerate the "whining or fighting or begging or making noise. I hate noise. They screech and cry and scream, and are oblivious to the damage they do to the property or peace of mind of others."

But far more common were the sentiments of childfree adults who truly enjoyed children. Like those who disliked children, they wanted to avoid the responsibility of raising them. But unlike the "child haters," they associated children with intimacy and play. "I love kids!" said Stephanie Borquist. "They're cute, smart, affectionate, and fascinating. Their unconditional love melts my heart. I enjoy playing with them, teaching them, and learning from them. I also relish handing them back to their parents at the end of the day. Being childfree, I get all the pleasure, none of the problems!" Jack Grade and his wife were both in the theater business and had a "great marriage," but they did not want children. "The idea of continual child energy (other than my own inner child) sounds like being trapped, buried alive." But he was fond of children. "My mind cries, 'Oh God, they're beautiful. Am I—are we missing the most meaningful event in life?'" Nevertheless, he made his choice. "Contrary to the American Dream, you can't have it all."

Many of the childfree were teachers or other professionals who worked with children. Sally Cort said, "It's not that I don't like kids—I teach junior high school and love it. But at 3:10 every day I send them home to their own mamas and I'm free to do as I please." Carolyn Macey takes "great joy in my work as a therapist—especially when my influence can make some child's life better." But like most of the childfree, she likes to "come home to peace and quiet and a relaxing night with my husband." Others were doting aunts and uncles or regularly "borrowed" the children of friends. "When we need a kid fix," said Maureen Arnold, "all we have to do is contact neighbors, friends, or relatives and babysit for a few hours." For Linda Barnett, "If a maternal instinct 'hits,'" she invites a friend's child over for the night. "After twenty-four hours I've had my instinct satisfied." Emma Stein McCoy resented the fact that "many people label me antichild. . . . Yeah, I hate kids, that's why I teach school." Lucy Warner, another teacher, wrote proudly, "I now have forty children and no stretch marks."

Some nonparents took seriously their role as nurturers of children in the wider world, as did many of the childless in earlier eras. They had a strong sense of responsibility for the children in their lives, and they represent the continuation of a long tradition of childless adults serving the needs of the community's children. Elizabeth Armstrong defended childless adults like herself in a 1993 article in the *San Francisco Chronicle*:

> Adults who do not have children can be as loving and as nurturing as parents. . . . We may not fit the traditional definition of family . . . but we aunts, uncles, teachers, counselors, neighbors, coaches, friends, big brothers and sisters are special kinds of family members to America's children.[38]

These voluntarily childless adults took seriously their responsibilities to children, while avoiding the burdens of parenthood. The childfree advocates who claimed that children were a great source of misery were right. Nearly all studies of psychological well-being concluded that couples with children were more depressed and agitated and less happy and satisfied than were those without children. This was as true in the baby-boom years as later. A 1965 study found that among 2,480 households in California, "parenthood detracts from both the physical and psychological health of husbands and wives, especially in younger couples," and concluded that "parenthood has a detrimental effect on both health and marital satisfaction" and that parents were "not as healthy or happy as the childless couples."[39]

Several respondents learned this lesson in their own childhood homes. It is interesting to note that among the younger letter writers, those under age thirty-five, the majority who wrote were infertile. Of the older respondents, those over age fifty-five who were of childbearing age during the baby-boom years when it was virtually unthinkable to be childless by choice, the majority were infertile or single. The vast majority of those in the middle, the group we would identify as "baby boomers," were childless by choice. They were the ones who grew up in the era of the idealized nuclear family. Several of these childfree baby boomers recognized the strains their parents suffered in their efforts to live according to the postwar ideology of domesticity. Marian Costello recalled that her father told all his daughters repeatedly that "children are a burden. He was unhappy in the city and felt trapped by his job and family. I know now that he does and always did love me deeply; nevertheless all of us absorbed that message—kids tie you down and mess up your life."

Maureen Arnold also remembered her childhood as a painful and difficult time. As the oldest of three sisters born to poor immigrant parents, she lived in a three-story walk-up on Chicago's South Side in a tiny apartment with no bath or shower. Her mother was ill, and she had much of the burden of caring for her siblings while her father struggled as a store clerk. With no car and no family vacations, her childhood in the 1950s was a far cry from the *Leave It to Beaver* ideal. She thought of having children "for about twenty minutes one day" as a teenager, but "that was the extent of my maternal yearnings. I had enough to do with elderly parents and 2 younger sisters that I felt were my responsibility to feed, clothe and shelter." Today she and her husband are happily married and "childfree" by choice. She is a housewife, and he works in computers. Their comfortable lifestyle is a marked contrast to her childhood. "We enjoy each other, the spontaneity of freedom from children, the good life of freedom from financial problems and Bob likes getting my attention all for himself."

Sally Cort had a similar story. She, too, watched her mother live out the prescribed housewife role, denying her own aspirations and resenting her children.

> One of the main reasons I don't want children is because of my own mother. . . . I think she always resented my sister and I (although she never said it to us) because she was a housewife for so many years and she would have rather been working. She always wanted to go back to college, too, but by the time my sister and I got out of high school she felt she was too old to go back. She told me once that she never wanted to have children. I never found out if she changed her mind or if we were "accidents."

Yet when Sally had a tubal ligation at age twenty-seven, instead of supporting her decision, "My parents absolutely had a fit when I told them. They just could not understand why I am so dead set against having children. In fact, very few people understand."

A Dark View of the World

One reason for many of the childfree respondents' preoccupation with their private lives was their sense that the larger world is a lost cause. Much of the optimism that fueled the baby boom had evaporated by the 1990s. A significant minority of the childfree who came of age since the 1960s believed that the world is a terrible place and that the best one can do is to look for meaning and fulfillment in personal experience. These women and men expressed such a deep sense of despair about the world that they did not want to bring children into it. Lynn Tosser is childless because "I would want my child to have clean air to breathe, clear water to drink, safe streets to walk on. The peer pressure kids had in my day is nothing compared to the present day." Camille Boise, born in 1943, is disturbed about "the world situation—which for people of my age was frightening and destructive. The cold war was flaming hot and the promise of a planet to live on was shabby." Lorraine Carlisle worried about "the seductions of drugs, liquor, sex and sexually-transmitted diseases for a child to deal with [and an] environmentally-compromised world full of disease, crowding and violence." Stephanie Borquist did not want to take the risk.

> It's such a gamble anyway. The kid could be defective or stupid. The kid could break your heart in so many ways by rejecting you to being hurt or killed. Very risky business. And expensive! What about the moral responsibility? . . . What if your kid turns out to be a racist or a robber, drug addict, killer? You *created* the monster. What about your child's consumption of scarce resources? . . . Bad news.

Eric Handle was deeply pessimistic about the future:

> It's obvious to me that the family along with almost every other facet of human endeavor is crumbling before us. . . . We've wasted vast amounts of our precious resources and now have put ourselves, literally, on the brink of extinction. . . . Life is going to get tougher and more people are going to suffer in the next ten to fifteen years than in all the years since the last biblical flood.

Nell Hyde is childless by choice because of

> the hideous state of the world. This is not a positive time to be alive. I have a constant feeling of foreboding and guilt and responsibility for the

events taking place globally, yet feel constant helplessness and powerless-
ness in the face of those atrocities. Sometimes I feel that we're hurtling
towards self-destruction, and no one wants to acknowledge that. It's an
uncomfortable world. To watch my child struggling in it would break my
heart.

Lee Bowman did not want to bring a child "into a world that's likely to go
splat within his or her lifetime."

Anita Freedman found it difficult "to listen to platitudes about 'mothers' (in a society that does not pay mothers living wages or high salaries,
does not offer much pre-natal care or parental leave, considers war to be
'fun' and sex 'dirty,' and still considers the female responsible for any
problems caused by a 'child')." Anita was among the most pessimistic of
the childfree. Her dark view of the world was grounded in her experience
as a child of Holocaust survivors. Her parents met in Auschwitz and survived, although most of their families were killed by the Nazis. "I grew up
knowing that the 'unthinkable' is real, and freedom should not be taken
for granted." In spite of her acute sense of society's hypocrisy, even Anita
was susceptible to the power of the domestic ideology of the 1950s: "By
the time I was in my early teens, I knew that the public images of 'home
life' were lies (though I still believed in some of the lies—I remember getting upset at my mother because she worked outside the home, instead of
staying home like the TV mom did)."

Such widespread pessimism reflects a profound change from the optimism of the early postwar years. Many of the children of the postwar era
grew up to reject the ideology of domesticity that shaped their parents'
lives. They also witnessed the collapse of postwar prosperity and a host of
new social ills. Nevertheless, the postwar parents and their childfree children shared one common goal: happiness in private life. The ideal of
togetherness against a hostile world prompted many of the parents of the
baby boomers to marry and have children. The ideal of togetherness
against a hostile world prompted many of their children to marry, but to
avoid having children. Although the childfree gave many different reasons
for their choice, most expressed a common theme: They wanted to find
happy, fulfilling lives in a private world of love, intimacy, and enjoyable
pursuits. Although the route to that desired life differed among them,
remaining childless was central to the effort. It is surprising that the values
they expressed were remarkably similar not only to one another, but to
those of the infertile women and men who desperately wanted children. At

first glance, the outspoken childfree seemed to express dramatically different values than did the desperately infertile who sacrificed so much in their pursuit of parenthood. But a careful examination of their letters revealed something much more intriguing. Ultimately, they wanted the same things: intimacy, happiness, and fulfillment in private life. For the childfree, those goals could best be achieved by *not* having children. For the infertile, the way to achieve those goals was to have children.

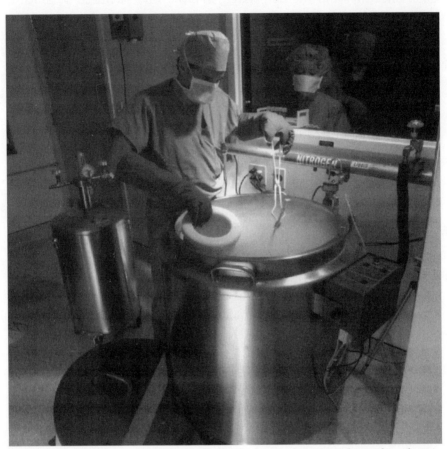

In today's world of new reproductive technologies, conception often takes place in the laboratory instead of the bedroom. *(Copyright © 1990 by Lou Manna. Used by permission)*

CHAPTER 7

Designer Genes: The Baby Quest and the Reproductive Fix
★☆

I asked God for a miracle. . . . Well, I did get my miracle. . . . He's the exotic vaca-tion I'll never take. The new house I'll never build. The jewels I'll never wear. . . . But for him I'd do it all again—gladly.

—Maureen Wendell, mother of a son conceived by the
costly GIFT procedure, 1993

There is a tremendous amount of medical help available and I have felt guilty not doing everything in my power to achieve pregnancy even though I have a nice life without children, even though it can cost years of time, even though treatment can run into the tens of thousands of dollars, and even though statistically an infertile couple has only a fifty percent chance of conceiving. . . . Still, there is tremendous social pressure to pursue this objective simply because we can. . . . The message to me was that of course a baby is priceless and therefore worth anything it takes to get one. . . . In the seventies when I was "coming of age," it was smart for a woman to seek the best way to bring out her best self. . . . Now, the same fervor that went into that fight is going into the importance of having children. This is the age of "family values." This is the thing to do now, the most important thing, the only important thing. . . . This is definitely the age of power motherhood.

—Margaret Lewis, infertile, 1993

Extra Money for Top Students . . . Must have placed at or above the 98th percentile on IQ test or college entrance exam. We will pay extra for extremely high IQ, out-standing achievements or evidence of creativity or giftedness.

—Advertisement for sperm donors, *Minnesota Daily,*
University of Minnesota, January 30, 1989

In-Vitro Fertilization Program seeking healthy young Scandinavian women ages 18–30, to donate eggs to Scandinavian couple who cannot otherwise achieve pregnancy. DONORS TO BE COMPENSATED for time and effort.
—Advertisement for egg donors, *Minneapolis Star Tribune,* May 24, 1994

Patricia Painter played by the rules. She worked hard, saved money, put herself through school, became a teacher, got married, and looked forward to living the American dream, which for her included children. When the expected reward eluded her, she felt betrayed. She had planned everything perfectly and never imagined that her body would malfunction. She and her electrician husband lived comfortably in a Los Angeles suburb and used birth control to prevent conception for the first five years of their marriage. When they decided to go off birth control, she got pregnant right away. To her astonishment, she miscarried.

> I absolutely could not believe that I miscarried. . . . It was really a horrible experience and just devastating. . . . I had always been the kind of person that got anything I wanted. I wanted to own a house so I worked two jobs and I went to school full time, and was able to save up enough money to buy a house. I wanted a career and a degree, and . . . I ended up with three teaching credentials and a master's degree. I wanted a husband and got a husband. . . . And there just seemed nothing that I couldn't do. I was living the American dream. And then, what a surprise, you know. Miscarriages do not happen to people like me. . . . I could not believe that this had happened.

When she miscarried a second time, "we got kind of crazy at that point."

According to the American ethos, if you work hard, earn a decent living, delay gratification, plan, and live by the rules, your life should be in your control. In the twentieth century, the work ethic has fed into the consumer ethic: Even if the job has few inherent satisfactions, doing the job should bring its reward in a home, leisure, consumer goods, and a fulfilling private life. Reproduction is linked to both the consumer and producer ethic. Children are both a reward for hard work *and* one of the few products that can still be created by the labor of one's own body. For most Americans, children are central to their vision of the good life; most polls show that children are still highly desired. In spite of the increasing visibility of the childfree, over 90 percent of American women who were surveyed in the 1980s considered childlessness to be undesirable for them and others.[1] By the late 1980s, the rate of childlessness had leveled off, the birthrate inched up, and a renewed interest in babies permeated the popular culture.

The New Pronatalism

On the heels of the childfree movement of the 1970s came what several observers identified as the new pronatalism of the 1980s. According to feminist author Susan Faludi, the renewed push toward parenthood took the form of a media blitz aimed at educated career women, warning them that if they delayed childbearing, they were likely to find themselves infertile. Few of the alarmists who pointed to a new "infertility epidemic" took note of studies showing a troubling trend in male fertility: the decline in the average sperm count by more than half in the past thirty years. Nor did they mention the fact that less-educated poor women were more likely than professional women to be infertile, as a result of pelvic inflammatory disease caused frequently by sexually transmitted diseases. Rather, many articles claimed that the alleged increase in infertility resulted from women postponing motherhood until they were in their thirties, when it might be too late to conceive.[2]

In 1987, NBC correspondent Maria Shriver called childlessness "the curse of the career woman." In the same year, *Life* published a special report entitled "Baby Craving." Headlines warned against "Having It All: Postponing Parenthood Exacts a Price" and bemoaned "The Quiet Pain of Infertility: For the Success-Oriented, It's a Bitter Pill." A columnist for the *New York Times* described the infertile woman as "a walking cliché" of the feminist generation, "a woman on the cusp of forty who put work ahead of motherhood." *Newsweek* noted the "trend of childlessness," and *Mademoiselle* warned, "Caution: You Are Now Entering the Age of Infertility."[3]

This media blitz of the 1980s was not lost on the childless. Margaret Lewis noticed a marked change in movie themes during the decade:

> The movies used to end when the couple fell in love. Now they end when the couple achieves parenthood. Anyone who doesn't have kids is portrayed

as selfish, cold, deprived, or pitiful. It seems as if all of Hollywood is having babies. I mean, Warren Beatty expounding on the virtues of fatherhood?! Really.

She observed that not only happy endings but also advertisements suddenly began to link children to consumerism and the good life: "The newspaper is filled with cute little 'Gap Kids' with little denim jackets."

Reminiscent of the early baby-boom days, babies, children, and parenthood began to permeate the nation's popular culture. Plots of movies and television shows and even popular songs revolved around the baby quest. Bonnie Raitt sang, "A friend of mine, she cries at night and she calls me on the phone/ Sees babies everywhere she goes and she wants one of her own."[4] Films like *Parenthood, Three Men and a Baby, Look Who's Talking, Mrs. Doubtfire, Made in America, Immediate Family,* and countless others focused either on babies and their charms or adults' preoccupations with having children and child rearing. The trend culminated in 1994 when Arnold Schwartzenegger, in *Junior,* gave birth to a baby himself! Unlike the earlier formulas, however, the traditional links between marriage, sex, and procreation no longer prevailed in these films. Single men raising babies, divorced fathers scheming to be with their children, single women having children, couples struggling with infertility, and even artificial insemination by donor became plot devices for comedies. The television character *Murphy Brown* sparked a national political debate when she became an unwed mother. Most striking about this new infatuation with having and raising children was that the marital imperative faded into the background. Whereas the romantic dyad for the childfree was the married couple, the romantic dyad featured in the new pronatalism was the parent and the child.

The new pronatalism took other forms as well. Almost as quickly as the population-control movement gained momentum, critics began to attack it. As early as 1977, James A. Weber complained about the "barrage of population control propaganda." Noting that the birthrate had already dropped below replacement level, he argued, "If the ZPGers [members of Zero Population Growth] were right, we should now be on the threshold of a new era of unprecedented plenty. In fact, the opposite is the case." Pointing to recession, pollution, and social problems, he blamed "a suicidal population theory" for the fact that "our posture in the world sinks lower." Sounding a theme reminiscent of Manifest Destiny, he hoped to "rekindle the instinctive appreciation and approval of population growth that has infused the country since its founding by showing how population growth is vital to the coming health and well-being of the American people."[5]

Ten years later, in 1987, Ben Wattenberg published his controversial pronatalist tract, *The Birth Dearth*. Sounding a eugenic theme, he warned, "I believe the demographic and immigration patterns inherent in the Birth Dearth will yield an ever smaller proportion of Americans of white European 'stock' . . . and this will likely cause more ethnic and racial tension and turmoil than would otherwise occur." He continued, "It will make it difficult to promote and defend liberty in the Western nations and in the rest of a modernizing world." Wattenberg's warning sounded a cold-war theme: that the communist nations were propagating at a higher rate and the "free world" would soon be reduced to a tiny minority of the world's peoples. At the same time he harked back to earlier national concerns: "'Manifest Destiny' was not the cry of a no-growth continent of old people." Wattenberg called attention both to the declining birthrate, which had dipped to fewer than two children per woman by the mid-1970s, and to the increase in childlessness. "I believe that most people—men and women—who freely decide not to have children will probably live to regret it." Critics claimed that Wattenberg raised "the 'yellow peril' argument all over again," and expressed deep-seated "collective fears of being swamped by external and internal enemies." Nevertheless, *The Birth Dearth* joined a chorus of voices calling for more American babies.[6]

As the politics of reproduction sparked public debate, articles in the popular press began to trumpet "The Coming Baby Boom." Demographers predicted a new epidemic of "fertility fever." As early as the 1970s, when the birthrate dipped to its lowest level ever, commentators began to predict that "pregnancy will once again become chic." For some, babies were already chic. As one young college-educated mother explained, "I married a man I thought was rather boring at first, but decided that having a family really sounded fascinating. I expected my friends to scoff but actually they think I've done something original, even quaint." Having a baby marked her as "the class bohemian."[7]

For this young woman, marriage was a means to an end. She married her "rather boring" husband to have a child, reversing the earlier romantic notion that the baby was the expression of the love of the couple. Doreen Welsh also considered marriage as a means to an end, the end being motherhood. Describing herself as divorced, "of Jewish descent . . . a professional classical symphonic musician," Doreen was looking for a man to achieve her goal.

> It is very difficult to find men interested in dating a 40 year old woman who wants to start a family. It puts me in a desperate condition. It is hard to be natural in meeting men, because I am on some kind of crash course deadline in creating a relationship and getting pregnant. . . . I still have a strong desire to have my own, natural child. I do not feel good about the thought of artificial insemination. I must be a traditionalist in wanting to have a partner to raise the child, and to share in my life. In addition, esoterically speaking, I want to choose the father of my child. . . . A desperation has overtaken my rational mind. I get strong urges to get pregnant during the middle of the month.

A few short decades ago, the desire for a partner and the ability to choose the father of one's child would not have seemed "traditionalist," "esoteric," or "irrational"; it would have simply been expected. But not any more.

In recent years, marriage has become a desirable but not necessarily a required precondition for motherhood. In the Black community, more children are born to single than to married women. In the White community, an increasing number of women are pursuing single parenthood through adoption, artificial insemination, and bearing children out of wedlock. The past decade also witnessed "a virtual baby boom in the lesbian and gay community," according to one observer. One study estimated that by 1988, between 1,000 and 3,000 children in the United States and Europe were born to lesbians using donor insemination.[8] Institutions responded to these trends. Adoption agencies began to allow single individuals to adopt, as they had in the early part of the century. And many infertility clinics and sperm banks began to inseminate single heterosexual women as well as lesbians. By the 1980s, single men and women, both gay and straight, found ways to become parents that previously had not been available.

The new pronatalism brought together advocates from the Left and the Right. Wattenberg's conservative warning about the "birth dearth" included a call for measures to enable more women to have children, such as on-site day care centers, parental leaves, and flexible work schedules—ideas that feminists had promoted for many years. And although the calls for "family values" emanated largely from the Right and condemned all nontraditional forms of sex and procreation, the lesbian and gay community, as well as single parents, drew upon similar rhetoric in their claims for legitimacy as parents and as families.

The movement for reproductive choice, although focused largely on the issue of abortion rights, also fed the new pronatalism and drew attention to the plight of the infertile. Resolve, a national organization serving infertile women and men, offered both support and advocacy for childless adults hoping to become parents. Feminists argued that women should not be forced to choose between parenthood and careers, claiming that women, like men, should have the opportunity to do both. On the opposite end of the political spectrum, the antichoice activists also heightened the public rhetoric around reproduction and sentimentalized babies anew. It is no wonder that infertile women like Margaret Lewis, surrounded by images of "power motherhood," felt that every political and cultural message, from the Left as well as the Right, urged her not to accept her childlessness but to fight against it tooth and nail.

Infertility and Reproductive Control

In this context, the old problem of infertility became a new kind of frustration. Many observers assume that infertility is on the rise. But there is no evidence that the proportion of infertile Americans has increased. There is evidence, however, that the number of people who are seeking treatment has risen dramatically. The number of visits to physicians for infertility treatment rose from 600,000 in 1968 to 1.6 million in 1984. The increase has been due, in part, to the huge baby-boom generation; the infertile among them are a large and visible group. But there are other reasons as well. Even if the chances for successful treatment are not much better than they were a half century ago, dramatic new technological interventions are now available. High-tech approaches, such as in-vitro fertilization (IVF, fertilization of the egg in a laboratory petri dish and then its insertion directly into the uterus), first successfully used in the birth of Louise Brown in England in 1978, appear to offer "miracle babies" to the childless. Treatments using assisted reproduction techniques jumped 30 percent from 1990 to 1991, even though the chance of ending up with a "take-home baby" from these procedures was only about 15 percent.[9]

The promise of a technological fix, combined with a faith in medical progress, led many Americans to believe that they could triumph over most physical limitations. Physicians have responded to the demand. Studies have shown that American physicians are more likely than British practitioners to resort to heroic measures for treating infertility, probably because their patients request such intervention.[10] But reproductive medicine, despite its many advances over the past century, remains an imperfect art, available only to those who can afford it. Nor does it guarantee success. Infertility treatment is a high-stakes gamble: It is possible to lose all the money, time, and effort invested and gain nothing in return. If all the efforts of modern science, human struggle, and economic sacrifice do not result in the desired child, the rage, desperation, and anguish can be overwhelming.

Because birth control and reproductive choice are widely taken for granted, the infertile experience extreme frustration. Reproductive choice is much easier to achieve if the goal is to avoid pregnancy. Contraceptive technologies offer a success rate of nearly 100 percent, and legal abortion provides a backup when birth control methods fail. But infertile couples who seek treatment have only a 50 percent chance for success in the 1990s, odds that have not dramatically improved since the 1950s.[11] The inability to "control" one's reproductive fate is among the most exasperating experiences of infertility, especially for those who have put so much effort into the struggle. As the reporter Susan Sward wrote of her struggle with infertility, "As an organized, energetic person, I was used to getting what I wanted in life most of the time. To a major extent, I was also used to feeling in control of my life and knowing what I did would produce results if I tried hard enough. When it came to making babies, I found I had a lot to learn."[12]

Those who become pregnant while using birth control tend to blame the technology. But infertility patients who do not conceive often blame themselves. They feel unable to control their bodies or their destinies, even with medical intervention. For Roberta O'Leary, "It gets more and more difficult to pick up the pieces after each failure. I also don't like the feeling of having no control over what happens." Amanda Talley "felt like a freak of nature . . . embarrassed and shameful. . . . I felt as though my body betrayed me." Dierdre Kearney explained, "My feelings of helplessness have been hard to handle. We humans like to have control over our own lives and the one thing we think we can control is our body." She has done everything to have a baby and

> still my body betrays me and deprives me of one of the things I want most in life. I cannot make my body do what I want. . . . I've heard some women say that being infertile makes them feel less like a woman. I've never really felt this. I guess, this has made me feel all too much like a woman because it's what makes me a woman that has caused my problem—PERIODS and

HORMONES! I just feel helpless in determining my own future. Sometimes I feel like a ship at sea and just when I am close to land, a huge wave washes me out to sea again.

The inability to control one's reproductive functions often leads to feelings of shame and worthlessness, especially for women. Maureen Wendell explained, "I began to feel defective, ashamed. I can't do a 'normal' biological function that most anyone else could do. I had to re-evaluate my life, my hopes, my dreams and my identity as a woman. I am blessed to have a very supportive husband but even with that I felt inadequate as a wife." Feelings of inadequacy were magnified by the association of fertility with sexuality. In a taped message, Patricia Painter used the language of sexual potency when describing her husband's healthy sperm. "My husband has this, you know, magnificent, I guess he's extremely virile. He has like super sperm. . . . Everybody from the lab technicians to the receptionist at the doctor's office was always so amazed at the amount and the virility of this sperm. It's like super-human sperm." When they accidentally spilled some of the semen sample, a physician replied:

> "It doesn't matter. He could impregnate the whole block with what's left in here. It's amazing." Which made me feel absolutely horrible because he couldn't impregnate me. Well, it was real obvious who had the problem in this relationship, as far as who was the one responsible for us not getting pregnant, and that was me. So I felt extremely terrible about that. This resulted in my being very embarrassed around people. I felt very defective. . . . It was just really such a blow. . . . I would get physically ill . . . 'cause I felt so defective and so embarrassed.

Laura Lerner also felt "abnormal," even though she was not infertile. But she was single, and her singleness deprived her of the opportunity to become a mother. "I am a woman. I am supposed to have children, right? What am I if I don't produce children?" She considered adopting as a single parent or trying donor insemination. But she could not bring herself to do it: "Withdrawing some sperm from the sperm bank sounds so cold and mechanical." Without children, she felt "unnatural. . . . I have had these damn menstrual cycles since age 11 and I have nothing to show for it. . . . I get so I hate the cycle when it comes. . . . I have the most trouble trying to determine why I am here. I feel very incomplete, and very abnormal."

Before she discovered she was infertile, Leila Ember felt that "Life was good! Most importantly I was in control of it!" When she did not get pregnant, however, she began treatment, even though she recoiled at the invasive procedures: "For a person who had never had so much as a band-aid applied to any part of their body I found it quite difficult to endure the poking and prodding and exploratory procedures which were both financially and emotionally expensive." But her body remained uncooperative. Infertility destroyed her peace of mind and self-confidence: "I remember sitting on the floor of my bathroom for what seemed like hours and sobbing, I'd look at my husband and begin to scream how sorry I was that I 'messed up again!'" Blaming herself, she wrote, "My biological clock isn't ticking; it isn't working at all!"

Many childless women who wanted children questioned their own womanhood. Suzanna Drew felt "less of a woman—somehow not complete." Kate Foley felt "barren." Paula Kranz described feelings of "failure . . . it's like an empty space within yourself that you can not fill." Marie Gutierrez blamed herself when her husband's semen analysis

> came back ok, then O Boy! All fingers pointed to me, *wow* was I ever so unhappy, people don't know what it is like to try and try and never succeed. . . . I told no one . . . we were both embarrassed, marked, hurt. My husband is a very supportive husband, a good man and tells me that he accepts whatever happens, but . . . I can't accept the fact that I feel like some sort of alien, all women who are "normal" have children.

Along with at least four other women and men who wrote, Marie offered to release her spouse from the marriage so that he could find a fertile partner and have children.

Not every infertile woman felt these feelings of inadequacy, but the sentiment was widely shared. Talia Herman was shocked that in her infertility group of ten women, all but she said they felt less complete as women.

> I have come to understand how far women *haven't* come in their acceptance of themselves. We still define our worth by the size, beauty, health of our families. . . . Women of past generations have had to break down societal stigmas. Our grandmothers perhaps went to work. Our mothers may have brought home more money than our fathers. How can women of my generation feel less complete because of societal pressures . . . ? Do men feel less complete? Do we love any differently?

Sheila Turner-Cohn noticed that physicians can contribute to the way women understand their infertility even by the language they use:

> It's interesting to me that my new gynecologist refers to my uterus and child-bearing inability as something separate from myself. When he examined me, he made the statement 'I don't know if *this uterus* could carry a baby.' I thought that was so strange, for him to put it that way. But when I thought about it, I decided that it was very enlightened of him to make it clear that it was my organs and not me as a person who lack this "ability." That's a key distinction, I think, because of how an infertile woman tends to globally perceive herself as a failure because she lacks this basic biological ability.

Her previous gynecologist infuriated her when he referred to "'some hapless soul who can't produce eggs of her own.' All I could do was repeat, 'Some hapless soul!' in disbelief. I really don't think he had a clue about why I was offended."

Although the women expressed more emotional pain over infertility, the men who wrote experienced similar feelings of inadequacy and loss of "manhood."[13] Dave Crenshaw felt like a failure, "alienated from the rest of society, as I knew I never could be one of them." Nothing could ever "replace the one thing I really wanted to be, a father to my own child." He questioned "what my function as a man was. . . . I felt I was no longer of any use to anyone for any reason . . . of no value to society as a whole, because we, childless people don't contribute to society what society holds so dear . . . children." Although his sterility resulted from a case of childhood mumps, he could not avoid blaming himself. He felt "bitterness. . . . I cannot get over the feelings that somehow I failed, and life passed me by. . . . I still have the guilty feelings of being inadequate."

Among the men who wrote, few actually discussed the question of masculinity, but those who did acknowledged that it was an issue. Joanne and Tom Paisley sent a tape in which Joanne described their response to the news about his negative semen analysis. It "did affect his image of manhood. . . . It was very difficult for Tom to accept that." Tom said simply, "We try to look at the bright side of things" and praised his wife for being so supportive. Lester Bernstein, on the other hand, acknowledged the blow to his masculinity with a sense of humor. When he was diagnosed as infertile, "that one term transformed this budding stud into a wimp." And when he learned that the quality of his semen was "borderline, I was shattered. My voice went up two octaves."

Parenthood and Identity

The comments of these infertile women and men indicate that for many, infertility meant more than an inability to produce children; it was also a blow to their sense of manhood or womanhood. In a society that often equates adulthood with parenthood, infertility affects personal identity as well as reproductive behavior. Childlessness involves at least two fundamental realities that are at odds with the adult norm: not having children and not being a parent. The two conditions are connected, but they are not the same.[14] Bearing and raising children pertain to behavior and private life; the status of being a parent has more to do with identity and public life. Although the voluntarily and involuntarily childless have different ideas about how to achieve happiness in private life, they share similar experiences as nonparents in the wider world. According to a 1979 study, most Americans ranked becoming a parent as the most significant marker of adulthood, more than marriage or getting a job.[15] Whether or not childlessness is chosen, it means the lack of a certain privileged adult status.

For some of the infertile, childlessness was more painful in public than in private. Margaret Lewis said, "So, how is a life without children? Honestly, not at all bad and actually pretty nice." But "it can be lonely," she admitted, not at home but in the social world where she and her husband felt "out of the 'mainstream' of the life of our peers. . . . This kind of exclusion has broken my innocence and my sense of trust in belonging in the world. I never felt like an outsider in any group and was always able to feel accepted on some level until now."

Many complained that the parents in their midst talked incessantly about their children. Margaret remarked, "At a cocktail party, the women will engage in baby talk the entire time, excluding the one (me) who has no children. Make no mistake: I like children and I like to hear about them. This is life, and children are a wonderful part of it. But I don't want to hear about that and only that for three hours." Stella Sims and her husband wondered

> if people lose their brains when they have children. It's as if these parents are incapable of discussing anything outside of their children. People who were formerly bright, charming and intelligent are now rendered conversationally incompetent when it comes to sports, politics or religion.

For many respondents, feeling "left out" was the worst part of being infertile. Sharon Stoner and her husband felt a profound sense of "isolation. . . . I just wish our society would not look upon us as incomplete people because we did not have children." Lydia Sommer wrote, "I think I am becoming more isolated each year—I have no connection with all these child-bearing women. I almost have no connection with myself anymore—I can't find a purpose in life. . . . It really gets depressing sometimes!" Tamara Afton found family get-togethers and holidays to be the most difficult. "Holidays only make me feel worse and more like a misfit." The Aftons now spend holidays with friends they met through Resolve, a national organization for infertile women and men. "We joke about a 'Misfit's Christmas' party."

This lack of connection, not "fitting in" as many described it, has little to do with children. It has much to do with adult identity and one's place in the world.[16] American society places a premium on parenthood. "What am I if not a parent?" wondered Corinne Gary. Tammy Bolen wrote that people treat her as if "I'm not grown up. Not mature, that's what people do. Grow up get married, have kids. Not me. I must not be grown up. What's wrong with me?" Not only full adulthood, but a measure of respectability is attached to parenthood. Daniel Steiner noticed a change in status when he and his wife had their first child after thirteen years of marriage. Their childlessness had marked them as "radical"—now they are "safely in the bosom of middle America!" He explained:

> Both of us are active in various social causes such as AIDS, homelessness, health care access, gay and lesbian issues, etc. . . . I sensed that people just sort of wrote us off as activist nuts. Now by deciding to have a child, people are all of a sudden very friendly towards us. "Ah-ha," I can hear them think, "Now you've decided to become a 'real' couple." What bullshit!!

Baby Craving

While some of the infertile explained their pain in terms of personal identity and adult status, others were simply desperate for a child. Many described their anguish not as a mere disappointment, but as a loss akin to the death of a loved one. Maureen Wendell described it as a deep sadness that continued even after she gave birth to a child:

The yearning inside to have a child is one I guess I'll never fully understand. Struggling with childlessness is a death that you never fully mourn,
a dream that never dies, a hope that never fades. . . . Infertility has
changed me. . . . There is not a part of my life or those who love me that
have not been affected by this.

Dave Crenshaw explained "how sterile people go on hurting, all their lives
. . . nothing ever takes away the feelings of loss . . . the hurt, and mind-
numbing pain."

One reason why infertility is so wrenching is that treatment holds out
the possibility of a "miracle cure," making it difficult to give up, grieve,
and find acceptance. To pursue medical intervention means to hold out
hope and experience disappointment month after month, while the possibility of pregnancy still exists.[17] Many infertility patients described the
experience as an "emotional roller coaster." Marie Gutierrez explained,
"After each surgery and taking the fertility drug Clomid still trying and
holding onto every good word from the Doctor that it could possibly happen this time, what a real drop in my Soul and a real let-down for my husband's ego, every test, every pill still no hope."

Amelia Monterey described the cycles of hope and disappointment. A
thirty-three-year-old medical secretary married fifteen years to a construction worker, she lives in a trailer house in rural Minnesota. Like many others,
she and her husband planned, dreamed, worked hard, saved, and assumed
that they would achieve their goals. "We're poor," she wrote, but they pursued every possible treatment available before they finally gave up, heartbro-
ken. Amelia wrote: "I've always been a caretaker. . . . I had no plans for
college or even a career. . . . My whole childhood was built on the dream of
becoming a wife and more—a Mother. I had no other life goals." When she
did not become pregnant,

> I tried EVERYTHING! I took Clomid, got [hormone] shots, took my [tem-
> perature] every morning for years and even put an experimental drug up my
> nose. . . . I even had major surgery. They removed part of my ovaries. . . .
> What I want to get across is the feelings and the heartbreak of all these years
> of poking and probing that I went through. Looking at that thermometer
> *every* morning and not seeing it rise. . . . I went through that hurt, ache and
> devastation EVERY month. . . . [It] was like killing a small part of my wom-
> anhood.

In a similar cycle of hope and devastation, Susan Delmont had eight miscarriages and one failed adoption attempt. "I feel like a failure," she wrote. The experience destroyed her self-confidence; she quit her job because she did not have "time enough to cry." She doubts her ability to raise a child. "I can't seem to apply for adoption. I don't know if I'm fit to be a mother or not, and I can't just say that I am. If God or whoever won't let me have my babies, why should an adoption agency?" Still, depressed as she was, she knew when she was getting the wrong advice from experts. One psychiatrist told her "just having 8 miscarriages couldn't make me as sad as I was. He was sure that my father sexually abused me as a child, and that my subconscious covered it up. Needless to say, I dumped him." But she was still left with her anguish. "I don't feel like I've had miscarriages, I feel like I've lost children. . . . I have 'phantom' children—you know, like an amputee has a phantom limb."

Rage

Along with pain and frustration, many infertile respondents expressed almost bottomless rage—at themselves, their bodies, and the fertile world. Carey Van Camp described feeling "almost hateful" and feeling "a burning rage inside me," especially toward pregnant women or infants. Lydia Sommer said infertility

came as a shock to us—like being punched in the stomach and not being able to catch your breath. . . . The world turns and we stand still. . . . I detest all pregnant women—whether they are my friends or not. They carry their pregnancy like a badge of honor, when they did nothing special to achieve it. Honestly, they make me sick. Sounds pretty bad, doesn't it? I'm becoming more cynical about it as I get older and my clock ticks away.

For many, the sight of their desired goal did not bring out warm feelings toward children. Rather, they felt hateful—even murderous. As Patricia Painter explained:

It was *so* painful to see anybody that was pregnant or had a baby. . . . I was the proverbial woman that was leaving the fertility doctor's office and saw the pregnant lady with two kids, a baby and a, you know, a toddler, in the crosswalks, and wanted to run over them all. God I felt *so* guilty for feeling that way until I got involved with Resolve. I really thought I was a horrible person. I thought God was punishing me or something. . . . I really wanted to run them over very badly with my car. . . . And I knew that every pregnant woman, every woman that had a new baby . . . got pregnant just to hurt my feelings. And God knows they did!

Patricia realized that her initial motivation for pursuing infertility treatment, her "love for children," virtually vanished. "I had a point where I could not see children at all. It was so painful." One friend, to protect her feelings when her toddler ran to the door, "looked around in her house, grabbed a newspaper, and put it in front of his face. Wasn't that nice? So I didn't have to see the kid. I thought that was nice. I'm sure my friends thought I was nuts." She even began to question her own sanity. "My values got real distorted and screwed up. . . . It felt very weird. . . . I had the ability to stand back and say, 'You're getting real strange, Patricia.' . . . And yet I couldn't seem to stop it. Kind of like trying to stop an avalanche, I think. The flood of emotion was so difficult."

Many of the desperately infertile expressed their most intense rage and disdain toward those who they believed neither wanted nor deserved their children, especially the young and the poor. Sonia Everly wrote, "It just doesn't seem fair . . . that young girls are getting pregnant when they have no desire to be parents." Daisy Posner's hatred went in all directions. As a nurse, she worked in labor and delivery. "I hated all the patients, even more so the ones with 3-4 kids who were on cocaine. I was sick with envy and hated God for being so unfair to me." In 1990, after infertility treatment, Daisy had a healthy daughter. But

> having one child isn't enough. . . . I still feel like a failure for all the miscarriages. I hate my body—it has felt empty and useless ever since my daughter was born. I hate reading about all the pregnant teenagers in the paper. . . . All my friends here are pregnant with their second child. It is all I can do to stay friendly with them—I hate them so much. . . . I pray all the time for another baby but God must hate me. He gives lots of babies to poor drug addicts and only one to me. . . . And I still hated my labor and delivery patients for having more kids. Needless to say I work elsewhere now . . . but I am still stuck in anger and despair.

Some infertile women expressed anger at women who had abortions. Paula Kranz felt "anger, bitterness and jealousy. . . . And then there are women out there being blessed with babies, and they are killing them with abortions." Dierdre Kearney wrote, "Each time I read of a child abuse case or of a woman having a third abortion, I cannot help but question, 'Why?'" But many infertile women saw abortion as a choice, much like infertility treatment. Karen Pasmore found it ironic that "so many women become pregnant without even thinking about it, many when they'd rather not," but she was nevertheless "strongly pro-choice. Many of my friends don't understand my position but if another woman becomes pregnant against her wishes, my infertility is not affected. I guess the grass is always greener."

Infertile women who had abortions themselves often felt guilty for years. Sue Kott got pregnant when she was twenty-five. Although she wanted to have the baby, her boyfriend wanted her to have an abortion. Two years later they married, and she has not been able to conceive again. She never forgave herself for the abortion. After years of infertility treatment, she is still childless, and her husband "refuses to adopt." Sonia Everly, on the other hand, has forgiven herself. Between her two marriages, she became pregnant while in graduate school and had an abortion.

> The abortion was traumatic, as it always is; never an easy decision, but the right one for me, and my partner, at the time. I obviously did not know that would be my only pregnancy. Would my choice have been different had I known? I think so, but I made my decision based on what I knew at that time. I still assumed I could become pregnant when I wanted to, when I was ready.

If abortion was difficult for some infertile women to accept, others found the fecundity of the poor unbearable. Some who believed that they had earned their right to reproductive self-determination were quick to deny the same right to others. Several shared the sentiments of Lisa Brown, who wrote, "I don't appreciate females having more kids than they can provide for and go on welfare. . . . I think there should be a law of 2 kids on welfare only. I think there should be sterilization inforced after the 2nd child."

Lisa's fury was directed toward the wrong target. Poor women on welfare were not responsible for her infertility, but she blamed them, rather than the real villains. In her case, as in many others, there were real villains. She was one of several respondents whose infertility resulted from severe damage to their bodies caused by sexual abuse when they were children. These respondents well understood the source of their problem, but did not express anger directly toward the men who raped them. None, in fact, mentioned whether their molesters had been apprehended. Thirty-one respondents, including two men, specifically mentioned abuse as a direct cause of their childlessness, ranging from emotional abuse to physical and sexual abuse.[18] The most horrifying were the stories of women like Lisa whose reproductive organs were damaged because they were raped when they were young children.

Lisa did not mention the rapes until the end of her letter. She began without a standard salutation, asking "if your some weirdo, getting off on others pain." She described years of infertility treatment, including several reconstructive surgeries; tubal pregnancies; and miscarriages. She and her husband tried to adopt, but they learned that it would take approximately ten years because they wanted a child under age two. At age forty-three, Lisa had lost her struggle to have a child and lost her marriage as well. She explained:

> When your husband goes out and gets a bar whore pregnate after 12 years of marriage and 4 miscarriages and 2 tubal pregnancies and the loss of 7 children, your mom says, "what do you expect? He wants kids, you can't give him any." So the marriage is gone and death looks good! What good am I to anyone? . . . Bitter? VERY! Being a female has not been fun for me. . . . Why did God see fit to take my kids but lets whores, child beaters and molesters have kids? And hurt or kill them?

Lisa was on the list for IVF when her husband "got a bar whore pregnate" and the marriage ended. "That was the hardest phone call I had to make in my life—calling and cancelling my only sure promise of a child." Although it was certainly far from a "sure promise," she was prepared to pay the $4,500 to try it. It was not until a brief postscript added after she signed her letter that she revealed the source of her difficulty: She was repeatedly raped by her step-grandfather and half-uncle from ages four through seven. "And by the way the rapes were performed (on the top of the bathroom toilet tank lid with my legs drawn up like I was squatting). It tilted my uterus so severely it caused all my future female problems."

Trudy Mayer, a White married factory worker, was also a victim of incest as a child and cannot carry a baby. She wrote three letters explaining her experience and her anguish, expressing anger not toward her molester but toward herself.

> When I first found out that I may never have a child I tryed to kill myself because I was raised to believe that women are to reproduce so that made me feel like if I can't do what God intend women to do then I didn't

belong. After that I felt very angry I was angry at me, at God at my Mother for having Me I was looking for some one to hate or blame I still have these feelings.

But the true villain remained unnamed.

Doctors and friends and family say oh just keep trying it will happen even my husband says we will just keep trying. Me I'm tired of it I want a baby but I don't want to keep going throw the hurt I have been pregnant seven times and each one I have lost and everyone says oh I understand but there is no way that they can understand what I go throu. I read the paper and see where some parents kill there kids or leave them in a trash can or something and stop and say to myself why would someone do such a thing to their own child but how can I understand I have never been in there shoes the same as you, you could never understand no matter how much you would like to.

She has seen specialists and had many surgeries, "so many that my stomach looks like a war zone." It was not until the end of her letter that she gave the reason for her misery: "I was molested very young . . . but it did not stop there it continued until I was 10 years old because I did not know that this was wrong."

Trudy did not name her abuser until her second letter: "I was molested when I was five years old by my father and it went on for years and I thought of suicide many of times through the years." She lived with her husband seven years before she finally married him

because if he can handle all these things we have been throu then I would be dum not to marrie him. . . . he has been at every doctors appointment been write there with every miscarriage he has cryed throu them with me he has been my clown but even with all this he new that he could leave and be with some one who can have children but he wanted to be with me even thou being with me hurts him a little of him dies every day because of are childless problem we have a specialist we go to and even with insurance it hurts the pocket book and we have looked in to adoption but they want you to be millionaire just to adopt a child this is what kills us every day a little to a time but what can you do.

In cases of sexual violence, the cause of infertility was grimly evident. But brutality surfaced in the letters of only a minority of respondents. In other cases, the very technologies that were developed to improve individual control over reproduction led to infertility. Ironically, many infertile individuals turned to medical experts to cure a problem that medical technology had created. Vivian Johnson discovered that her tubes were scarred from her previous use of an intrauterine device (IUD), and surgery did not correct the problem. Ultimately, high-tech reproductive medicine overcame the problem created by high-tech contraception: She had twins from her first IVF attempt. Karen Pasmore had a problem shared by tens of thousands of her peers; she was infertile because her mother was treated with diethylstilbestrol, or DES, during pregnancy. The drug was used widely in the 1940s and 1950s to prevent miscarriages.[19] In college, "DES became the specter in my life that it remains today." She turned to invasive high-tech infertility treatment, with no luck. Lorraine Pascasio was luckier. She, too, was a DES daughter. Initially she felt, "I'm defective . . . Damaged goods." But she finally had a "miracle baby" and wrote her story for the *Ladies Home Journal*.[20]

The Promise of a Technological Fix

To gain control over their uncooperative bodies, infertile women and men often turn to the medical profession, which ironically involves losing even more control. But getting professional assistance is also taking action. While some of the infertile respondents took a "wait and see" approach, many more turned to medical intervention as soon as they perceived that they might have a problem. Sometimes they demanded treatment even when their physicians were not convinced that intervention was necessary, or they changed physicians if they were not satisfied with the way they were treated.[21]

Amanda Talley was "going to leave everything in the doctor's hands, and I was very, very happy." The physicians found nothing wrong after six months of tests and suggested that she and her husband simply try on their own for a while. Since many of the infertile ultimately conceive on their own, this was not unfounded advice. According to a congressional study, "Time is the greatest, and certainly the cheapest, cure for infertility."[22] But Amanda insisted on treatment.

> I was very upset. . . . I could not possibly wait even six months to go for treatment. . . . We had to convince the doctor to start treating me. He was hesi-

tant about it because he thought that I didn't need it, but I was very, very impatient, and I had to. . . . So we talked him into it, and he started me on Pergonal the following month.

Pergonal, a powerful fertility drug that stimulates ovulation, required that her husband learn to give her the daily injections. "He was very, very shaken up by it, but he knew that this was what he had to do, and he was going to do it. He wanted a baby just as much as I did. The needles weren't so bad. It was an exciting time because I was very optimistic that this was going to work."

Some observers of the infertility industry complain that patients, particularly women, are exploited and manipulated by a powerful and intimidating medical establishment who rob them of their money, dignity, and decision-making capabilities. But the evidence suggests that most infertility patients, like Amanda, made active decisions at every juncture and did their best to remain in charge of their medical care.[23] They became careful consumers of infertility and adoption services, as well as trusting and cooperative patients who put their faith in the experts. This dual identity was not easy and called for major decisions about how much of their time, bodies, financial resources, and emotional well-being they were willing to sacrifice in their efforts to become parents and how much of their own judgment they were willing to relinquish to the experts.

Kathy Quell took her health care into her own hands before succumbing to major medical intervention. After she was diagnosed with endometriosis, she had laser surgery that was only partially successful. The endometriosis had started to invade organs outside the reproductive tract. "At this point my doctor suggested that I have a 12 inch section of my bowel removed if I really wanted to get pregnant. Then the [endometriosis] would be completely removed from my body. We really did want to get pregnant, but not so bad that I wanted to start chopping up the rest of my body." She then joined an endometriosis support group and through research learned that she might control the condition with diet. After two years on a new diet, exercise regimen, vitamins, and treatment for allergies, both she and her husband improved their overall health. Her endometriosis apparently disappeared, and then they tried IVF. She became pregnant on her first attempt and gave birth to twins.

Although there is no guarantee that do-it-yourself treatment will work, Kathy combined her own health care with high-tech medicine and took control of her treatment. Angela Carter took charge by discarding physicians until she found the one she liked. "I am on my third doctor [in two years] because the first two were only going down their infertility check lists and not listening to me as a person. I felt like I was on a conveyor belt. The third doctor listens and is willing to discuss options which is a help." Similarly, when Joyce Williams expressed reluctance about taking fertility drugs, her physician "hit the ceiling," and she "checked him off," along with medical treatment altogether. She eventually ended up with adopted as well as biological children.

The Cost of the Baby Quest

The baby quest is largely driven by demand and supply, like any other market system. Although the "market" is an odious concept when human lives are concerned and baby selling is almost universally considered to be an abomination, there is no avoiding the fact that babies—or, more precisely, reproductive and adoption services—are bought and sold. The infertility industry is a $2 billion a year business.[24] Each try at IVF, for example, can cost anywhere from $6,000 to $13,000. Susan Sward spent $15,000 on more than forty visits to the fertility clinic, plus three unsuccessful IVF attempts and five unsuccessful artificial inseminations before she finally became pregnant. Annie and Tony Hillman spent over $20,000 for their IVF baby.[25] Vivian Johnson and her husband finally gave birth to twins conceived by IVF, after spending four months and $5,000. Vivian was luckier than Rose Norsika, a lesbian who, with her partner of twenty-two years, "spent twelve years and several thousands of dollars trying to get pregnant with artificial insemination. It was a long hard journey for both of us," and they never managed to conceive.

Angela Carter and her husband spent three hundred dollars per month on treatment for several years, but they stopped short of IVF, which they could not afford. Marie Gutierrez and her husband were unable to follow through with treatment because the clinic required payment "up front" at each visit. She spoke for many when she complained that

> already this year alone my husband and myself have paid dearly with our savings and simply ran out of money, which really disappoints both of us, we both have full time jobs but the cost of infertility treatments are so costly we just can't afford it, and both of our clocks are ticking soon to be 30 years. And

it hurts terribly. . . . I will strive with all my heart and Soul to make this dream my reality. My husband and I did not chose this pain, but maybe some of the Clinic's can understand that we *infertile people* need more affordable care. . . . I could get treatments I need and deserve if they were affordable for all.

Like Marie Gutierrez, Kendra Groneman and her husband were unable to afford the costly treatment. Because their insurance would not cover the treatment, each insemination would cost them $150, plus $1,500 for the Pergonal, in addition to the fees for all the tests. "We discontinued treatment terrible hurt and discouraged." Although they were still young, they feared that they would never achieve parenthood. "I'm 25 and my husband will be 24, my clock won't tick forever. Then people say you can always adopt," but she worried about the cost and the shortage of healthy White infants. For White couples who turn to adoption for the same reasons that they seek infertility treatment—their desire for a healthy newborn who resembles them—the costs of adoption can be as prohibitive as infertility treatment. Kendra Groneman believed that the system discriminated against people of modest resources and exploited the desperation of the infertile: "I feel like infertile couples are being punished for not being able to have children by charging outlandish fees for us to adopt a baby that needs a good home with people that will love them. Tell me who is making out here? These agencies are."

Sometimes couples chose between infertility treatment and adoption by considering the costs and risks of both strategies. Most infertile couples are not wealthy, and most insurance companies only partially cover treatments. High-tech interventions like IVF can cost thousands of dollars per attempt, and pursuing a course of treatment can quickly become a $40,000 decision.[26] Dierdre Kearney and her husband were a White middle-class couple in their early thirties with college degrees who were living in a small town in Tennessee. Their opportunities for pursuing parenthood were limited by their resources. They tried to conceive for four of their five years of marriage. "I think we have experienced every emotion and feeling one can in dealing with this situation. We have also been through every fertility test there is." Her husband was on medication for three years, and his problem was corrected. She had four surgeries, medication, fertility drugs, and artificial insemination using her husband's semen. "The only option left for us is IVF. We do not have the money; what savings we have is going toward adoption." They hope to adopt within a year. "It is very expensive to adopt plus the strain and waiting are a continuation of the strain and waiting we've already endured." Sue Kott echoed the same sentiment when she wrote that she and her husband have tried everything except IVF, which they cannot afford. "At $5,000 a try with less than 30% success rate you have to be rich to have a baby that way."

Adoption was not always an option. For Dave Crenshaw, who is sterile, infertility treatment would not help and adoption was beyond his means. He found the adoption process not only expensive, but humiliating and invasive. "The poorest person in the world can give just as damn much love, caring, etc. to an adopted child, as someone whom can buy their way through the system. . . . Some of us quit as we feel our Rights as Human beings are being violated." Money was not the only obstacle to adoption. Janet Dewey and her husband also wanted to adopt, but "no adoption agency in the U.S. would consider us due to our age and religion (excess of the former and absence of the latter)."

Institutional policies, especially insurance coverage, often made the difference between infertility treatment, adoption, or permanent childlessness. Roberta O'Leary and her husband had insurance that covered only four tries at any one procedure, so they tried Clomid, then Pergonal, and artificial insemination with the husband's semen four times without success. They finally decided to try IVF before their insurance expired. The grueling routine required a great deal of time and a willingness to go through extremely invasive procedures. In addition to the physical and emotional impact of hyperactive ovaries caused by the hormone supplements that are used to stimulate the ovaries to produce eggs, there were "three injections a day. . . . Time became an issue as I would need daily Ultrasounds to monitor the progress of the eggs. I wasn't real excited but decided to try anyway." At the time of the surgery, there were thirty-one eggs to harvest, but twenty-eight were immature and one was damaged; only two were mature, and neither one was fertilized. As the O'Learys prepared for their second attempt, they noted that their treatment would have been impossible without good insurance coverage and jobs with flexible hours.

For couples whose insurance covered unlimited infertility treatment, money was not an issue, and medical treatment was less costly for them than was adoption. But pursuing infertility treatment with unlimited insurance coverage did not guarantee success. Patricia Painter still had "unexplained infertility" and no children after years of treatment that cost her insurance company $300,000 before she and her husband decided to stop treatment. Similarly, Penny Singer and her husband considered themselves fortunate because their "insurance has paid for everything at about $100,000 a year (three years now)." In spite of the strain on their marriage, which became "shaky to say the least," and the torture to Penny's body, "a thousand tests, some have been so painfull," the Singers felt that continuing treatment was their only option, given their financial situation. "We tried adopting, it comes down to you pay about $15,000 or wait about 12 years—they visit your house several times to check a million things—we both decided not to pursue it." Because they did not have the $15,000 to adopt, and adoption was not covered by health insurance, their insurance company paid twenty times that amount for treatment that was ultimately unsuccessful.

Maureen Wendell did not have comprehensive insurance that covered the costs of treatment, "so materially we've sacrificed much." She and her husband paid for several expensive procedures, including two attempts at gamete intra-fallopian transfer (GIFT), in which "harvested" eggs and sperm are inserted directly into one of the fallopian tubes, before she gave birth to a healthy son, who she described as "a miracle." She also understood that by pursuing costly treatment, they made a consumer choice: "He's the exotic vacation I'll never take. The new house I'll never build. The jewels I'll never wear. . . . But for him I'd do it all again—gladly."

Infertile people like Maureen invested their money in medical treatment that held out the promise of achieving a new status—parenthood—and the happy domestic life with children they desired. Maureen's child was an expensive proposition, even before he was conceived. But ultimately she made the same sacrifices, or consumer choices, that all parents make to one extent or another. For the infertile who poured their resources and energies into treatment, the desired child became the source of personal pleasure, family status, leisure enjoyment, even consumer indulgence: the "cute little 'Gap Kids' with little denim jackets" that Margaret Lewis described. The childfree made a different choice, but for essentially the same reasons. They, too, used their resources to achieve the status and private lives they wanted. They chose to spend their time and money on other sources of personal enjoyment, such as travel, nice homes and furnishings, leisure pursuits, and other pleasures. As different as their reproductive goals appeared, they all invested their resources and energies in creating a personal life that would provide them with the domestic intimacy, status, leisure pursuits, and rewards they desired.

Although children are costly sources of satisfaction, like consumer goods and leisure pursuits, the comparison ends there. Whether or not children are commodified, they are certainly not commodities. No disappointment caused by the inability to purchase a particular item or adventure can compare with the heartache and anguish of infertility for those who are desperate for a child. It is not simply that the infertile often pay and pay but never get the desired goods, it is also that the pain they experience is unlike any other. Because the pain and frustration continue as long as the possibility for parenthood exists, many of the infertile described their quest for a child as an "obsession." Both the nature of infertility treatment and the adoption system contribute to their obsession because of the huge amount of time and energy required in the effort. Like many other respondents, Lester Bernstein discovered quickly that once he and his wife began the grueling routine of treatment, "infertility had taken over our lives."

The Lure of a Cure

For many of those who decided to pursue treatment, the baby quest took on a momentum all its own, and it became difficult to know when to stop.[27] Like compulsive gamblers or the architects of the Vietnam War, the greater the investment and loss, the more desperate the need to keep trying for success so the sacrifice would not be in vain. As one infertility specialist explained, "The door never, ever completely closes on an infertile couple. There's always the latest snazzy technique to rekindle hope. They can end up at the end of the line childless and financially depleted."[28] If a shred of hope remained, many infertile respondents found it difficult to give up. After seven years of treatment and no results, Marie Gutierrez wrote, "I can't give up now, We've come too far we have never been quitters so I guess we will hang in there."

Treatment is so intense and all-consuming that it can become a full-time job in itself. News anchor Connie Chung made headlines when she announced that she was taking an "infertility leave" to pursue the baby quest full time.[29] Because of the enormous commitment of time, energy, money, and emotion, the decision of whether to begin or stop treatment or to pursue adoption was torturous for many infertile respondents. For those who pursued infertility treatment, the decision to stop was sometimes more difficult than the decision to begin.

Karen Pasmore finally decided to abandon the "medical merry-go-round," but not until she and her husband had exhausted themselves and their resources. After Clomid, intrauterine insemination, and laparoscopic surgeries, they tried Pergonal.

We are already deep in debt and we decided this would be our last ditch effort. I was so desperate to try this that I was positive it would work, and that I could deal with the consequences later. Pergonal is the big gun of fertility drugs and has numerous side effects and cautions. It is also a very demanding schedule—you must be available for daily blood tests and ultrasounds, carefully monitored so as not to do permanent damage to your ovaries. We live hours away from the office so I needed to make arrangements to stay near the city. Pergonal also must be injected daily. Usually the spouse does the injections but since my husband had to stay here to work, I injected them myself which was harder than I expected. . . . When the time was right, the insemination was performed, and by some lousy twist of fate, I got my period two days later, more than two weeks early. So after all it was a waste of time AND MONEY.

The Pasmores gave up treatment after that, but Karen has not come to terms with the situation. "I have all these miserable feelings inside and I don't know how to deal with them."

Myra Olivia and her husband tried infertility treatment for more than a decade and finally gave up. "After 11 years, the quest became too hard for me. I don't regret quitting the fight, but I know that this emptiness will go with me to the grave." Sheila Turner-Cohn finally gave up treatment because three years of IVF resulted in the growth of ovarian cysts.

The decision to stop treatment was extremely difficult—more so for me than for my husband. He saw it as very clear cut—the treatments were jeopardizing my health and had to stop. However, I saw it as giving up and I'm the type of person who doesn't like to give up on anything I want to achieve.

Turning her creative impulses from high-tech reproduction to high-tech production in her work helped to ease her pain. "Sometimes I jokingly say to myself that my computer is my 'electronic womb,' because of the creative products I produce with it."

Doris Malory was married for five years before she came out as a lesbian. Although she and her former husband decided not to have children, she and her current partner, Susan, tried to have a child. "About a year after we met, I started on this journey, which still finds me childless, and frustrated, with a lot of money spent." Although some lesbians have arranged nonmedical inseminations with the semen of friends or acquaintances, "we never considered anything other than using an unknown donor through my ob-gyn." Artificial insemination (AID) by donor was difficult because Doris had endometriosis and she was not ovulating. So she started taking Clomid. "Wait about two weeks—get a period, be disappointed. Talk about an emotional roller coaster." This went on for a year, which took a huge emotional and financial toll. "I took last summer off—the emotions and $$$ were getting to me. (The AID runs $600 per month—I took a second job to help pay for it.)" Finally she became pregnant, but miscarried. "Susan and I were both crushed. . . . My system was pretty goofed up after the D and C [dilation and curettage], so I had to take Provera to get a period." Still, she did not give up. "I'm taking Clomid now in preparation for AID again later this month." After investing so much in the effort, Doris is struggling to quit as if she were trying to break an addiction, with her partner in the role of co-dependent:

> I find myself setting deadlines I then break such as 'I'm only going to try 2 more times.' Susan doesn't want to try much longer— she's four years older than me and feels she's getting too old to entertain thoughts of a baby. So I worry there will come a time when I'll have to decide between staying with her and having a child.

The Emotional Dangers of Technological Intervention

One risk of medical technology is that it can heighten the stakes, extend the possibilities endlessly, and transform a reproductive experience in unpredictable ways. For Kristina Shubert, high-tech medical intervention was a mixed blessing. It transformed what certainly would have been a first-trimester miscarriage into "the loss of twin girls at birth," and for all her suffering she was still childless. After an ectopic pregnancy and surgery, "I was devastated. . . . That is when my depression and obsession truly began." She became "obsessed with having a baby." When she miscarried, "I felt that I emitted a force that was destructive to life. A woman is made to create life, but I couldn't. I wasn't good enough." When she got pregnant again, an ultrasound showed that she had "stuck twin syndrome," in which one fetus got too much blood and the other did not get enough. The ultrasound also showed that the twins were both female, and Kristina and her husband gave them each names. But the smaller fetus was at risk. The only way to save it was to withdraw amniotic fluid as it built up, to prevent premature labor.

Kristina immediately went on leave from her job. "I was totally entrenched in the situation at work. So, it was difficult to just not go back and finish what I had been doing." But she gave up her job to stay at home, have a uterine monitor twice a day, and have amniotic fluid withdrawn at the physician's office twice a week. "This was painful, but I was most concerned about the possibility that it could cause me to lose the babies."

The ultrasound images had the psychological effect of transforming the tiny, fragile, and damaged embryos into full-fledged babies. They saw the fetuses twice a week on the ultrasound screen, "so we got to bond with them. . . . We were in love with our babies. Tom read stories to them every night and we decided to decorate the nursery in a celestial theme—moons and stars." But they lived in "a constant state of anxiety." They did not want any discouraging news. One physician told her the prognosis was "hopeful at best. . . . I was devastated. I was fighting for their lives and they were telling me it wasn't going to work. I needed their positive support."

In her twenty-fifth week of pregnancy, in September, Kristina entered the hospital. She was to stay there until she delivered in January, four months later. "I was prepared to spend the holidays in the hospital." But her stay was much shorter than expected. The larger of the two fetuses died that day. "Carla was dead! . . . Helen—she was still alive. She became my world in that moment—my only reason to live." They decided the only possibility of saving the other twin was to deliver the fetus then, undeveloped and weighing less than a pound. "I knew it was very, very early for her to be born" at 25 weeks of pregnancy. Kristina had a caesarean and the baby was born alive: "Her skin was gray and she was extremely tiny (11 inches long, 15 ounces). But she was alive!" When the second twin died, "I could hardly stand to live." The twins were buried in "identical little doll dresses and doll diapers" because they were too tiny for baby clothes. At the funeral, the Shuberts put up a pink granite stone marked "Our twin angels." Kristina's recovery was terrible: The placenta "was imbedded in the walls of my uterus and [the physician] had to rip it out." Kristina got an infection and remained in the hospital eleven days. For her, the experience was devastating.

> I know what it feels like to want to die. I didn't understand suicide before. . . . I knew that I had better get some help before I did kill myself. I wanted to be with my babies that bad. Everyone said that they are in God's hands. I don't trust God with them—look what happened to me! I don't know anything

anymore. I don't know if there's a God and I don't know why I'm here on this earth.

She is now on a prescription antidepressant; "that is probably what is keeping me alive and sane."

For Kristina, technological intervention was not successful. In fact, it made her physical and emotional condition much worse than it would have been had she simply miscarried. She would still have her job and her body might not have been so badly damaged. And she might have been spared some of the trauma. Joan Morgan had a similar experience, although infertility was the result, not the cause, of the intervention. She became pregnant while living with her husband in France. Her pregnancy was uneventful until her eighth month, when a pregnant friend showed her a photograph taken of her fetus during an ultrasound. Joan thought it would be "fun" to have a similar photograph as a souvenir of her pregnancy, so she requested an ultrasound from her physician. The ultrasound revealed fluid on the fetus's brain. Although the extent of damage to the brain was unclear, the physician persuaded Joan to abort the fetus. Because it was the eighth month, they decided to kill the fetus with an injection and induce labor, so Joan would deliver a stillborn infant. The entire ordeal was so traumatic and upsetting for Joan that she became suicidal. In addition to the emotional devastation, the delivery was painful and complicated and left her with part of the placenta embedded in the uterus. After several additional surgeries, the condition is still not corrected. Her reproductive organs are so severely damaged that it is unlikely she will be able to get pregnant again. For Joan, what began as a lark, an elective ultrasound to get a "souvenir," ended up as a tragedy.

Of course, medical intervention can be beneficial. But there are no guarantees, and the process is often stressful. Infertility treatment can be a major ordeal involving at least two and sometimes more individuals. Whether infertility treatment is carried out on one or both bodies, the couple's sex life and intimate relationships are inevitably affected. Sonia Everly described the routine of

charting my temperature, taking the hormone, having intercourse at ovulation, then running in to his office within six hours of intercourse to see if I still had live sperm in my cervical mucus. . . . Again the monthly routine of temperatures, douching, intercourse, doctor's visit . . . ad nauseam. This is not romantic stuff. And each month I had the same result: nothing.

With artificial insemination with the husband's semen, conception takes place in the clinic, not in the bedroom. For Sonia,

> This meant that on my "fertile day" and the day after, my husband would go to the medical clinic and leave them a sperm sample. . . . I would arrive at the lab in time to snatch up the sample (no pun intended) and transport it to my doctor's office down the street. I would be whisked into the exam room, and the sperm (in a syringe) would be inserted directly into my uterus. This was not un-painful. The doctor couldn't use any lubricant in case it had a negative effect on the sperm, which made it more uncomfortable. . . . Needless to say, sex became a chore rather than a wonderful thing. I became quite anti-sexual, actually. I felt constantly invaded by the doctor, who was of course trying to help, and having sex when I wasn't in the mood, just because I was ovulating. These things I was willing to do. But my husband and I didn't talk between us about how we felt.

After many months of treatment, the Everlys ended up with no child—and divorced.

Sonia's experience was typical of many respondents. Daisy Posner recalled, "The pursuit of a child has hurt our marriage also. Everything is so orchestrated and timed. I haven't had desire in years. Every month I say 'why bother,' but if I don't try I feel worse for missing a chance." Carey Van Camp complained, "It's hard making love on command—actually sex becomes an *exercise* and love has nothing to do with it, when one is trying to make a baby." For Tess Printer, sex "became so routine that it was almost like taking medicine." Kristina Shubert wrote that infertility treatment was "disastrous to our sex life. . . . My husband didn't like to perform on demand and a hysterical, desperate woman is not much of an aphrodisiac." Karen Pasmore explained, "Sex has become very difficult. I associate making love with making babies and I can't do one or the other." Joseph Loren described the "loss of pleasure in our lovemaking, my needing to perform on demand, the stress associated with sex for the 'wrong' reasons. . . . We tried to get pregnant with a vengeance," but gave up after three months. Lester Bernstein joked about the strains infertility treatment places on marriage:

> Whatever romance was left in our sex life dwindled as we began to exchange our bodily fluids with the medical laboratory instead of each other. For me, this meant developing a relationship with a glass jar. . . . This, of course, was very unnatural. I started getting erections at recycling centers.

Third Parties to Conception

Along with the decision about whether to pursue infertility treatment and when to stop, infertile couples had to decide whether to pursue conception with the help of a donor or to try to adopt a baby. Reproduction achieved with the sperm or egg of another person is usually considered part of reproductive "medical technology," but in many ways it is closer to adoption. Sperm donation is simpler than egg donation and is usually anonymous. Egg donation can also be anonymous, as the advertisement quoted at the beginning of this chapter suggests. But it can also involve a "surrogate" (a woman who provides the egg and carries the pregnancy), as in the notorious case of "Baby M." Controversies over the rights of surrogates versus "contracting parents" have stymied courts and traumatized parents on all sides of the issue.

AID became part of the medical repertoire when Dr. William Pancoast and Dr. Addison Davis Hard collaborated to inseminate an unconscious woman in the 1880s. But it first became widely available and controversial in the 1930s. The process carried such a stigma of dubious legitimacy that it remained a highly secret matter. In the 1950s, a judge ruled in a custody case involving a child conceived by AID that the woman had committed adultery because she had given birth to a child whose father was not her husband, even though she never had sex with any man except her husband.[30] Although that was an extreme case, until fairly recently most clinics would not perform insemination unless a legally married couple requested it and the husband signed forms agreeing to be the child's legal father. These policies not only reflected the prevailing morality, they also protected infertility physicians, who feared they would be sued for child support if the husbands ever denied paternity.

The procedure has become much more respectable, and it is now available to single women, whether heterosexual or lesbian. But its most common use is among married couples, and it still involves secrecy and controversy over whether children should be informed; about the screening of donors; about who should have access to insemination; and about whether the donor's semen should be mixed with the husband's, a practice some physicians use so that husbands can think the child may be their own biological offspring. Although some practitioners think that semen mixing offers a psychological benefit, critics claim that it is dishonest, does not allow a man to come to terms with his infertility, and encourages unnecessary fantasies about biological parenthood. According to one study, secrecy became an "obsession" for couples using AID. The authors concluded that efforts to hide AID were unhealthy and detrimental to the parents and children alike.[31]

The selection of donors also perpetuates certain eugenic theories. Whereas donors are usually screened for inheritable diseases, most are selected on the basis of their academic achievement. They are usually medical students, or at some centers, undergraduates with B (3.0) or better grade-point averages. Since the genetic basis of grade-point averages is questionable at best, the sociologist Barbara Katz Rothman sarcastically dubbed these specimens the "3.0 sperm." Nevertheless, the qualities of sperm donors are a matter of controversy. The notorious commercial "genius sperm bank" in California offers to sell the sperm of Nobel laureates and noted scientists to parents who are hoping for genius offspring. Some sperm banks offer forty dollars per donation from male students who do well on standardized tests, with bonuses for extremely high achievers, as the advertisement at the opening of this chapter suggests. These methods of selection do not guarantee genetic "superiority," and the system is vulnerable to abuse. One physician so abused the system that he used his own semen to inseminate dozens of women at his clinic, creating a community filled with genetic half siblings.[32]

Adoption

Before the development of reproductive technologies, adoption—formal or informal—offered infertile couples their best chance of parenthood. Today, contrary to the widespread belief that the childless "can always adopt," adoption can be as costly, tortured, and uncertain a path for would-be parents as is infertility treatment. Several developments have made it increasingly difficult to adopt children. With the easing of the stigma of single parenthood, more and more mothers are raising children born out of wedlock and hence fewer children are available for adoption. Legal abortion has also reduced the number of available infants. And the costs and rigorous screening procedures contribute to the difficulties of adoption.

In addition, the informal channels of child sharing that prevailed in the preindustrial era have largely evaporated. In the nineteenth and early twentieth centuries, formal legal adoption replaced more flexible systems of apprenticeship, servitude, and caretaking. In some communities, however, especially those characterized by strong ethnic, religious, or kinship ties, informal child sharing or "child-keeping" practices have continued into the late twentieth century. Although these communities are often poor, poverty is not necessarily the primary motivation for child sharing. "It is part of our culture," according to the Black sociologist Robert B. Hill.[33]

Typical of this pattern was the case of Penny and John Majors, a Black couple who desperately wanted children. John was a postal carrier, and Penny was a teacher; they lived in a large and comfortable home that they owned in a Black neighborhood of a large city. In the 1950s, when they discovered that they were unable to have their own biological child, they took a special interest in a six-year-old neighborhood girl, the daughter of a White mother and a Black father. When the child's parents split up, her mother decided that the girl would have a more stable life with the Majors. Although they were not related to the child by blood, the Majors raised her as their own. The girl's mother stayed in touch with her daughter, sent money, and visited frequently. Long after the child grew up, graduated from college, and became a successful professional journalist, she considered "Aunt Penny" and "Uncle John" to be her parents, along with her biological mother and father.

Although no formal adoption took place, the "fictive kinship" between the Majors and their child functioned in much the same way as "open adoption" does today, with adoptive and biological families known to and remaining in contact with each other. Open adoption is relatively new to the adoption establishment, but it mirrors practices that have prevailed in many communities for generations and that are still standard in some places. Estelle Pozak discovered this system to be alive and well in an Inupiat village in Alaska, where she has lived since 1972. She tried to get pregnant during a brief marriage and considered single parenthood after her divorce. Raised a Roman Catholic from a "very Italian background," she hoped for children, and as time went on, "I heard that famous biological clock ticking." She contemplated adoption, but when she realized that she had a number of children in her life and often in her home, she felt that adoption was unnecessary.

At forty-five, as a successful journalist, Estelle was satisfied with her life. But her neighbors, the indigenous people of her village, were worried about her.

People here feel you are deprived if you do not have children. It is culturally acceptable to give children away for adoption to relatives who cannot conceive if you already have some. These adoptions are open, with the child knowing from day one who his/her "real" parents are. Often these "adopted" children will acknowledge their "real" brothers and sisters and continue the formation of extended kinship networks. As I aged in this town, people offered me children with some regularity. I have a good reputation here and people felt they were offering me a very precious gift since I had no children of my own. In cases like this, having a marriage partner is not considered necessary. In fact, having a child to take care of you becomes even more important if you are not married. People here eventually accepted that I was not interested in adopting any children. Since I have always been heavily involved with children in my work, this was considered an acceptable substitute.

Although Estelle never adopted, neither was she "childless." She is virtually surrounded by children; many frequently stay in her home. "My life is fuller than I ever thought it could be."

In many communities, particularly among certain nationalities, immigrant groups, and communities of color, these child-sharing practices remain viable. But childless Americans of all backgrounds who do not live in places where these practices are common turn not to kin or neighbors, but to legal and medical institutions, in their efforts to bring children into their homes. Because the typical private home is expected to "produce" and rear its own offspring, few informal channels are available to the childless who want children. Thus, the childless must seek assistance from public institutions—medical, legal, and social—to achieve their goals in the most private arena of life.

Compared to infertility treatment, formal adoption is less stressful physically, but it can be equally draining emotionally and financially, and the outcome is just as uncertain. With the demand for adoptive babies so much greater than the supply, the decision to pursue adoption involves not only the pragmatic concerns about cost, time, and energy and the likelihood of success, but also soul-searching about whether the prospective parents would be happy with a child that is not biologically related to either of them. Would they accept a child who did not resemble them, was racially different, was older, or had special needs? For some, like Amanda Talley, adoption was not an option: "I have a problem dealing with the fact that a child wouldn't be my biological child." For others, like Patricia Painter whose infertility treatment was unsuccessful, the decision was not so obvious. It was difficult to let go of the hope for a biological child, and she had to consider the pros and cons: "My husband has these beautiful blue eyes, I so much wanted those in a child. And I have nice hair. So I wanted those in a child. Of course, with my luck they would have my small, brown eyes and my husband's prematurely gray hair! So there's no guarantees." Some respondents resented comments they heard suggesting that simply because they were infertile they should be willing to raise a child with needs beyond the routine challenges that parents face when raising biological children. Fertile couples, they noted, are not asked why they do not seek to adopt children who are different or have difficulties. In addition to their feelings about these issues, some felt uncomfortable with the politics and economics of adoption.

Some prospective parents had no qualms about adoption but found the process daunting. Joseph Loren and his wife pursued adoption after unsuccessful infertility treatment. They decided "not to pursue the more sophisticated technological possibilities of conception; both because we didn't want nor have the money to invest in that, but also because a biological child wasn't that important to us." John explained, "We were not committed to, or necessarily interested in a Caucasian infant, nor were we interested in 'buying' a baby through an adoption agency." Like other hopeful parents who wrote, they wanted a baby placed with them "because of the love and nurturing we could give a child, not because of the size of our bank account." They ended up with a private adoption and described "the beauty and grace with which our son's biological parents relinquished him." But their efforts to build their family continued to be plagued by heartbreak. During the three years after they adopted their son, they had two failed adoptions and two miscarriages and felt "a growing anger." They experienced "the sting of being dependent upon the whims and judgments of the strangers who determine whether or not we are capable parents, and whether or not we are able to manage an expansion of our family."

Like infertility treatment, adoption is often a struggle with a small chance of success. Sandy Herman was among the lucky ones. She and her husband were "chosen by a 16 year old to be the parents of her child," and they are now awaiting their second adoption. "Our daughter is a very special gift to us and we have no regrets finally giving up trying to have a biological child." But not all the adoption stories ended so happily. With so much demand and so little supply, there is great potential for corruption. Dierdre Kearney wanted a child desperately, but was horrified when confronted with a black-market baby-selling scheme. A woman in her church told Dierdre and her husband of a young woman who was pregnant with her fourth child and was looking for adoptive parents. "She has had no pre-natal care and she wants $8,000 'to help her buy clothes and get back into life.'" When Dierdre said that this was illegal, the woman "said her sister had paid $17,000 to a girl for a baby." They argued about the morality and legality of the situation.

> This woman even had the gall to say our lawyer was giving us 'bad advice' by telling us not to get involved. She said this was a real 'steal' and we'd probably never get a baby though an agency. She also implied we didn't really want a baby or we'd do whatever it took, regardless of the legality of it. Needless to say, I was hurt as well as mad. I had two migraine headaches that week thanks to that stressful situation.

Dierdre's anger extended to the pregnant teenager as well: "This girl can have babies like rabbits and obviously doesn't want them or love them. She's not getting prenatal care and she's willing to sell her baby for new clothes. Yes, situations like this really make me question and wonder 'why?'"

For some who adopted children, the pain did not necessarily end with parenthood. Carol Hall, like some of the other adoptive parents who wrote, treasures her children but still feels the pain of infertility.

> We have 2 beautiful adopted boys . . . and love them dearly. Being unable to conceive I think is the worst thing a woman can experience. Sometimes the emptiness is really great. Even with my 2 boys sometimes it comes on fast and you really have to take hold and try to control. But my 2 boys are everything to me if I didn't have them I am sure I would have gone crazy a long time ago.

Carla Edmonds has two children, one biological and one adopted. She confessed that as much as she loves both children, she feels differently about the one who was adopted:

> I love my adopted daughter very much—but I am honest enough to admit that much as I love her, she is still the living representation of a dream that I had to give up—*painfully*! . . . I love my two girls uniquely—*differently*. I can't believe I'm the only biological/adoptive parent who feels this way. . . . I've never seen this point of view in print anywhere. So much of what is written about adoption is syrupy tripe. It *is* an exciting, difficult, rewarding, ambivalence-producing thing. I've *never* been sorry we adopted [her]—but I still grieve for the children I *would* have given birth to had I been able. Life is complex!

Albert Kingman has two adopted children and believes he is a "wonderful father." Yet he still feels "deeply hurt by the news that I had no sperm at all." Because he was unable to produce biological offspring, "I've missed part of life's key experience. The part I've had may be 98 percent of being a parent, or possibly 120 percent—but it is definitely different. As I look at [my children] . . . I see life, I see joy, I see response to me as a father, but I never see my nose, my hair, my eyes."

For married people, who make up the vast majority of adoptive parents, as well as infertility patients, the decision to adopt involves both partners. If the spouses do not agree, the impact on the relationship can be devastating. Studies have shown that husbands are usually more reluctant to adopt and are more eager to have biological children than are wives. Although many women respondents wanted to experience pregnancy and birth and wished for biological children, their responses confirm the findings of others that wives were more eager to pursue adoption when infertility treatment did not work. Daisy Posner complained, "My husband won't think of adoption because 1) he thinks we haven't tried all the surgical/medical options 2) he wants the baby to be *his*. It isn't *his* body that gets stuck with needles and operated on. . . . He also won't go to an infertility support group." Some marriages did not survive the strain. Betty Jones's husband "refused to adopt. . . . I knew I was able to love any child. He said he could only love his own." They ended up divorced. Betsy O'Connell got pregnant, but when amniocentesis showed "that everything possible was wrong with the baby," she had an abortion. Her physicians advised her not to try to have another child. Her husband disagreed with this decision and would not consider adoption. Their marriage also ended in divorce.

The decision to adopt required agreement not only on whether to adopt, but on how and who to adopt. In the baby-boom era, most adoption agencies tried to "match" children to adoptive parents as closely as possible and to hide the fact of adoption, so the nuclear family would appear to be a biologically based unit. In recent decades, in spite of the controversy that continued to swirl around cross-racial adoption, many adoptive families began to include individuals of different colors and nationalities. Cross-racial and cross-national adoptions have increased both the possibilities for adoption and the soul-searching that many prospective adoptive parents undergo.[34]

Isabel Root, aged fifty-two, is a teacher who loves children and does not care what they looked like. She was a nun from age sixteen to twenty-eight.

When she left the convent and married at age thirty, "all I wanted from then on was a child of my own." In the 1970s, when she and her husband tried to adopt a child of color internationally, they faced hostility from all sides, including White acquaintances as well as Black social workers who had condemned the adoption of Black infants by White parents. Sensitive to these concerns, she explained,

> My doctor, who is Irish, was very disturbed that we wanted a dark South American baby. I did tell him I was requesting no black blood. At that time I felt I couldn't handle a child growing up and asking me why I didn't let him or her have black parents. Today I'd have ten black children and answer that question with, 'Black, purple or polka-dotted, I'm your mother and you're stuck with me.' I was more sensitive in the 70s.

While waiting for news from the agency, Isabel learned from her physician of a teenager who was pregnant and considering giving up the baby for adoption. "I asked if I could come right over and beg her on my knees for her baby." But she worried,

> Would she give it up? (I wouldn't) (I couldn't). Will she keep it? (I would). How could they make her? What were they using to influence her? A career? Freedom to be a child? Freedom from a burden? She was only 17. What was the bribe? Would they promise her child a good home? What made her make a decision I couldn't ever make? I thank God she did. I thanked God every day, all day, for months when that baby came home with me. . . . She was like a gift. And to this day it is my only thought every day, all day, "She is my gift."

Isabel wanted any child she could get, regardless of racial background. But other respondents found the idea of cross-racial adoption intolerable. When Lydia Sommer discovered that her adopted baby was biracial, the issue of race overshadowed everything else, and she gave her back to the agency. Lydia is a White thirty-three-year-old account specialist in a large advertising agency, and her husband is a thirty-five-year-old attorney. For six of their seven years of marriage, they pursued infertility treatment, but they stopped short of IVF, "drained emotionally and financially." They adopted a daughter in 1991.

> But after she was with us for 2 months we realized that she was bi-racial—she did not appear so at birth. Our birth mother had lied to us about the father. We struggled with this but after some gut-wrenching introspection came to

see that we were not prepared for the challenge of raising a bi-racial child. We loved Sarah dearly and with all our hearts, but knew that there was another couple out there who *was* prepared for this. We gave our daughter everything we had while she was ours, and finally relinquished custody back to the agency. They found another family for Sarah and we pray that she is loved as we loved her. Our hearts are still broken, and we feel so betrayed—why did this happen to us? After all of our sorrow over infertility we brought home a baby who was not destined to be ours. The agency treated us miserably and gave us no support whatsoever—we are very bitter over that. They took our money and refused to help us—we sought counseling on our own prior to relinquishing custody. We wanted to be sure we were doing the right thing. I guess we'll never be fully at peace, but we just knew that we would never be at peace if we could not truly accept our daughter's heritage. . . . I pray for her every night. We are still pursuing adoption and hope that soon we will have a child.

The voluntary return of a child to an adoption agency was extremely rare. Much more common was the loss of an adopted child to the child's biological kin. A strong emphasis on biological connection has fueled not only the infertility industry, but adoption policies. In many celebrated cases, biological kin have been awarded custody of children even if they never knew the child and even when custodial parents have raised a child from birth. The possibility that a child might be taken away caused a tremendous amount of anxiety among the adoptive parents or those considering adoption who wrote letters for this study. Dorothy Norwich and her husband went through painful infertility treatment before they tried to adopt. Finally they became foster parents to a four-year-old girl who was physically, emotionally, and sexually abused. It is a long-term placement and they are trying to adopt the girl they call "our child" after raising her for two years. But the child's birth mother will not sign over custody. Like many children, the girl is caught between adults who are competing to be her legitimate parents. Dorothy is angry that "judges today are . . . putting children back with their *Birth Mother!* Regardless of the past. I have learned that a Birth Mother does not make a Mommy." But unlike the informal practices of the past, the legal system today requires that the child "belong" to one designated family, and Dorothy and her husband anxiously await the court's verdict.

The waiting, struggling, and suffering became too much for some would-be parents, and they came to accept their childlessness. Some found that the process left them with a new philosophy toward life and children. Flo

Hartman looked back on her struggle to have a child. She felt that her child-lessness "contributed to the end of two marriages and has denied me full adult membership in my own clan, my own tribe: The Family of Women." She had several miscarriages, but her husband would not adopt because he "couldn't love a child that wasn't 'his.'" He "would not consider adoption but wanted me to have every drug [and] surgical procedure known at that time. Risks be damned!" She came to recognize the dangers of pursuing the baby quest "at any cost: so medical technology rushes in at great expense in dollars. Then attorneys rush in and courts—to determine who owns the child. And every day already birthed children go without food and shelter. Women maim themselves, risk themselves to give birth." She finally realized that her two decades of teaching in the public schools meant that she was not really childless: "5,000 kids ought to be enough fulfillment for any woman."

Science and Religion

Today, the involuntarily childless have several routes to parenthood: medical, legal, low-tech, or high-tech. Scientific advances have vastly expanded the reproductive technologies available, but for some infertile women and men, religious faith is as important as it was for their colonial forebears three centuries ago. When Grace Kamali and her husband learned that he had a low sperm count, "We both accepted this for what it was worth, and moved forward with our lives." After ten years of marriage, however, they began wishing for "the pitter patter of tiny little feet around the house." At that point, this middle-class Black couple turned to God:

> I asked my husband if he really wanted a child, and if so I would pray for us (I had never prayed for a child before). My husband said he did, so I prayed to God with all my heart and soul. . . . I truly put the situation in God's hands. . . . Praise God! I hope that this will be an inspiration to other couples that are childless. I pray that they will try God as opposed to subjecting themselves to costly, and sometimes risky and disappointing methods of conceiving.

As a lifelong Baptist, she had always believed in the power of prayer, and her prayers were answered. They now have a baby daughter. Grace and her husband decided to put their trust in God, rather than in the physicians, and for them it apparently worked.

According to recent estimates, approximately a third of infertile couples will conceive with no medical intervention, compared to half of those who pursue treatment.[35] Whether or not prayer has anything to do with it, infertile couples may wonder whether the odds of success with treatment are that much better than the odds without it. For the spiritually inclined like Grace, prayer is a less costly and perhaps equally effective route to their reproductive goal. Considering the fact that stress affects fertility, it is likely that for believers, prayer calms the nerves and reduces stress. Grace was by no means alone in her turn to prayer. Many of the infertile wondered, like the Puritan poet Ann Bradstreet centuries before, what sins they had committed that might have rendered them childless—and they turned to their faith for a cure. Leila Ember felt "guilt and unworthiness. . . . God was punishing me for waiting and (foolishly) taking the PILL during the first six months of my marriage." Judy Voler "felt angry at God and blamed him. Once I stopped blaming God, I took the blame on myself. . . . What was wrong with me? Wasn't I as good a woman as they?" For those who blamed themselves, praying for forgiveness may have eased their torment.

Noreen Cooper and her husband were New Age spiritualists who decided to hedge their bets. She is Protestant, her husband is Jewish, but they turned to Native American traditions in their quest. After years of infertility, they went to New Mexico and purchased a Hopi fertility doll and then pursued high-tech infertility treatment. They conceived their daughter through IVF. Crediting their success to "modern technology and ancient mysticism," they called the child their "Hopi baby."

For others, it was not so easy to reconcile high-tech medical intervention with personal faith. Anita Rosaldo, a thirty-year-old Latina and a devout Catholic, was faced with a dilemma over treatment. She had one miscarriage and one premature stillbirth, and her physicians recommended that she take powerful fertility drugs that might cause multiple births. "My dilemma as a Catholic [is] having to abort one child to save the others," which is against her religion. Her priest advised, "Leave it in God's hands, trust in Him." Others gave up their religion, rather than give up infertility treatment, but kept their own private faith. Roberta O'Leary explained, "The Catholic Church of course disagrees with any fertility intervention. This stance confuses us and we tend to ignore their views. It has made us less involved with our church and the Catholic faith. We continue to pray at home and look for God's guidance."

Practicing Catholics were not the only ones who found it difficult to reconcile infertility treatment with the doctrines of their faith. Observant Jews also had to come to terms with some difficult reproductive issues. Traditional Jewish law requires that men have children; reproduction is not required of women. In ancient times, when men had multiple wives, not all the wives had to bear children as long as at least one did. Today, of course, the requirement that men have children means that their wives must, too. But some infertility treatment requires practices forbidden by Jewish law, such as masturbation. To reconcile these conflicting religious laws, some rabbis have interpreted the laws to suggest that masturbation for the goal of reproduction is not "wasted seed" and that all infertility treatments, as well as adoption, are legitimate means of achieving the higher goal of continuing the Jewish people.[36] Among the religiously observant respondents of many different faiths, most found ways to reconcile their reproductive efforts with their beliefs and turned to prayer as well. Whether through organized religion, private faith, or New-Age mysticism, many people held their beliefs at the center of their quest. Technological intervention has not fully replaced the spiritual route to reproductive goals.

The Obsession with Reproduction

For some people who wrote, the baby itself became the spiritual quest, the only thing that would give life meaning. The extreme desperation of some of the childless respondents led them to subordinate everything else in life to the baby quest—even life itself. Serena Whitman wrote that she is so obsessed with having a child that she intends to commit suicide if she is not married and a mother by the time she is forty. She is currently thirty-seven and single. In her fourteen-page single-spaced typed letter, she described a life preoccupied with achieving marriage and motherhood. She decided against single parenthood and pursued marriage as a means to an end, the end being motherhood.

For a self-described "child of the sixties" looking for the nuclear family ideal, the "sexual revolution" placed many obstacles in Serena's path. She got pregnant in college, had an abortion, and has felt bad about it ever since. From a boyfriend she acquired several sexually transmitted diseases, and from an IUD, she developed PID (pelvic inflammatory disease). Later she lived with a man in a commune for several years in a nonmonogamous relationship. "Sex was great," but he did not want children, so she left him. The next man in her life wanted children, but not a relationship. "Our initial discussions about having a kid were to co-parent rather than to be in a relationship with each other. What he wanted was for a woman to have a child for him, and give it to him. Unfortunately we got rather attached to each other." After an ectopic pregnancy, they broke up. "I often get very depressed when my period comes, another month of failure. I used to really enjoy sex and liked to do it often. Since that pregnancy, the only time I have orgasms is when I am ovulating. I cannot become sexually aroused without thinking about getting pregnant."

A few relationships later, Serena met a man who "didn't bother to tell me he had a vasectomy until we had been seeing each other for 4 months. . . . I was annoyed at wasting my time." After this long and painful history, she has only one goal. "At this point I don't want to have sex except to get pregnant. I don't feel very confident about finding someone to share my life with. I don't even know if I am physically capable of having children." She now has PID and a fibroid pressing on her one functioning fallopian tube and ovary.

> Intercourse is painful. Having a husband and children are the two most important things in life to me. I have made a decision that if I still don't have those things when I am 40 years old, I don't want to live any longer. The idea of spending 30 or more years without children or a husband is intolerable.

Serena refuses to compromise on either the reproduction or the mate. "For me, the actual process of pregnancy, giving birth and breast feeding are very important—I don't consider adoption adequate." She does not have the financial resources to be a single parent and rejects artificial insemination because "I believe that it is essential to know the father of my child (and for the child to know the father as well). . . . I believe that babies should come from good, hot sex with someone you love." She also has specific criteria for her marriage partner:

> I don't feel that what I want in a partner is unreasonable, but it is difficult to find someone. I want someone who also wants a life-long relationship and family. Has interests in science, medicine and computers. Likes food, healthy

eating habits, but enjoys all the wonderful variety we are so fortunate to have here in California (and it would be nice if he liked to cook, but not essential). Must read, liking science fiction would be nice. Spiritual, but not into mainstream religion or astrology. Active, into hiking and backpacking—that is my very favorite type of vacation and something I very much want to share with my family.

As for religious compatibility, "For me, the Grateful Dead is a spiritual experience I need to share with my mate."

Serena has a tall order to fill, a private life with all the details worked out and a child at the center. She represents an extreme, of course. But her life incorporates many of the contradictory trends that have shaped the culture of reproduction since the 1960s: the new sexual freedom with all its pleasures and risks, the persistence of the nuclear family ideal, the firm belief that one should be able to construct the private life of one's dreams, the spiritual quest that transcends organized religion, and the obsession with reproduction. Serena claimed that she would rather end her life than transform her dreams to conform to her reality. Perhaps she will change her mind before reaching her fortieth birthday.

The American obsession with reproduction has a long and complex history. New possibilities for achieving procreative goals, along with greater acceptance of a wide range of family structures, have added new layers to the experience of childlessness. The more options that appear possible and legitimate, the more forcefully Americans pursue their dreams and the less willing they are to accept a reality that differs from their desires—even if their desires change. The stakes have become so high that sometimes the children born to the previously infertile face unreasonably high expectations to fulfill their parents' hopes. Kate Foley explained that after years of longing for a child and feeling "ashamed" about her infertility, when the child finally arrived, "you just want everything to be perfect. Perfect child, perfect parent, every material thing a child could ever dream of—it's hard to relax, be human, let the child be her little imperfect self."

Continuity and Change

The pursuit of happiness over the past century has taken a decidedly private turn. Although the family has always been central to American national identity, it originally held a place in political ideology as the place where citizens were nurtured. Private life served public life by sending forth productive individuals to build the nation. In the twentieth century, that process has reversed. Now public life largely serves the needs of private life. The family no longer produces goods or even citizens; rather, it consumes. Although society remains vastly interested in the reproduction of its citizens, its citizens have largely given up on public life. Reproductive goals now reflect individual desires for the good life, and Americans expect the nation's institutions to help them achieve those goals.

Although this intense quest for private fulfillment represents a trend that has accelerated since World War II, it has its roots deep in the nation's past. From the era of early nationhood, when George Washington described "the sequestered walks of connubial life" as the place where "permanent and genuine happiness is to be found,"[37] Americans have directed their pursuit of happiness largely toward private life. But many have balanced that quest with an equally powerful engagement in community and civic enterprises. That is why, until quite recently, childless Americans who dedicated themselves to public pursuits found a respected place in the cultural landscape. Today the voluntarily childless have gained a different kind of legitimacy, based on the widespread belief in the individual choice of personal lifestyles. Even that legitimacy is offered grudgingly in a pronatalist society that equates adulthood with parenthood. The childless who carve out active public lives in lieu of parenthood do so in spite of, rather than because of, the cultural norms and expectations that surround their endeavors. At the same time, the involuntarily childless have gained a new kind of sympathy, grounded in the idea that only the family life of one's choosing can confer happiness. In accord with that belief, personal and societal resources are poured into the effort to enable the infertile to procreate.

The emphasis on private life is not so much a rupture with the past as it is an intensification of a trend. As public life in the United States has atrophied, the private side has loomed larger and larger. Reproduction, accordingly, has become a matter of increasingly high private stakes. But the public stakes in reproduction have not diminished. With private life so evidently detached from civic concerns, why are public institutions and politicians still so preoccupied with individual reproductive behavior? In this matter, too, the historical record is instructive. Since the early national period, reproductive manipulation has served public as well as private ends. Americans of today may either cringe or cheer at the news that postmenopausal women can now give birth to babies; that grand-mothers bear their grandchildren for their infertile offspring; and that sci-entists inject sperm into eggs, "harvest" ova, and clone gametes. But the "brave new world" of reproductive engineering must have raised as many eyebrows over a century ago with such experiments as artificial insemina-tion or the eugenic breeding practiced by Oneida Perfectionists. And the same thin odds that sparked hopes a century ago in the childless who pur-chased Lydia Pinkham's Vegetable Compound, with its promise of "a baby in every bottle," now lure today's infertile to the IVF clinics, with their dismal 80 percent failure rates.[38] The means and technology have changed, but the belief that scientific progress will enable individuals, as well as the society, to manipulate procreative behavior is more powerful than ever.

It is small wonder, then, that as Americans look to the home for per-sonal happiness, they turn to experts to help them achieve their repro-ductive desires. These expectations are embedded in our national ideals. What has evaporated, however, is the optimism and civic engagement that once connected private to public life. Today, individuals look to social institutions to help them achieve private goals, while social institu-tions look to the family to fix the nation's ills. Parenthood looms larger and larger as a force for good or evil. Ideas about parental worthiness still overshadow the true needs of children. For more than a century, institu-tional and political policies and practices have operated on the assump-tion that if the "right" people became parents—those with the "right" genes, background, race, or income—children's needs would be met auto-matically. That presumption has proved tenacious, even though it has never been supported by evidence.

Along with the desire to control and manipulate human reproduction, beliefs about parental worthiness also have a long history. Manifest Des-tiny no longer permeates political rhetoric or explicitly provides the foun-dations for social policies concerning reproduction. But eugenic ideas are still salient, as is evident in the media blitz surrounding the publication of an old-fashioned eugenic polemic like The Bell Curve, by Richard J. Herrnstein and Charles Murray, in 1994. Parental worthiness, based on alleged genetic superiority or economic status, affects decisions ranging from the selection of donor sperm for artificial insemination to custody cases of children with more than one set of "parents." Political debates continue to rage over whether welfare policies should cap benefits after two children and whether poor women should be coerced into using some form of birth control. Parents are still expected to solve the nation's ills by instilling "family values" in their children, while legislation geared toward providing support for families, such as parental leaves and government-sponsored day care, continue to meet with defeat. The nation still expects the family to operate as an autonomous unit that builds society from the bottom up by rearing its citizens, even though it has never functioned in that capacity and cannot do so without institutional support.[39] Today, the family is at the receiving end of the nation's woes, but it is still expected to provide the fix.

The lion's share of that burden falls on women. Although the majority of all women hold jobs outside the home and much lip service is paid to shared reproductive and child-rearing responsibilities, procreation still falls largely within the female domain. Women are still much more likely to be infertility patients than are men (even though men are just as likely to be infertile); there are more available treatments for female reproductive problems; women's bodies are likely to be the ones that are poked, prodded, and pumped with hormones, even if they are fertile and the problem resides with their male partners. They are also more likely to suffer the stigma of childlessness and to be driven to distraction by their inability to achieve their reproductive goals. Women are both more tormented by infertility and more vehemently committed to voluntary childlessness than are men. The fact that reproduction remains primarily a woman's problem is due less to women's biological capacity for pregnancy and more to the cultural norms that still place motherhood at the center of female identity.[40]

The childless do not have different values than the rest of the society. But they articulate their hopes and dreams because they are so often frustrated in their pursuit of happiness. Increasingly, parents and nonparents alike hope to find meaning, status, and happiness in their private lives, removed from the civic and economic arena. The particular reproductive culture that has emerged in the late twentieth century is grounded in a society that looks to the family to solve its problems, but offers the family little in the way of support. Yet many Americans believe that the only place they can find true happiness is in private life. This belief places an overwhelming burden, as well as an overwhelming sense of expectation, on individual procreative behavior. Because the larger society appears out of control and beyond their ability to influence, Americans pursue their reproductive goals with fierce determination. Now that medical, legal, technological, and cultural developments hold out the promise of reproductive self-determination, procreation appears to be one of the few areas of life within a person's control. As long as public life appears bankrupt and alienating, Americans with or without children will continue their pursuit of happiness in the most private areas of life. And as long as Americans care more about each other's reproductive behavior than about each other's children, our private obsession is likely to remain.

Appendix:
A Note on the Sample of Letters
★☆

The letters used in this study, unless otherwise indicated in the endnotes, were gathered using an author's query sent to newspapers and journals across the country. The query letter, addressed to the editors, asked individuals who had experienced childlessness at some point in their lives to write to me about their experiences and feelings. The letter specifically invited responses from men and women, of all ages, ethnic groups, marital status, and sexual orientation, childless for any reason, temporarily or permanently. I indicated the nature of the project and promised anonymity. Cynthia Richter, who provided the research assistance for this part of the project, sent the query to all newspapers with a circulation of over 50,000, as well as to publications that target particular ethnic communities, women, gays and lesbians, and the childless. She made sure that each response was answered and kept track of each respondent who wrote more than once. She organized, tallied, and helped to categorize and analyze the contents.

We had no way of knowing which journals published the query, but more than five hundred people wrote back from all over the country. These respondents do not constitute a random sample or a representative sample of the childless. But no in-depth study of the childless to date has been "representative." The studies I have examined, mostly written since the 1970s, have been primarily qualitative rather than quantitative. Those based on census or other aggregate data have not investigated motives or feelings because the data do not reveal such information. Among the qualitative studies done in recent decades, some have examined men and women, some only women, and some only couples. Some have considered childlessness by choice, others infertility, and others both. But in almost every case, the studies have been based on in-depth interviews with fewer than one hundred subjects, mostly White women or couples.

For example, Carolyn M. Morell's *Unwomanly Conduct: The Challenges of Intentional Childlessness* (New York: Routledge, 1994) was based on interviews with 34 married women who are childless by choice; Mardy S. Ireland's *Reconceiving Women: Separating Motherhood from Female Identity* (New York: Guilford Press, 1993) was based on interviews with 105 childless women; Susan S. Lang, for her book *Women Without Children: The Reasons, the Rewards, the Regrets* (New York: Pharos Books, 1991), interviewed 63 women aged 36 to 100, childless for a variety of reasons, mostly White and middle class, drawn from her personal network; Elaine Campbell, for *The Childless Marriage: An Exploratory Study of Couples Who Do Not Want Children* (London: Tavistock Publications, 1985), interviewed 44 women and 34 of their husbands contacted through a medical clinic in a Scottish city; Diana Burgwyn interviewed 100 married and divorced voluntarily and involuntarily childless people for her book, *Marriage Without Children* (New York: Harper & Row, 1981); Arthur L. Greil interviewed 22 married infertile couples in western New York and studied 449 health histories from an infertility clinic for his book, *Not Yet Pregnant: Infertile Couples in Contemporary America* (New Brunswick, N.J.: Rutgers University Press, 1991); and Marian Faux did 43 in-depth interviews with ambivalent or voluntarily childless women, along with 20 additional questionnaires, for her book, *Childless By Choice: Choosing Childlessness in the Eighties* (Garden City, N.Y.: Anchor Press, 1984). Margarete Sandelowski, for her book *With Child in Mind: Studies of the Personal Encounter with Infertility* (Philadelphia: University of Pennsylvania Press, 1993), interviewed 48 infertile women and 94 couples. These and other studies appear in the footnotes of this book. They are excellent and worthwhile studies, and I have drawn on them extensively.

My own sample differs in several ways. The number of respondents is larger and more diverse than the samples used in most other primarily qualitative studies. But because I did not conduct interviews, I had much less control over the information I received. At the same time, the anonymity of writing enabled some respondents to articulate thoughts and feelings they would not have expressed in face-to-face interviews. The questions and categories were generated by the respondents, not by me. Some of the replies were brief and cursory, but many others were lengthy, continuing for several pages. A few respondents sent tapes rather than letters. Many people wrote twice or three times, often responding to our follow-up letters in which we requested additional information. But respondents did not all provide the same information.

Some gave their age, ethnic background, religion, or occupation, but many did not. It is therefore not particularly useful to use percentages when referring to the number of people in certain categories because only a small percentage of the total included that information. Similarly, if, say, a dozen respondents wrote about the experience in a particular way, it does not mean that none of the others shared those feelings. It means, more likely, that many more did. For that reason, if a particular experience or attitude appeared in a significant number of letters, I interpreted that fact as a signal that the comments did not represent unique or idiosyncratic experiences.

The people who chose to respond did so because they felt a particular need or desire to express their feelings about this issue. Therefore, it is likely that the sample is skewed toward those with particularly strong feelings or significant experiences related to their childlessness. Of the total number of respondents, 89 percent were women; 11 percent were men. In terms of age, 69 respondents were under age 35, 255 were between 35 and 55, 52 were over 55, and the rest did not mention their ages. According to race, 138 described themselves as White, 7 as Black, one as Puerto Rican, two as Asian, three as Mexican American, 2 as Hispanic, 2 as Native American, and three as "multiracial" or of a "different race." The rest did not mention race. A significant minority mentioned their sexual orientation: 14 indicated that they were gay or lesbian, 7 men and 7 women; 65 women and 7 men described themselves as heterosexual; 2 women and 1 man said they were celibate. The rest did not mention their sexual orientation. In terms of marital status, 164 women and 20 men mentioned that they were married, 51 women and 5 men said they were divorced, 14 women and 2 men noted that they were remarried, 32 women and 8 men said they were single, 2 women and 1 man stated that they were widowed, and 7 women described themselves as partnered.

Few mentioned their religious background. The largest number of those who did were the 43 respondents who identified themselves as Catholic and the 12 who said they were Jews. Nine described themselves as Protestant, and several others mentioned other religious affiliations, including Episcopalian (2), Methodist (5), Christian (2), and Pantheist (1). These numbers probably do not reflect the respondents as a whole; those who mentioned their religion were more likely to discuss it in terms of their experience of childlessness. The respondents also appeared to be a highly educated group, as one might expect from those who would choose to answer an author's query. Only 4 mentioned that they had attended high school; 50 mentioned college and 37 cited postgraduate work. The rest did not mention education.

A total of forty-six occupational categories were mentioned in the letters, with small numbers in each. The largest occupational categories mentioned were those of teacher (37), writer or editor (16), manager/administrator (11), nurse (11), physician (4) or other medical professional (8), housewife (3), artist (5), psychologist or counselor (7), lawyer (7), secretary (7), factory worker or other unskilled or semiskilled work (11), and psychologist (9).

I found a number of experiences and feelings repeated in the letters. The repetition of specific words, phrases, or images to describe the experience of childlessness signaled shared cultural meanings. If a significant number of respondents used similar language or described similar concerns, attitudes, or experiences, I looked carefully at those descriptions and at the consistency of language to guide my analysis of childlessness. For example, 3 men and 32 women mentioned feeling incomplete as a man or a woman, and that child-lessness affected their feelings of manhood or womanhood. Among those who were childless by choice, 3 men and 13 women mentioned the need to care for their "child within" or to raise themselves and care for themselves before they could contemplate having children. Also among the voluntarily childless, 4 men and 36 women specifically discussed "freedom" in their choice not to have children or used the term "childfree"; 11 described moth-erhood as a full-time job, requiring full attention; 61 women and 3 men men-tioned that they had chosen to undergo sterilization surgery; and 9 mentioned physicians who refused to perform or resisted performing the surgery. Among all those who wrote, 33 women and 2 men specifically men-tioned abuse they had experienced as children as reasons for their childless-ness; 7 mentioned incest, 22 mentioned physical abuse, and 5 mentioned emotional abuse. At least 8 said that the world was a terrible place for children.

Many described feeling marginalized and stigmatized: 12 described being treated rudely because of their childlessness, and 12 specifically mentioned the stigma of "selfishness" that attached to the childless. In terms of a "maternal instinct," 11 said they had none, and 3 said they did; 16 discussed their ambivalence about having children. Among the infertile, 66 infertile women described infertility treatment as a major physical and emotional ordeal, 15 explained how and why they decided to give up trying to conceive, 22 respondents discussed the pain and torment of infertility, 25 wrote about the costs, 12 women wrote about their husbands' refusal to pursue medical treatment, 3 women did not or would not see a physician, 8 described infertility treatment as a "roller coaster" or "merry-go-round," 10 described the effects of infertility treatment on their sex lives, 12 described accepting or coming to terms with their infertility, 7 mentioned holidays and family reunions as being particularly painful, and 11 specifically mentioned faith or prayer as a response to their childlessness. Of the total, 13 mentioned negative or eugenic attitudes toward parents who were poor, young, unwed, or on welfare, and 6 specifically mentioned their "biological clocks." In terms of health history, 31 women mentioned having abortions, 8 having had two and 3 having had three or more, and 28 mentioned miscarriages, 8 having had two and 14 having had three or more. Among those who were temporarily childless, 18 had one biological child, 11 had two, and one had three or more; 25 had adopted children; 11 had one, 12 had two, and 2 had three or more. In terms of concern about overpopulation, 45 women and 17 men mentioned population and environmental concerns in their letters.

Virtually every letter contained deep, personal feelings about the experience of childlessness, and many, many issues were mentioned that I was unable to include in the book. I did, however, attempt to provide a fair representation of the most frequently expressed attitudes, experiences, and feelings of the childless women and men who provided me with a window into their lives.

Notes
★☆

Introduction. The Public and Private Stake in Reproduction

1. I am grateful to Julia Mickenburg who searched and compiled the lists of various forms of publicity surrounding the Baby M controversy. See also "Regulating the Baby Makers: From Baby M to the Present" (Monticello, Ill.: Vance
   Bibliographies, 1991), for a twenty-eight-page bibliography on the subject.
2. Prithwis Das Gupta, *Future Fertility of Women by Present Age and Parity: Analysis of American Historical Data, 1917–80 (Current Population Reports*, Special
   Studies, Series P-23, No. 142), (Washington, D.C.: U.S. Department of Commerce, Bureau of the Census, 1985): 8.
3. See Elaine Tyler May, *Homeward Bound: American Families in the Cold War Era*
   (New York: Basic Books, 1988).
4. None of the respondents is identified by his or her real name in the book.
   Quotes are attributed to fictionalized names; the same pseudonym is used consistently for each respondent. Ethnicity or nationality implied in the original
   names has been preserved. Any persons who are quoted without citation are
   respondents from the query. For a profile of the respondents, see the Appendix.
5. See, for example, Arthur L. Greil, *Not Yet Pregnant: Infertile Couples in Contemporary America* (New Brunswick, N.J.: Rutgers University Press, 1991). For a
   personal account of the pain of infertility, see Anne Taylor Fleming, *Motherhood Deferred: A Woman's Journey* (New York: Putnam's 1994) and the excerpt
   from that book, "Sperm in a Jar," *New York Times Magazine*, Sunday June 12,
   1994, 52–55.
6. Although many respondents did not identify themselves according to marital

status or sexual orientation, 14 respondents identified themselves as gay or lesbian (7 men and 7 women). See the Appendix for elaboration.

7. The question of whether gay men or lesbians are "fit" for parenthood continues to be debated in the courts. Recently, for example, a Virginia court denied a lesbian mother custody of her biological son, but the Virginia Court of Appeals overruled the lower court's decision and the mother regained custody. See "Homosexuality Does Not Make Parent Unfit," *New York Times*, June 22, 1994, A8.

8. Personal letter to the author, quoted by permission, dated November 10, 1993.

9. A Hamms poll, June 19, 1992, reported that 61 percent supported *Roe v. Wade*, which made abortion legal; a Fuji Tape "Voices of Young America 2" Public Opinion Survey of eighteen to twenty-four year olds in 1992 reported that 64 percent were pro-choice; and the Gallup Poll Monthly, June 1991, reported that polls from 1975 to 1991 showed that the majority were in favor of legal abortion. See Dennis A. Gilbert, *Compendium of Public Opinion* (New York: Facts on File, 1988).

10. One study, Lois Wladis Hoffman and Jean Denby Manis, "The Value of Children in the United States: A New Approach to the Study of Fertility," *Journal of Marriage and the Family* 41 (August 1979): 583–96, showed that few Americans considered children to be an economic utility in the 1970s. See also Viviana A. Zelizer, *Pricing the Priceless Child: The Changing Social Value of Children* (New York: Basic Books, 1985).

11. There are huge literatures on infertility, voluntary childlessness, adoption, and reproductive technology. But no study has investigated all these aspects of childlessness together as part of the changing culture of reproduction in the United States, and no study of the childless has approached the subject historically. A book by Margaret Marsh and Wanda Ronner, *The Empty Cradle*, which traces the social and medical history of infertility, is forthcoming from Johns Hopkins University Press.

12. Rates of lifetime childlessness are difficult to compare accurately over time because of how the statistics have been gathered. Some studies have looked only at White women or at ever-married women, and still others have defined "permanently childless" women as those who had no children at age thirty-five—a highly inaccurate calculation. However, aggregate statistics do reflect changes over time. See U.S. Department of Commerce, Economics and Statistics Administration, Bureau of the Census, *Fertility of American Women: June 1990* (Series P-20, No. 454) (Washington, D.C.: U.S. Department of Commerce, Bureau of the Census, 1990), 12–22; see also Clyde V. Kiser, Wilson H. Grabill, and Arthur A. Campbell, *Trends and Variations in Fertility in the United States* (Cambridge, Mass.: Harvard University Press, 1968), 163.

13. This finding conforms to those of other studies that have examined satisfactions derived from having children. "Stimulation and fun" rank with "primary group ties and affection" at the top of the list. See, for example, Hoffman and Manis, "The Value of Children."

14. Of those who indicated their level of education, only 4 respondents said they had no more than some high school education, 50 said they had some college education, and 37 said they had some postcollege education. See the Appendix.

15. See Hoffman and Manis, "The Value of Children"; Judith Blake, "Is Zero Preferred? American Attitudes Toward Childlessness in the 1970s," *Journal of Marriage and the Family* 41 (May 1979): 245–57; Rose Brewer, "Theorizing Female-led African-American Families," in Bette Dickerson, ed., *Female Headed Households: African-American Women's Perspectives* (Beverly Hills, Calif.: Sage, forthcoming 1995).

Chapter 1. Barren to Infertile: Childlessness Before the Twentieth Century

1. Quoted in Wendy Martin, *An American Triptych* (Chapel Hill: University of North Carolina Press, 1984), 25; see also Laurel Thatcher Ulrich, *Goodwives* (New York: Knopf, 1982), poem quoted on p. 162; Colonel Luther Caldwell, ed., *An Account of Anne Bradstreet the Puritan Poetess and Kindred Topics* (Boston: Damrell & Upham, 1898); and Jeannine Hensley, ed., *The Works of Anne Bradstreet* (Cambridge, Mass.: Belknap Press, 1967).

2. Cotton Mather, *Ornaments for the Daughters of Zion* (1st ed. 1692; reprint of 1741 ed.; Delmar, N.Y.: Scholar's Facsimiles & Reprints, 1978), 67.

3. Quoted in Martin, *American Triptych*, 25.

4. Robert Hutchinson, ed., *Poems of Anne Bradstreet* (New York: Dover, 1969), 179–80.

5. Birth control methods were not nearly as effective as they are today, but they were used to space children and to avoid pregnancy. For a discussion of birth control methods that were available at the time, see Linda Gordon, *Woman's Body, Woman's Right: Birth Control in America*, rev. ed. (New York: Viking Penguin, 1990), chap. 2; see also Catherine M. Scholten, *Childbearing in American Society, 1650–1850* (New York: New York University Press, 1985), 8–22.

6. Jacqueline Jones, "Race, Sex, and Self-Evident Truths: The Status of Black Women During the Era of the American Revolution," in Ronald Hoffman and Peter J. Albert, eds., *Women in the Age of the American Revolution* (Charlottesville: University Press of Virginia, 1989), 293–337.

7. Ulrich, *Goodwives*, 156–63; quote on p. 161.

8. Quoted in Scholten, *Childbearing in American Society*, 8.

9. Phillippe Ariés, *Centuries of Childhood: A Social History of Family Life* (New York: Vintage Books, 1962), 268.

10. Laurel Thatcher Ulrich, *A Midwife's Tale: The Life of Martha Ballard, Based on Her Diary, 1785–1812* (New York: Knopf, 1990), 12.

11. Viviana A. Zelizer, *Pricing the Priceless Child: The Changing Social Value of Children* (New York: Basic Books, 1985), 8–31, quote on 25.

12. Philip J. Greven, Jr., "Family Structure in Andover," *William and Mary Quarterly*, 3rd ser., 23 (1966): 239–56. See also Greven, *Four Generations: Population, Land and Family in Colonial Andover, Massachusetts* (Ithaca, N.Y.: Cornell University Press, 1970). In seventeenth-century New England, the population grew mainly from births, rather than from migration. Fertility in the middle colonies was also high compared to Europe because the colonists had a higher marriage rate and married at an earlier age, thus extending the childbearing years. The pattern was different in Maryland, where population growth did not result from births until the late 1680s. It was not until the early eighteenth century that the majority of the adult White population in Maryland was born in the colony. This difference was due to the profoundly different mission and migratory pattern of the settlers in the Chesapeake. Unlike New England, men came to Maryland primarily for economic, not religious, reasons, and women followed them to find husbands. There were far more men than women, which meant that virtually every woman would marry. But these women married late because most—85 percent—came as indentured servants and owed their masters a number of years of service. If they married during their term of service, their husbands had to purchase their remaining time. Since few men could afford to do so, most servants had to wait to marry. But not all waited to have children: Over 20 percent of the female servants bore children out of wedlock between 1658 and 1705 in one Maryland county. In contrast, few children were born out of wedlock to women who were not servants because these women were free to marry the fathers. About one-third of all immigrant women were pregnant at the time of marriage, however, twice the rate of English women. See Robert V. Wells, "Family Size and Fertility in 18th Century America: A Study of Quaker Families," *Population Studies* 25 (April 1971):73–81, which looks at family size among the Quakers; Lois Green Carr, Russell R. Menard, and Lorena S. Walsh, *Robert Cole's World: Agriculture and Society in Early Maryland* (Chapel Hill: Institute of Early American History and Culture, University of North Carolina Press, 1991), esp. chap. 5; Lois Green Carr and Lorena S. Walsh, "The Planter's Wife: The Experience of White Women in Seventeenth-Century Maryland," *William and Mary Quarterly*, 3rd ser., 34 (1977): 542–71; and Julia Cherry Spruill, *Women's Life and Work in the Southern Colonies* (New York: Norton, 1972).
13. Benjamin Coleman, *The Duty and Honour of Aged Women* (Boston: B. Green, 1711, from Women's Collection Microfilm Series), 28.
14. Mather, *Ornaments for the Daughters of Zion*, 99–101.
15. Quoted in Scholten, *Childbearing*, 14–15.
16. Steven Mintz and Susan Kellogg, *Domestic Revolutions: A Social History of American Family Life* (New York: Free Press, 1988), 12.
17. Carol F. Karlsen, *The Devil in the Shape of a Woman: Witchcraft in Colonial New England* (New York: Vintage Books, 1989), 144.
18. Lyle Koehler, "The Case of the American Jezebels: Anne Hutchinson and Female Agitation during the Years of Antinomian Turmoil, 1636–1640," *William and*

Mary Quarterly, 3d ser., 31 (1974): 55–78; and Karlsen, *Devil*, 16–20. Although most midwives and healers were widely respected and never accused of heretical practices, female medical practitioners in Europe, as well as in America, were subject to persecution as witches. See Gordon, *Woman's Body*, 31–32.

19. Karlsen, *Devil*, 6–7.
20. John Demos, *Entertaining Satan* (New York: Oxford University Press, 1982), 327; Ulrich, *Goodwives*, 157–59; and Karlsen, *Devil*, 20, 144.
21. Demos, *Entertaining Satan*, 327.
22. Ibid.; Karlsen, *Devil*, 52–57.
23. Joy Barbre, "From 'Goodwives' to Menoboomers: Reinventing Menopause in American History" (Ph.D. diss., American Studies, University of Minnesota, 1994); and Karlsen, *Devil*, 119.
24. Demos, *Entertaining Satan*, 62.
25. John Demos, *A Little Commonwealth* (New York: Oxford University Press, 1970).
26. Ulrich, *Goodwives*, 156–59; see also Lawrence Stone, "Family History in the 1980s: Past Achievements and Future Trends," *Journal of Interdisciplinary History* 12 (Summer 1981): 51–87.
27. John Robinson, quoted in Robert Griswold, *Fatherhood in America: A History* (New York: Basic Books, 1993), 10; see also Phillip J. Greven, *Child-Rearing Concepts, 1628–1861* (Itasca, Ill.: F. E. Peacock, 1973).
28. See, for example, Phillippe Ariés, "The Family and the City in the Old World and the New," and John Demos, "Images of the American Family Then and Now," both in Virginia Tufte and Barbara Myerhoff, eds., *Changing Images of the Family* (New Haven, Conn.: Yale University Press, 1979), 29–41, 43–60. For a discussion of early American inheritance practices, see Toby L. Ditz, *Property and Kinship: Inheritance in Early Connecticut, 1750–1820* (Princeton, N.J.: Princeton University Press, 1986). See also "Bonds of Apprenticeship, 1655–1705, Kent County, Maryland, 1655," in Donald M. Scott and Bernard Wishy, eds., *America's Families: A Documentary History* (New York: Harper & Row, 1982), 160. Even if both parents were alive, a child might be placed in another home, voluntarily or by the civil or religious authorities. Since child rearing was an important community responsibility, parents who were "adjudged incapable of supporting and bringing up such child or children, by reason of his, her, or their idle, dissolute, and disorderly course of life, or that they neglect to take due care of the education and instruction of such child or children in Christian principles, that then it shall and may be lawful . . . for the churchwardens of the said parish . . . to bind out, or put out to service or apprenticeship, such child or children." From the Laws of Virginia, February 1727, excerpted in Scott and Wishy, *America's Families*, 159.
29. Scholten, *Childbearing*, 8–22; "The Declaration, Dying Warning, and Advice of Rebekah Chamblit" (Boston, 1733), in Scott and Wishy, *America's Families*, 22. On birth control in preindustrial Europe and America and on child-spacing efforts, see Gordon, *Woman's Body*, esp. chap. 2.

30. Scholten, *Childbearing*, 13–15; quote on p. 15. For additional excerpts from Elizabeth Sandwith Drinker's diary (1758–1807), see Cecil K. Drinker, *Not So Long Ago: A Chronicle of Medicine and Doctors in Colonial Philadelphia* (New York: Oxford University Press, 1937).

31. Mintz and Kellogg, *Domestic Revolutions*, 12; for a classic article on Puritan sexuality, see Edmund S. Morgan, "The Puritans and Sex," *New England Quarterly* 15 (December 1942): 591–607. See also Edmund S. Morgan, *The Puritan Family* (New York: Harper & Row, 1966).

32. Nancy F. Cott, "Eighteenth-Century Family and Social Life Revealed in Massachusetts Divorce," in Nancy F. Cott and Elizabeth H. Pleck, eds., *A Heritage of Her Own: Toward a New Social History of American Women* (New York: Simon & Schuster, 1979), 107–35, quotes on 119.

33. John Demos, "The American Family in Past Times," *American Scholar* 43 (1974): 424–26.

34. From *Records and Files of the Quarterly Courts of Essex County, Massachusetts* (Salem, Mass., June 1682), in Scott and Wishy, *America's Families*, 96.

35. Demos, *Little Commonwealth*, 94–95.

36. For discussions of early American medical practices, see Paul Starr, *The Social Transformation of American Medicine* (New York: Basic Books, 1982), chap. 1; Judith Walzer Leavitt, *Brought to Bed: Child-Bearing in America, 1750–1950* (New York: Oxford University Press, 1986), chaps. 1 and 2; Ulrich, *A Midwife's Tale*; and Whitfield J. Bell, Jr., "A Portrait of the Colonial Physician," in Judith Walzer Leavitt and Ronald L. Numbers, eds., *Sickness and Health in America: Readings in the History of Medicine and Public Health* (Madison: University of Wisconsin Press, 1978), 41–53. The quote from Franklin is from "Benjamin Franklin to a Friend," June 25, 1745, in Scott and Wishy, *America's Families*, 55.

37. Ulrich, *Midwife's Tale*, 171–72; Charles W. Bodemer, "Natural Religion and Generation Theory in Colonial America," *Clio Medica* (Amsterdam: B. M. Israel) 11, no. 4 (1976): 233–43.

38. Ulrich, *Midwife's Tale*, 12–56, 171–72.

39. Nicholas Culpeper, *A Directory for Midwives; or a Guide for Women* (London: John Streater, 1671), 68–78 (Book 3: "Of What Hinders Conception, together with its Remedies"), 89–99 ("What Hinders Conception"); and Part 2, pp. 130–40 ("Of Barrenness and Wont of Conception").

40. Fertility was high compared to the West Indies, where half the colonial families in the 1720s had no children. The island colonies had few women, either European or African, and fewer children were born to each woman. At any given time, from one-fourth to one-half of all White island families had no children. By comparison, in New York at the same time, only one in five families had no children. Because slavery was particularly brutal on the islands, the death rate among Africans was extremely high and the population was replenished by the slave trade, rather than by reproduction. Infant mortality was also higher on the islands, and the few White children who survived there were likely to be sent back to England for schooling. See Robert V.

Wells, "Household Size and Composition in the British Colonies," *Journal of Interdisciplinary History* 4 (Spring 1974): 543–70.

41. See John D'Emilio and Estelle Freedman, *Intimate Matters: A History of Sexuality in America* (New York: Harper & Row, 1988), chaps. 3 and 4.

42. John Adams, "Fourth Annual Message to Congress, Washington, D.C., November 22, 1800," in Janet Podell and Steven Anzovin, eds., *Speeches of the American Presidents* (New York: Wilson, 1988), 33.

43. Thomas Jefferson, "First Inaugural Address, Washington, D.C., March 4, 1801," in Podell and Anzovin, eds., *Speeches of the American Presidents*, 39.

44. Andrew Jackson, "Second Annual Message, Dec. 6, 1830," in Fred L. Israel, ed., *The State of the Union Messages of American Presidents, 1790–1966*, vol. 1 (New York: Chelsea House, 1966), 335.

45. J. Hector St. John de Crèvecoeur, *Letters from an American Farmer*, enlarged French ed. (1787), frontispiece. This frontispiece, entitled *Ubi panis, et libertas, ibi Patria*, was designed by C. Bornée and engraved by P. Martini. See illustration at the beginning of chap. 1.

46. The structure of the family actually changed little, although the ideology of the home and the functions of the household changed dramatically. For an excellent discussion of family structure, see Steven Ruggles, "The Transformation of American Family Structure," *American Historical Review* 99 (February 1994): 103–28. See also Christine Stansell, *City of Women: Sex and Class in New York, 1789–1860* (New York: Knopf, 1986).

47. *The American Spectator, or Matrimonial Preceptor. A Collection (with additions and variations) of Essays, Epistles, Precepts, and Examples, relating to the Married State, from the most celebrated Writers, Ancient and Modern, adapted to the State of Society in the American Republic* (Boston, Manning & Loring, for David West, proprietor of the copyright, 1797), 285–86.

48. Miriam Anne Bourne, *First Family: George Washington and His Intimate Relations* (New York: Norton, 1982), 106–7.

49. Quoted in Bourne, *First Family*, 107.

50. M. J. V. Smith, "The Father Who Was Not a Father," *Virginia Medical Monthly* 103 (January 1976): 14–22. I am grateful to Richard D. Amelar, M.D., for calling this article to my attention.

51. M. L. Weems, *Hymen's Recruiting Sargeant, or, the New Matrimonial Tat-Too for the Old Bachelors* (1821), 12–14.

52. Karen Lystra, *Searching the Heart: Women, Men, and Romantic Love in Nineteenth-Century America* (New York: Oxford University Press, 1989), 77–78; Anthony Rotundo, *American Manhood: Transformations in Masculinity from the Revolution to the Modern Era* (New York: Basic Books, 1993), 158. The historian Robert Griswold noted that "the paternal dominance and evangelical authority that infused Calvinist visions of family life in the seventeenth century eroded in the eighteenth century, as they were slowly replaced by an emphasis on more affective, less instrumental family relationships. Hierarchy and order, the watchwords of older forms of paternal dominance, gave way to a growing emphasis on

mutuality, companionship, and personal happiness." Quote is from Griswold, *Fatherhood in America*, 11.

53. Yasuhide Kawashima, "Adoption in Early America," *Journal of Family Law* 20 (1981–82): 677–96.

54. Jamil Shaheen Zainaldin, "The Origins of Modern Legal Adoption: Child Exchange in Boston, 1851–93" (Ph.D. Diss., University of Chicago, 1976), 6–7, 12–13, 24–26, 96; Stephen B. Presser, "The Historical Background of the American Law of Adoption," *Journal of Family Law* 11 (1971): 465.

55. Jamil S. Zainaldin, "The Emergence of a Modern American Family Law: Child Custody, Adoption, and the Courts, 1796–1851," *Northwestern University Law Review* 73, no. 6 (1979): 1038–89; cases cited and quotes on pp. 1052–55.

56. Temporary Home for the Destitute, *Annual Report* (1859), quoted in Zainaldin, "Origins of Modern Legal Adoption," 315.

57. Zainaldin, "Origins of Modern Legal Adoption," 99–103.

58. Diary of Sally Hitchcock Bliss, entries from October 7, 1828, and February 15, 1829, American Antiquarian Society, Worcester, Mass. I am grateful to Nancy Cott for alerting me to this diary and to Karin Gedge, who generously shared her notes from her research.

59. Starr, *Social Transformation of American Medicine*; quote is from Alexander Hamilton, *A Treatise on the Management of Female Complaints* (New York: Samuel Campell, 1792), 108–9.

60. See Adrian W. Zorgniotti, "Spermatozoa Count: A Short History," *Urology* 5 (May 1975): 672–73; and Starr, *Social Transformation of American Medicine*, 36.

61. Hugh Smythson, *The Compleat Family Physician; or Universal Medical Repository Containing the Causes, Symptoms, Preventions and Cures of all the Maladies to which Human Nature is Subject from Birth to the Grave* (London: Harrison & Co., 1781), 433–34.

62. See Starr, *Social Transformation of American Medicine*, chap. 3. For an excellent discussion of the development of infertility treatment, see Margaret Marsh and Wanda Ronner, *The Empty Cradle* (Baltimore, Md.: Johns Hopkins University Press, forthcoming). I am grateful to Margaret Marsh for sharing her work in progress.

63. See Elaine Tyler May, "Artificial Insemination: The First Debate," in William Graebner, ed., *True Stories of the American Past* (New York: McGraw-Hill, 1993), 74–87; and Anne Lockhart Needham, "Artificial Insemination and the Emergence of Medical Authority in Twentieth-Century America" (senior thesis, Harvard University, 1988).

64. D'Emilio and Freedman, *Intimate Matters*, 58; and Joan M. Jensen, *Loosening the Bonds: Mid-Atlantic Farm Women 1750–1850* (New Haven, Conn.: Yale University Press, 1986), 20–27.

65. Increasing uses of birth control and abortion resulted in greater intervals between births, and as children spent more years living with their parents, child rearing, rather than childbearing, became the most time-consuming part of a woman's life. See Mintz and Kellogg, *Domestic Revolutions*, 51–54; and

D'Emilio and Freedman, *Intimate Matters*, 58. See also Gordon, *Woman's Body*, 24–61.

66. Daniel Scott Smith, "Family Limitation, Sexual Control, and Domestic Feminism in Victorian America," in Cott and Pleck, *Heritage*, 222–45. Quotes from Henry Adams drawn from J. C. Levenson et al., eds., *The Letters of Henry Adams*, 6 vols. (Cambridge, Mass. Harvard University Press, 1988), 2:233, 1:504, 2:316. For a discussion of Adams's childlessness and his references to his work as his "offspring," see T. J. Jackson Lears, *No Place of Grace: Antimodernism and the Transformation of American Culture, 1880–1920* (New York: Pantheon, 1981), 266–69. I am grateful to C. Joshua Borowicz for alerting me to this material and for sharing his own work on the subject.

67. For a classic study of the origins of racial attitudes, see Winthrop Jordan, *White Over Black: American Attitudes Toward the Negro, 1550–1812* (Chapel Hill: University of North Carolina Press, 1968).

68. Ellen Rothman, *Hands and Hearts: A History of Courtship in America* (New York: Basic Books, 1984).

69. Charles E. Rosenberg, "Sexuality, Class and Role in 19th-Century America," in Elizabeth H. Pleck and Joseph H. Pleck, eds., *The American Man* (Englewood Cliffs, N.J.: Prentice Hall, 1980), 219–54, quote is on p. 226; see also Michael Gordon, "The Ideal Husband as Depicted in the 19th Century Marriage Manual," in *American Man*, 145–57; Ben Barker-Benfield, "The Spermatic Economy: A 19th-Century View of Sexuality," in Michael Gordon, ed., *The American Family in Social-Historical Perspective* (New York: St. Martin's Press, 1973), 336–72; Nancy F. Cott, "Passionlessness: An Interpretation of Victorian Sexual Ideology, 1790–1850," in Cott and Pleck, *A Heritage of Her Own*, 162–81; Carol Groneman, "Nymphomania: The Historical Construction of Female Sexuality," *Signs: Journal of Women in Culture and Society* 19 (Winter 1994): 337–67; and Kevin Mumford, "'Lost Manhood' Found: Male Sexual Impotence and Victorian Culture in the United States," *Journal of the History of Sexuality* 3, no. 1 (1992): 33–57.

70. Robert Dale Owen, *Moral Physiology, or, A Brief and Plain Treatise on the Population Question*, 5th ed. (New York: Wright & Owen, 1831).

71. Charles Knowlton, *Fruits of Philosophy, or the Private Companion of Young Married People* (London, n.d.), 33–36, excerpted in Erna Olafson Hellerstein, Leslie Parker Hume, and Karen M. Offen, eds., *Victorian Women: A Documentary Account of Women's Lives in Nineteenth-Century England, France and the United States* (Stanford, Calif.: Stanford University Press, 1981), 190–92; and D'Emilio and Freedman, *Intimate Matters*, 59–60.

72. D'Emilio and Freedman, *Intimate Matters*, 57–66; Linda Gordon, *Woman's Body*, 52–60.

73. See Beverly Hungry Wolf, *The Ways of My Grandmothers* (New York: Morrow, 1980), 202–3; and Virgil J. Vogel, *American Indian Medicine* (Norman: University of Oklahoma Press, 1970), 165–66, 238–44.

74. D'Emilio and Freedman, *Intimate Matters*, 63–66; and James C. Mohr, *Abortion*

in America: The Origins and Evolution of National Policy, 1800–1900 (New York: Oxford University Press, 1978), chaps. 1 and 4; see also Carl N. Degler, At Odds: Women and the Family in America from the Revolution to the Present (New York: Oxford University Press, 1980), chap. 9; C. P. Frost, "Report of a Trial for Criminal Abortion," American Medical Monthly and New York Review 14 (September 1860): 196–97, 201–2, reprinted in Hellerstein et al., eds., Victorian Women, 201–2. See also Janet Farrell Brodie, Contraception and Abortion in Nineteenth-Century America (Ithaca, N.Y.: Cornell University Press, 1994).

75. See Linda K. Kerber, Women of the Republic: Intellect and Ideology in Revolutionary America (Chapel Hill: University of North Carolina Press, 1980).

76. Quoted in Lee Virginia Chambers-Schiller, Liberty, A Better Husband: Single Women in America, The Generations of 1780–1840 (New Haven, Conn.: Yale University Press, 1984), 59–62.

77. Lydia Maria Child, The Mother's Book, 2nd ed. (Boston: 1831), pp. 1–5, excerpted in Hellerstein et al., Victorian Women, 242–44.

78. See Gerda Lerner, The Grimke Sisters from South Carolina, Pioneers for Women's Rights and Abolitionism (New York: Schocken Books, 1971); and Lois W. Banner, "Elizabeth Cady Stanton: Early Marriage and Feminist Rebellion," in Linda K. Kerber and Jane DeHart-Mathews, eds., Women's America: Refocusing the Past (New York: Oxford University Press, 1987), 201–12.

79. Rotundo, American Manhood, 140–46; Ik Marvel, Reveries of a Bachelor (New York, 1851), 19–28, excerpted in Scott and Wishy, America's Families, 228.

80. Mary Wollstonecraft to Jane Arden (1782 or 1783) in Collected Letters of Mary Wollstonecraft, ed. Ralph M. Wardle, 1979, excerpted in Bridget Hill, ed., Eighteenth Century Women: An Anthology (London: Allen & Unwin, 1984), 79.

81. Journal of Louisa May Alcott, February 14, 1868, cited in Chambers-Schiller, Liberty, A Better Husband, 2–3; see also Ednah D. Cheney, Louisa May Alcott: Her Life, Letters and Journals (Boston, 1889), 266–75, excerpted in Hellerstein et al., Victorian Women, 338–40.

82. Quoted in Chambers-Schiller, Liberty, 55.

83. Ibid., 2–3; quotes on pp. 18, 55. By the twentieth century, the trend in singlehood reversed. Among women born at the turn of the century, 8 percent remained single, but among the next generation born in the teens and twenties, less than 5 percent remained single. In other words, the percentage of women who remained single was more than twice as high among those coming of age in the mid-nineteenth century than among those who reached adulthood in the mid-twentieth century. See Daniel Scott Smith, "Family Limitation, Sexual Conduct, and Domestic Feminism," 224.

84. Excerpted from Edward Deming Andrews, The People Called Shakers: A Search for the Perfect Society (New York: Dover, 1963), pp. 253, 256, in Scott and Wishy, America's Families, 338. See also D'Ann Campbell, "Women's Life in Utopia: The Shaker Experiment in Sexual Equality Reappraised, 1810–1860," New England Quarterly 51 (March 1978): 23–38; and Stephen J. Stein, The Shaker Experience In America (New Haven, Conn.: Yale University Press, 1994).

85. Orson Pratt, "Celestial Marriage Explained," in *The Most Holy Principle: Vol. I: The Law and the Testimony*, excerpted in Scott and Wishy, *America's Families*, 342; Joan Iversen, "Feminist Implications of Mormon Polygyny," *Feminist Studies* 10 (Fall 1984): 505–36; and Joan Smyth Iversen, "A Debate on the American Home: The Antipolygamy Controversy, 1880–1890," *Journal of the History of Sexuality* 1 (1991): 585–602. On Ellen Whittaker, I am grateful to Dawn Pulsipher for sharing her unpublished paper, "From Monogamy to Polygamy: The Stories of Ellen Whittaker and Mary Ann Wilson," University of Minnesota, 1994.

86. Quote is from Allan Estlake, member of the Oneida Community, in *The Oneida Community: A Record of an Attempt to Carry Out the Principles of Christian Unselfishness and Scientific Race Improvement* (London: George Redway, 1900), 94. See also Lawrence Foster, *Religion and Sexuality: Three American Communal Experiments of the Nineteenth Century* (New York: Oxford University Press, 1981); and Lawrence Foster, *Women, Family and Utopia: Communal Experiments of the Shakers, Oneida Community and the Mormons* (Syracuse, N.Y.: Syracuse University Press, 1991).

87. See Gordon, *Woman's Body*, 93–113, for an excellent discussion of voluntary motherhood.

88. Deborah Gray White, *Ar'n't I a Woman? Female Slaves in the Plantation South* (New York: Norton, 1985), chap. 2; and Herbert G. Gutman, *The Black Family in Slavery and Freedom, 1750–1925* (New York: Pantheon, 1976), 75–80.

89. See, for example, Herbert Gutman and Richard Sutch, "Victorians All? The Sexual Mores and Conduct of Slaves and Their Masters," in Paul A. David, ed., *Reckoning With Slavery: A Critical Study of the Quantitative History of American Negro Slavery* (New York: Oxford University Press, 1976), 134–60; see also Frederick Bancroft, *Slave Trading in the Old South* (Baltimore, Md.: J. H. Furst, 1931); and Gutman, *The Black Family*, 75–80; see also Captain Theophilus Conneau, *A Slaver's Log Book, or 20 Years' Residence in Africa* (original 1826; Englewood Cliffs, N.J.: Prentice Hall, 1976), 64–67. In some areas, particularly in northern areas of the South where the soil was worn out, slave breeding was the principle economic activity. One observer noted that in Maryland and Virginia, "slaves were seldom kept in these States for the sake of raising crops, but crops were often cultivated for the sake of raising slaves." See Bancroft, *Slave Trading in the Old South*, 74–87. On the slave-trading business, see Thomas R. Dew, *Review of the Debate in the Virginia Legislature of 1831 and 1832* (original 1832; Westport, Conn.: Negro University Press, 1970), 47–69; and Richard Sutch, "The Breeding of Slaves for Sale and the Westward Expansion of Slavery, 1850–1860," in Stanley L. Engerman and Eugene D. Genovese, eds., *Race and Slavery in the Western Hemisphere: Quantitative Studies* (Princeton, N.J.: Princeton University Press, 1975), 173–210.

90. Gutman, *The Black Family*, 75–80.

91. Mintz and Kellogg, *Domestic Revolutions*, 73.

92. Rose, "Look for some others for to 'plenish de earth," Manuscript Slave Narra-

tive Collection, Federal Writers' Project, 1941, vol. 17, Texas Narratives, part 4, pp. 174–78, Library of Congress, Washington, D.C., in Kerber and DeHart-Mathews, *Women's America*, 98–100.

93. On some plantations, a newborn's mother got a small pig or a new frock when the child was a year old. Because infant mortality was high among babies of field hands, one owner offered incentives: "for every baby that had been properly attended to, thirteen months old and in sound health, he rewarded the mother with a muslin or calico frock." See Bancroft, *Slave Trading in the Old South*, 86; see also Gutman, *The Black Family*, 75–80.

94. Letters, such as these, are rare, since slaves were generally forbidden to learn how to read or write and could correspond only if a White person wrote the letter for them. This quote is from Maria Perkins to her husband Richard Perkins, October 8, 1852, Ulrich B. Phillips Collection, Yale University Library, New Haven, Conn.; it is also in Kerber and DeHart-Mathews, *Women's America*, 97.

95. Frances Anne Kemble, *Journal of a Residence on a Georgian Plantation in 1838–39* (New York: Knopf, 1961). See also Gutman, *The Black Family*, 76–77.

96. See Brenda Child, "A Bitter Lesson: Native Americans and the Government Boarding School Experience, 1890–1940" (Ph.D. diss., University of Iowa, 1993). One excellent documentary film account is *In The White Man's Image* (produced by WGBH Boston for *The American Experience*, 1992).

Chapter 2. The "Race Suicide" Panic: Eugenics and the Pressure to Procreate

1. Theodore Roosevelt, quoted in Linda Gordon, *Woman's Body, Woman's Right: Birth Control in America*, rev. ed. (New York: Viking Penguin, 1990), 133, 139–40; and "Mr. Roosevelt's Views on Race Suicide," *Ladies Home Journal*, February 1906, 21. Roosevelt published extensively on the subject; see, for example, Roosevelt, "Race Decadence," *Outlook* 97 (1911): 763–69; and Roosevelt, "Women's Rights; and the Duties of Both Men and Women," *Outlook* 100 (1912): 262–66; see also Ethel Wadsworth Cartland, "Childless Americans," *Outlook* 105 (1913): 585–88.

2. See Gordon, *Woman's Body*, 48, 150–51; Peter G. Filene, *Him/Her/Self: Sex Roles in Modern America*, 2nd ed. (Baltimore, Md.: Johns Hopkins University Press, 1986), 41; Royal S. Copeland, M.D., "Alarming Decrease in American Babies," *Ladies Home Journal*, July 1922, 37ff; and "Letters to the Editor," *Ladies Home Journal*, April 1906, 2.

3. Daniel J. Kevles, *In the Name of Eugenics: Genetics and the Uses of Human Heredity* (New York: Knopf, 1985), 44–58; and Harry H. Laughlin, "The Eugenics Record Office at the End of Twenty-Seven Months of Work," Report no. 1, June 1913, from Social Welfare History Archives, University of Minnesota, Eugenics Collection.

4. Kevles, *Eugenics*, 61–63.

5. "A College Baby Crop," *Good Housekeeping*, June 1911, 738–39; on singleness among women's college graduates, see Gordon, *Woman's Body*, 136; quote is from Roswell Hill Johnson, "To Urge the Good to Marry," *Literary Digest*, March 28, 1914, 693–94.

6. Quoted in Donald M. Scott and Bernard Wishy, eds., *America's Families: A Documentary History* (New York: Harper & Row, 1982), 466.

7. A. D. Hard, M.D., "Artificial Impregnation," *Medical World* 27 (April 1909): 163–64. All quotes and descriptions of the event are taken from this article.

8. On sterility due to the lack of female orgasm, see Th. H. Van De Velde, M.D., *Fertility and Sterility in Marriage: Their Voluntary Promotion and Limitation*, trans F. W. Stella Browne (New York: Covici-Freide Medical Books, 1931), 169–70. See also Thomas Laqueur, *Making Sex: Body and Gender from the Greeks to Freud* (Cambridge, Mass.: Harvard University Press, 1990).

9. Augustus K. Gardner, A.M., M.D., *The Causes and Curative Treatment of Sterility, with a Preliminary Statement of the Physiology of Generation* (New York: De Witt & Davenport, 1856), 160–63; and Dr. William A. Alcott, *The Young Woman's Book of Health* (New York: Miller, Orton, Mulligan, 1835), 224.

10. See Victoria Bissell Brown's biography in progress, "The Young Jane Addams," which I am grateful to Brown for sharing with me.

11. All quotes from readers who responded to the article by Dr. Hard are from Letters to the Editor, *Medical World* 27 (May, June, and July, 1909).

12. A. D. Hard, M.D., Letter to the Editor, *Medical World* 27 (July 1909): 306.

13. Charlotte Perkins Gilman, "Race Improvement," *The Independent* 66 (March 25, 1909): 629–32; on Gilman, see Sara Evans, *Born for Liberty* (New York: Free Press, 1989), 154–55.

14. Lydia Kingsmill Commander, *The American Idea: Does the National Tendency Toward a Small Family Point to Race Suicide or Race Development?* (New York: Barnes & Co., 1907), 97–98, 207, 221.

15. Gordon, *Woman's Body*, 110.

16. See, for example, Diane Paul, "Eugenics and the Left," *Journal of the History of Ideas* 45 (1984): 567–90; Kenneth M. Ludmerer, "American Geneticists and the Eugenics Movement, 1905–1935," *Journal of the History of Biology* (1977): 337–62; Kevles, *Eugenics*, 63–90. See also Molly Ladd-Taylor, *Mother-Work: Women, Child Welfare, and the State, 1890–1930* (Urbana: University of Illinois Press, 1994).

17. Richard Jensen, "Family, Career, and Reform: Women Leaders of the Progressive Era," in Michael Gordon, ed., *The American Family in Social-Historical Perspective* (New York: St. Martin's Press, 1973), 267–80.

18. On Boston marriages, see John D'Emilio and Estelle Freedman, *Intimate Matters: A History of Sexuality in America* (New York: Harper & Row, 1988), 191–93. See also Brown, "The Young Jane Addams"; Estelle B. Freedman, *Maternal Justice: Miriam Van Waters and the Female Reform Tradition, 1887–1974* (Chicago: University of Chicago Press, forthcoming), chap. 8. Along with Van Waters, the

nineteenth-century pioneer woman physician Elizabeth Blackwell and her sister adopted children, as did such twentieth-century women as Assistant U.S. Attorney General Mabel Walker Willebrandt, the psychologist Jessie Taft and her life partner Virginia Robinson, and others who could afford to do so. It became much more difficult for single women to adopt children after World War II.

19. George B. H. Swayze, M.D., "Reluctant Pregnancy," *Medical Times*, November 1909, 321–25; quote on p. 321.

20. See article and discussion, S. Pozzi, "On the Surgical Treatment of a Most Frequent Cause of Dysmenorrhea and Sterility in Women," *Transactions of the American Gynecological Society* 34 (1919): 360–75.

21. Editorial, "Is the Human Race in Peril?" *The Independent* 65 (December 31, 1908): 1626–28; Editorial, "Our Duty to Posterity," *The Independent* 66 (February 4, 1909): 269–71.

22. George J. Engelmann, M.D., "The Increasing Sterility of American Women," *Journal of the American Medical Association* 37 (1901): 890–97.

23. Ibid. Responses were included at the end of the article.

24. A. J. Rongy, M.D., "Primary Sterility in Women: A Study Based Upon 120 Cases," *Medical Record* 79 (February 18, 1911): 291–99; 1914 study cited in Linda Gordon, *Woman's Body*, 202; see also Allan Brandt, *No Magic Bullet: A Social History of Venereal Disease in the United States, 1880–1980* (New York: Oxford University Press, 1985).

25. Margarete J. Sandelowski, "Failures of Volition: Female Agency and Infertility in Historical Perspective," *Signs: Journal of Women in Culture and Society* 15 (1990): 475–99. Sandelowski found that "the failure to reproduce at all or insufficient numbers was increasingly viewed as a consequence of the failure to want to reproduce. . . . A constant theme in medical and prescriptive literature on women's health and fertility was that expanded education and women's ambitions perverted their biological destiny" (pp. 484–85). See also Sandelowski, *With Child in Mind: Studies of the Personal Encounter with Infertility* (Philadelphia: University of Pennsylvania Press, 1993).

26. In the mid-1940s, the rate of childlessness among Black women began to decline, largely as a result of improved health care. See Prithwis Das Gupta, *Future Fertility of Women by Present Age and Parity: Analysis of American Historical Data, 1917–80* (Current Population Reports, Special Studies, Series P-23, No. 142), (Washington, D.C.: U.S. Department of Commerce, Bureau of the Census, 1985), 6–8.

27. On the campaign for maternal health, see Molly Ladd-Taylor, "'My Work Came Out of Agony and Grief': Mothers and the Making of the Sheppard-Towner Act," in Seth Koven and Sonya Michel, eds., *Mothers of a New World: Maternalist Politics and the Origins of Welfare States* (New York: Routledge, 1993), 321–42. One study of trends among White Americans concluded that "substantial variations in childlessness were due largely to voluntary choice on the part of many American women, particularly in the North Atlantic region. In other areas, such as the agricultural South, almost all childlessness was probably

involuntary." This statement suggests that among Whites as well as Blacks, poverty and rural life in the South, where health care was limited, led to increases in infertility. Stewart E. Tolnay and Avery M. Guest, "Childlessness in a Transitional Population: The United States at the Turn of the Century," *Journal of Family History* 7 (Summer 1982): 200–29.

28. George J. Engelmann, M.D., "The Increasing Sterility of American Women," *Journal of the American Medical Association* 37 (1901): 890–97.

29. Linda Gordon, *Woman's Body*, 99.

30. Franklin Martin, M.D., "Transplantation of Ovaries," *Transactions of the American Gynecological Society* 33 (1908): 489–521. A number of physicians were skeptical of these experiments, and by 1922 Martin himself concluded that ovarian transplantation was not a feasible cure for sterility.

31. Edward Reynolds, M.D., "The Theory and Practice of the Treatment of Sterility in Women," *Journal of the American Medical Association* 35 (January 11, 1913): 93–101.

32. Charles G. Child, Jr., M.D., "Sterility in the Female: A Report of Operative Cures," *Transactions of the American Gynecological Society* 45 (1920): 129–40.

33. A. Koplowitz, M.D., "Sterility in Women," *Medical Journal and Record* 119 (March 19, 1924): 300–304. See also Frederick C. Holden, M.D., "Are the Operative Procedures Done for Dysmenorrhea and Sterility Justifiable in the Light of Developmental Study?" *Transactions of the American Gynecological Association* 44 (1919): 271–80.

34. Letter from C. F. C., Oklahoma, "Sterility," in "Questions and Answers," *Hygeia* 3 (September 1925): 540.

35. John Osborn Polak, M.D., "A Study of the Pathology in Its Relation to the Etiology with the End Results of Treatment of Sterility," *Transactions of the American Gynecological Society* 41 (1916): 588–620.

36. Reynolds, "Theory and Practice of the Treatment of Sterility in Women."

37. Mrs. B. R. G., "Childless," *Good Housekeeping*, April 1911, 532; Mrs. H. P. L., Letter to Editor, *Good Housekeeping*, July 1911, 21–22.

38. Arno Dosch, "Not Enough Babies to Go Around," *Cosmopolitan*, September 1910, 431–39.

39. Letters quoted are from Molly Ladd-Taylor, *Raising a Baby the Government Way: Mothers' Letters to the Children's Bureau, 1915–1932* (New Brunswick, N.J.: Rutgers University Press, 1986), 63, 65–66, 68.

40. Ida M. Tarbell, *The Business of Being a Woman* (New York: Macmillan, 1912), 5, 19, 44–48, 75. Emphasis added.

41. H. C. Potter, "Mother and Child," *Harper's Monthly Magazine*, December 1901, 102–4.

42. E. S. Martin, "Children As An Incentive," *Harper's Weekly*, December 10, 1904, 29–31.

43. "The Refusal to Multiply," *Living Age* 279 (November 29, 1913): 566–69; "The Extinction of the Upper Classes," *Living Age* 262 (August 7, 1909): 346–55.

44. Editorial, "Is the Human Race in Peril?" *The Independent* 65 (December 31,

1908): 1626–28; Editorial, "Our Duty to Posterity," *The Independent* 66 (February 4, 1909): 269–71.

45. Sarah Trent, *Women Over Forty* (New York: Macaulay, 1934), 87.

46. See Viviana A. Zelizer, *Pricing the Priceless Child: The Changing Social Value of Children* (New York: Basic Books, 1985), esp. chap. 2.

47. Judith Walzer Leavitt, *Brought to Bed: Child-bearing in America, 1750–1950* (New York: Oxford University Press, 1986), 23–27, 267–68.

48. Edward S. Martin, "The Luxury of Children," *Harper's Monthly Magazine,* August 1903, 402–10.

49. Louis I. Dublin, "Babies," *American Magazine* 127 (January 1939), 68.

50. Letter from "Old Subscriber," Letters to the Editor, *Good Housekeeping,* April 1911.

51. See Elaine Tyler May, *Great Expectations: Marriage and Divorce in Post-Victorian America* (Chicago: University of Chicago Press, 1980), esp. chap. 4; see also Lary May, *Screening Out the Past: The Birth of Mass Culture and the Motion Picture Industry, 1890–1929* (New York: Oxford University Press, 1980).

52. Quoted in Linda Gordon, *Woman's Body,* 140–41.

53. Case D492, 1920, Los Angeles County Archives, in Elaine Tyler May, *Great Expectations,* 1. Name has been modified.

54. This series of letters and comments are all taken from Letters to the Editor, *Good Housekeeping,* April 1911 through April 1912.

55. Anonymous, New York City, "A Woman's Reason," *The Independent* 62 (April 1907): 780–84.

56. See Ladd-Taylor, "'My Work Came Out of Agony and Grief'"; see also Ladd-Taylor, *Raising a Baby the Government Way;* Ladd-Taylor, *Mother-Work.* On the struggles of fathers, see Robert Griswold, *Fatherhood in America: A History* (New York: Basic Books, 1993), esp. chaps. 2 and 3.

57. James G. Powers, quoted in May, *Great Expectations,* 88–89. Such sentiments prevailed well into the twentieth century. In 1931, a typical medical textbook claimed that "normal women . . . have a deep urge for children," but "in the man it can hardly be said that there is a fundamental urge towards fatherhood." Van de Velde, *Fertility and Sterility in Marriage,* 167, 81.

58. Leta S. Hollingworth, "Social Devices for Impelling Women to Bear and Rear Children," *American Journal of Sociology* 22 (July 1916): 19–29; see also Ellen Peck and Judith Senderowitz, eds., introduction to *Pronatalism: The Myth of Mom and Apple Pie* (New York: Crowell, 1974).

59. Julie Berebitsky, "'To Raise as Your Own': The Growth of Legal Adoption in Washington," *Washington History* 6 (Spring–Summer 1994): 5–26.

60. See Lary May, *Screening Out the Past;* and Elaine Tyler May, *Great Expectations,* chap. 4.

61. Thomas Arkle Clark, "A Home Without Children May Still Be A Home," *American Magazine,* August 1927, 44–46.

62. Alfred C. Kinsey et al., *Sexual Behavior in the Human Female* (Philadelphia: W. B. Saunders, 1953), 314–21; Kristin Luker, *Abortion and the Politics of Moth-*

erhood (Berkeley: University of California Press, 1984), 40–49; D'Emilio and Freedman, *Intimate Matters*, chap. 11; James C. Mohr, *Abortion in America: The Origins and Evolution of National Policy, 1800–1900* (New York: Oxford University Press, 1978); see also Rickie Solinger, *The Abortionist: A Woman Against the Law* (New York: Free Press, 1994).

63. See Solinger, *The Abortionist*. Of the 42 women over age fifty-five who wrote in response to the author's query for this study, 27 were infertile. Of the 16 letters from fertile, childless women, 5 mentioned their abortions; 3 of the 5 had more than one abortion. This number undoubtedly underrepresents the proportion of women who had abortions, since they were asked only to write about their experience of childlessness, not their medical, reproductive, or sexual history. Those who mentioned abortions did so in the context of telling their stories; it is likely that many more had abortions but did not mention them in their letters. See the Appendix.

Chapter 3. Unfit for Parenthood: Class, Race, and Compulsory Sterilization

1. See Philip R. Reilly, M.D., J.D., *The Surgical Solution: A History of Involuntary Sterilization in the United States* (Baltimore, Md.: Johns Hopkins University Press, 1991), 140; and Linda Gordon, *Woman's Body, Woman's Right: Birth Control in America*, rev. ed. (New York: Viking Penguin, 1990), esp. chap. 14.

2. Robert Latou Dickinson and Clarence James Gamble, "Human Sterilization: Techniques of Permanent Conception Control" (Princeton, N.J., and New York: Birthright, Inc. and Sterilization for Human Betterment, 1950), 30, in Clarence Gamble Papers, Francis A. Countway Library of Medicine, Rare Books and Manuscripts Collection, Harvard University School of Medicine, Boston (hereafter Gamble Papers, Countway Library); and Reilly, *The Surgical Solution*, xiii, 84–90, 96. See also Thomas S. Shapiro, *Population Control Politics: Women, Sterilization, and Reproductive Choice* (Philadelphia: Temple University Press, 1985).

3. Sanger quoted in Gordon, *Woman's Body*, 282.

4. Correspondence is from Papers of the Margaret Sanger Research Center, Countway Library.

5. See James W. Trent, *Inventing the Feeble Mind: A History of Mental Retardation in the United States* (Berkeley: University of California Press, 1994).

6. See Gordon, *Woman's Body*, 269.

7. Quoted in Reilly, *Surgical Solution*, 19–21.

8. Quoted in E. P. Bicknell, "Custodial Care of the Adult Feeble-Minded," *Journal of Psycho-Asthenics* 1 (December 1896): 51–63.

9. Daniel J. Kevles, *In the Name of Eugenics: Genetics and the Uses of Human Heredity* (New York: Knopf, 1985), 107; Reilly, *Surgical Solution*, 13–25; on

imprisonment of women for sexual misbehavior, see Estelle B. Freedman, *Their Sisters' Keepers: Women's Prison Reform in America, 1830–1930* (Ann Arbor: University of Michigan Press, 1981); Estelle B. Freedman, *Maternal Justice: Miriam Van Waters and the Female Reform Tradition, 1887–1974* (Chicago: University of Chicago Press, forthcoming). See also William Goodell, M.D., "Clinical Notes on the Extirpation of the Ovaries for Insanity," *American Journal of Insanity* 38 (January 1882): 295; Dr. W. H. Hammond, "Castration Recommended as a Substitute for Capital Punishment," editorial in support, *Journal of the American Medical Association* 18 (April 16, 1892): 499–500; Julius Paul, Ph.D., "The Psychiatrist as Public Administrator, Case in Point: State Sterilization Laws," *American Journal of Orthopsychiatry* 38 (1968): 76–82.

10. Molly Ladd-Taylor also found this connection in "The State Regulation of Reproduction: Maternal and Infant Health Legislation and Compulsory Sterilization Laws, 1900–1930," unpublished conference paper, 1989. I would like to thank her for sharing this work with me. See also Molly Ladd-Taylor, *Mother-Work: Women, Child Welfare and the State, 1890–1930* (Champaign: University of Illinois Press, 1994).

11. See Christine Stansell, *City of Women: Sex and Class in New York, 1789–1860* (New York: Knopf, 1986); Kathy Peiss, *Cheap Amusements: Working Women and Leisure in Turn-of-the-Century New York* (Philadelphia: Temple University Press, 1986); Regina G. Kunzel, *Fallen Women, Problem Girls: Unmarried Mothers and the Professionalization of Social Work, 1890–1945* (New Haven, Conn.: Yale University Press, 1993); and Ruth M. Alexander, "'The Only Thing I Wanted Was Freedom': Wayward Girls in New York, 1900–1930," in Elliott West and Paula Petrick, eds., *Small Worlds: Children and Adolescents in America, 1850–1950* (Lawrence: University of Kansas Press, 1992), 275–95. For a discussion of the increasing intolerance for nonmarital sex, see Joan Jacobs Brumberg, "'Ruined' Girls: Changing Community Responses to Illegitimacy in Upstate New York, 1890–1920," *Journal of Social History* 18 (1984): 247–72.

12. Reilly, *Surgical Solution*, 136.

13. Reports are in Gamble Papers, Countway Library.

14. Kevles, *In The Name of Eugenics*, 74–75, quote on p. 97.

15. Charles E. Rosenberg, "Charles Benedict Davenport and the Beginning of Human Genetics," *Bulletin of the History of Medicine* 35 (May–June 1961): 266–76, quotes on pp. 269, 271, 275.

16. Reports from institutions collected in Correspondence File, Gamble Papers, Countway Library.

17. Reilly, *Surgical Solution*, 25, 74.

18. Ibid., 28–29.

19. Quotes are from Ibid., pp. 44–45, 111, 118.

20. Kevles, *In the Name of Eugenics*, x, 72–77.

21. Ibid., 101; other supporters included lawyers, judges, journalists, and wealthy philanthropists like Mrs. E. H. Harriman and John D. Rockefeller, who sup-

ported the Eugenics Record Office at Cold Spring Harbor. See Reilly, *Surgical Solution*, pp. 13–18, 34–35, 42.

22. Laughlin had a mild seizure disorder, which may help explain his interest in eugenics and his childless marriage. See Reilly, *Surgical Solution*, 56–58.

23. Ibid.

24. Story of Dorris Buck Figgins and quote are in "Virginia Lawmakers Appalled to Find Law for Sterilizing 'Misfits' Still on the Books," *Los Angeles Times*, February 24, 1980, 14. See also Shapiro, *Population Control Politics*, 3.

25. Oliver Wendell Holmes, "Opinion of the Supreme Court of United States, Delivered by Mr. Justice Holmes" (May 2, 1927), reprinted in Harry H. Laughlin, *The Legal Status of Eugenical Sterilization* (Washington, D.C.: Eugenics Record Office of the Carnegie Institute of Washington, 1930), 50–52; Reilly, *Surgical Solution*, 68–72, 86–88, 117.

26. See, for example, Mark H. Haller, *Eugenics: Hereditarian Attitudes in American Thought* (New Brunswick, N.J.: Rutgers University Press, 1963).

27. Reilly, *Surgical Solution*, 68–72, 93–98, 110.

28. "Sterilization of Unfit Urged for Better Race," unpaginated clipping from Minneapolis *Star*, May 11, 1938, in Eugenics Collection, Social Welfare History Archives, University of Minnesota.

29. Charlotte Perkins Gilman, "Progress Through Birth Control," *North American Review* 224 (December 1927): 622–29; and Gordon, *Woman's Body*, 307–35. In spite of the discrediting of intelligence tests, some eugenic thinkers in the 1990s still use them to claim genetic superiority of some groups over others. See, for example, Richard J. Herrnstein and Charles Murray, *The Bell Curve: Intelligence and Class Structure in American Life* (New York: Free Press, 1994).

30. "Human Sterilization Today," publication of the Human Betterment Foundation, Pasadena, California, c. 1937, in "Sterilization" clipping file, Schlesinger Library, Radcliffe College, Cambridge, Mass.(hereafter called Schlesinger Library); and Reilly, *Surgical Solution*, 84–90, 125.

31. See, for example, Steven Noll, "Incapable of Leading a Clean and Proper Life: The Case of Willie Mallory and Eugenic Sterilization in Virginia before Buck"; Edward Larson, "Women in the Southern Eugenics Movement"; and Nicole Rafter, "Eugenic Criminology in the Progressive Era," papers presented at the annual meeting of the Organization of American Historians, April 16, 1994, Atlanta, Ga.

32. Reilly, *Surgical Solution*, 29–35, 84, 93–94, 187.

33. Letter from Mrs. Paul C., November 14, 1946, St. Paul, Minnesota, in Hjalmar Petersen's Papers, Minnesota Historical Society. I am grateful to Jennifer Delton for sharing this document with me from her research.

34. See William Ray Van Essendelft, "A History of the Association for Voluntary Sterilization: 1935–1964" (Ph.D. diss., University of Minnesota, 1978); and Shapiro, *Population Control Politics*.

35. Dickinson and Gamble, "Human Sterilization" (1950), 3–31, and Ethel Beckwith, "Admit State Sterilizes Girls," *The Herald*, October 7, 1951, unpaginated

clipping, both from Clarence Gamble Papers, Countway Library; and Reilly, *Surgical Solution*, 149–51, emphasis in original.

36. Clarence J. Gamble, M.D., "Trends in State Programs for the Sterilization of the Mental Deficient," paper presented at the First International Congress on Mental Deficiency, Boston, May 21, 1948 (notes on the meeting are also included), in Gamble Papers, Countway Library; and Reilly, *Surgical Solution*, 98–103.

37. On the 120 rule, see Gordon, *Woman's Body*, 431. In addition, according to guidelines dated May 8, 1948, signed by Malcolm T. MacEachern, M.D., associate director, American College of Surgeons: "In all cases of sterilization the following procedure is required: 1) A complete history of the patient. . . . 2) Recorded consultation of two other members of the medical staff. . . . 3) Sterilization operation to be done only for pathological conditions which might endanger the health or life of the mother and never for social or personal reasons. 4) Careful record of operation. . . . 5) All cases of sterilization to come up for review and analysis by the medical staff," document in Gamble Papers, Countway Library; see also Ad Hoc Women's Studies Committee Against Sterilization Abuse, "Workbook on Sterilization" (Bronxville, N.Y.: Sarah Lawrence College, Women's Studies Department, 1978); Reilly, *Surgical Solution*, 146–48. Mrs. Stein reported that she had four complicated pregnancies, one miscarriage, toxemia, hemorrhages, kidney infections, and high blood pressure, but was denied sterilization because she was younger than age thirty and did not have five children; see "Woman Sues Mt. Kisco Hospital After being Denied Sterilization," *New York Times*, May 12, 1970, in Sterilization File, Schlesinger Library. Mrs. Florence Cafarelli also sued a community hospital for refusing to sterilize her; see "Sterilization, Aim of Suit, Is Granted," *New York Times*, 1971, unpaginated, undated clipping in Sterilization File, Schlesinger Library.

38. Letter to Mr. Alfred Lee, Michigan, April 20, 1948. Gamble said that it is possible to reverse sterilizations in 9 of 14 cases, which shows that "in the very rare case in which unexpected recovery occurs and children are desired a high proportion can have their fertility restored"; see Letter to the Editor, *Time*, February 3, 1948, and Letter to the Editor, *Newsweek*, November 29, 1949, all documents in Gamble Papers, Countway Library.

39. Mr. Sam M., St. Petersburg, Florida, to Clarence Gamble, September 2, 1949, in Gamble Papers, Countway Library.

40. In a draft of a flyer, Gamble wrote, "Selective Sterilization means the VOLUNTARY STERILIZATION of men and women so they may live safely outside of institutions—live without danger to themselves or to the community"; in Gamble Papers, Countway Library.

41. Mrs. Mary B. (Mrs. John T.) P., January 7, 1957, to Clarence Gamble, Gamble Papers, Countway Library.

42. The clippings quoted are all in the Gamble Papers, Countway Library.

43. Stern argued for training, rather than sterilization, but recognized that the costs

might be prohibitive: "The scalpel is cheaper than the school." Curiously, Stern was not altogether against sterilization. Like many postwar Americans, she put her faith in the experts: "The decisions should be made by qualified experts and only after careful consideration of the individual case. If a person is clearly unable to take care of children properly, then, and only then, might sterilization be considered justifiable." Edith Stern, "Should Anybody Be Sterilized?" *Woman's Home Companion*, undated, unpaginated clipping, Gamble Papers, Countway Library.

44. Gerard Piel, chairman, Board of Editors, *Scientific American*, October 25, 1949, to Gamble; Jack Alexander, associate editor, *Saturday Evening Post*, January 28, 1948, to Gamble; and Janet Baird to Gamble, April 19, 1948. Baird added a note that suggested how Gamble financed his own campaign from his personal fortune: "In the meantime the larder is low and I shall greatly appreciate $300 on account." All correspondence in Gamble Papers, Countway Library.

45. Christopher Tietze to Gamble, December 13, 1948, in Gamble Papers, Countway Library. Tietze demonstrated his own racial bias while recognizing the sensitivity of the issue: "If Baltimore or another Southern city is selected I suggest that the investigation be limited to the white population. Most of our tests are standardized on white persons. The apparent percentage of colored mental defectives is high but the interpretation of this finding has been the subject of much discussion and criticism. In addition, families tend to be more unstable among Negroes and information on parentage may be unreliable in an appreciable proportion of cases among the latter."

46. Reilly, *Surgical Solution*, 148; see also Shapiro, *Population Control Politics*.

47. Committee for Abortion Rights and Against Sterilization Abuse (CARASA), "Sterilization: It's *not* as simple as 'tying your tubes,'" 1982, Sterilization file, Schlesinger. In one of the most notorious cases of mass sterilization abuse, in Puerto Rico more than one-third of the women were sterilized, most of them in their twenties. They "chose" sterilization, but abortion was illegal, and sterilization was cheap and available, subsidized by the U.S. government. Joan Kelly (professor of history, City University of New York, and member, Women's Studies Ad Hoc Group Against Sterilization Abuse), "Sterilization and Civil Rights," *Rights* (September–October 1977): 9–11. See also Sterilization File, Schlesinger Library. Another federally funded study found that Black and Hispanic women were more likely to be sterilized than White women in the same programs. See Denaton Vaughan and Gerald Sparer, "Ethnic Group and Welfare Status of Women Sterilized in Federally Funded Family Planning Programs, 1972," *Family Planning Perspectives* 6 (Fall 1974): 224–29. Judge quoted in Shapiro, *Population Control Politics*, 90–91; *Boston Globe*, July 27, 1981, quoted in Reilly, *Surgical Solution*, 163.

48. Nadine Brozan, "The Volatile Issue of Sterilization Abuse: A Tangle of Accusations and Remedies," *New York Times*, December 9, 1977, B14; Judge Gisell quoted in Shapiro, *Population Control Politics*, 4–6, 91.

49. "Dickinson's Human Sterilization Techniques of Permanent Conception Control

by Clarence James Gamble and Alan F. Guttmacher" (rev. ed., 1958), unpublished manuscript, Gamble Papers, Countway Library.

50. Judges approved sterilizations for African American welfare recipients who they described as "worthless parents." See "Judge Issues Plea for Sterilization," clipping from Raleigh, North Carolina, *News and Observer,* April 10, 1949, which reported, "Another plea for sterilization of 'worthless parents' was made . . . today by Judge H. Winfield Smith in reviewing the case of a Negro woman, Eloise Lane Thomas . . . charged with disorderly conduct. Evidence was presented showing that the woman drank frequently, neglected her three illegitimate children. Testimony indicated the State pays more than $40 monthly for the support of two of the children. . . . 'The people are disgusted at paying taxes for the support of children of worthless parents,' said Judge Smith." Clipping from Clipping File, "Sterilization," Schlesinger Library.

51. Vilma Di Biase, director of counseling, Crittenton Hastings Clinic, Brighton, Mass., quoted in Sarah Wernick, "The Personal Dilemmas of Sterilization," *Boston Magazine,* December 1980, 116ff. One physician in support of Dr. Pierce wrote, "One way to decrease future welfare roles (sic) is the deliberate prevention of future welfare recipients. Sterilization is the answer, and just exactly as the obstetrician in South Carolina recommends." See clippings from *Medical Tribune,* October 10, 1973, and November 21, 1973, and Nancy Hicks, "Sterilization of Black Mother of Two Stirs Aiken, S.C," *New York Times,* August 1, 1973; see also *Civil Liberties* 308, p. 1, all clippings in Sterilization File, Schlesinger Library.

52. Physicians quoted in Charles Ludlow, "Truth About Sterilization: Ethics, Racism, Rights at Issue in Alarming Reports," *Dawn Magazine,* October 27, 1973; B. Drummond Ayers, Jr., "Racism, Ethics and Rights at Issue in Sterilization Case," *New York Times,* Monday, July 2, 1973; "Sterilized: Why?" *Time,* July 23, 1973, p. 50, all in Sterilization File, Schlesinger Library. The most frequent targets were Medicaid patients who were giving birth. Quoting a federal judge: "Mrs. Waters was actually refused medical assistance by her attending physician unless she submitted to a tubal ligation after the birth." From *Relf vs. Weinberger et al.*: Civil Action nos. 73-1557 and 74-243, U.S. District Court for the District of Columbia, March 15, 1974. Federal funding worked to make the poor choose sterilization, rather than abortion, which was reimbursed only 50–80 percent. The incentives also promoted unnecessary hysterectomy, which paid $800 to surgeons, rather than tubal ligation, which paid only $250. See Joann Rogers, "Rush to Surgery," *New York Times Magazine,* Sunday, September 21, 1975, 40.

53. Quotes and discussion in Kay Mills, *This Little Light of Mine: The Life of Fanny Lou Hamer* (New York: Dutton, 1993), 21–22, 276.

54. The targeting of African American women is well documented. See, for example, U.S. Department of Health and Human Services, Public Health Service, Centers for Disease Control (CDC), Division of Reproductive Health, *Surgical Sterilization Surveillance: Tubal Sterilization and Hysterectomy in Women Ages*

15–44, 1970–1980 (Atlanta, Ga.: CDC, September 1983), 5. The report found that the mean age for sterilization remained constant at around thirty, rates for Black women were higher than those for White women, and Black women tended to be younger than White women when sterilized. On the case of the Relf sisters, see Ayers, "Racism, Ethics and Rights at Issue in Sterilization Case," in Sterilization File, Schlesinger Library.

55. The judgment required that all persons who were sterilized had to be notified and offered "medical, surgical and psychological assistance." The state agreed to try to contact all persons and to provide modest compensation. See Reilly, *Surgical Solution*, 156; see also Richard D. Lyons, "Virginia Is Sued by Victims of Involuntary Sterilization," *New York Times*, December 30, 1980, Sterilization file, Schlesinger Library. In a similar case, a panel of three appellate judges ruled that former members of a North Carolina eugenics board could be sued for ordering the sterilization in 1968 of a thirteen-year-old mentally retarded girl. See *New York Times*, "Ruling Permits Woman to Sue Over Sterilization," Sunday, May 2, 1982, 25, Sterilization File, Schlesinger Library. See also Gordon, *Woman's Body*, 431–36.

56. Unpaginated, undated clipping from *ACLU News*, Sterilization File, Schlesinger Library.

57. Judge quoted in Shapiro, *Population Control Politics*, 90–91; *Boston Globe* article of July 27, 1981, quoted in Reilly, *Surgical Solution*, 163; Gordon, *Woman's Body*, 431–36.

58. Alexander Cockburn, "Beat the Devil: Welfare, Norplant and the Nazis," *The Nation*, July 18, 1994, 79–80. See also V. Burke, *Time-Limited Welfare Proposals* (Washington, D.C.: Congressional Research Service, 1993); and Linda Gordon, *Pitied But Not Entitled: Single Mothers and the History of Welfare* (New York: Free Press, 1994).

59. For an excellent study of these policies, see Sally J. Kenney, *For Whose Protection? Reproductive Hazards and Exclusionary Policies in the United States and Britain* (Ann Arbor: University of Michigan Press, 1992), quote of Betty Riggs on p. 303. Quote of Betty Moler is from "Four Women Assert Jobs Were Linked to Sterilization," *New York Times*, January 5, 1979, A21.

Chapter 4. The Baby Craze: The Rise of Compulsory Parenthood

1. Surveys taken in 1941, 1945, 1955, and 1960 indicated that *zero* percent said no children was the ideal family size; only 2 percent of Whites and 7 percent of non-Whites said that they wanted no children themselves, and only 1 percent of wives aged eighteen to thirty-nine said that they wanted no children. Pascal K. Whelpton, Arthur A. Campbell, and John E. Patterson, *Fertility and Family Planning in the United States* (Princeton, N.J.: Princeton University Press, 1966), 33–34, 162–63; and Wilson H. Grabill and Paul C. Glick, "Demographic

and Social Aspects of Childlessness: Census Data," *Milbank Memorial Fund Quarterly* 37 (1959): 60–86, see poll on p. 61.

2. For a discussion of the demographic upheavals of the postwar years, see Elaine Tyler May, *Homeward Bound: American Families in the Cold War Era* (New York: Basic Books, 1988), 136–37.

3. See May, introduction to *Homeward Bound,* for a discussion of various theories of postwar demographic changes.

4. Pamela Moore added a postscript to her letter: "Despite my own regret over having an abortion, I am pro-choice. Not all women want children as ardently as I did and not all are in a position to care for them. Abolishing safe abortions will mean many women who make one 'mistake' as I did, will also become childless, or some will die in back alleys." See also Rickie Solinger, *The Abortionist: A Woman Against the Law* (New York: Free Press, 1994).

5. "To the Young," aired in 1942 under the sponsorship of the United States Office of Facts and Figures, quoted in John Morton Blum, *V Was for Victory: Politics and American Culture During World War II* (New York: Harcourt Brace Jovanovich, 1976), 28. See also Robert B. Westbrook, "'I Want a Girl, Just Like the Girl that Married Harry James': American Women and the Problem of Political Obligation in World War II," *American Quarterly* 42 (December 1990): 587–614.

6. Joseph Adelson, "Is Women's Lib a Passing Fad?" *New York Times Magazine,* Sunday, March 19, 1972, 94.

7. Susan Hartmann, *The Home Front and Beyond: American Women in the 1940s* (Boston: Twayne Publishers, 1982), 7, 164.

8. Louisa Randall Church, "Parents: Architects of Peace," *American Home,* November 1946, 18–19.

9. Ronald R. Rindfuss and James A. Sweet, *Postwar Fertility Trends and Differentials in the United States* (New York: Academic Press, 1977), 191; and Ira S. Steinberg, *The New Lost Generation: The Population Boom and Public Policy* (New York: St. Martin's Press, 1982), 3. The conformity to patterns is described in John Modell, Frank Furstenberg, Jr., and Douglas Strong, "The Timing of Marriage in the Transition to Adulthood: Continuity and Change, 1860–1975," in John Demos and Sarane Spence Boocock, eds., *Turning Points: Historical and Sociological Essays on the Family,* supplement to the *American Journal of Sociology* 84 (1978): s120–s150.

10. J. Edgar Hoover, "The Twin Enemies of Freedom: Crime and Communism," address before the 28th Annual Convention of the National Council of Catholic Women, Chicago, November 9, 1956, in *Vital Speeches* 23 (December 1, 1956), 104.

11. John D. Durand, "Married Women in the Labor Force," *American Journal of Sociology* 52 (November 1946), 217–23.

12. "Books Versus Babies," *Newsweek,* January 14, 1946, 79; Mildred Gilman, "Babies: Quantity or Quality?" *American Mercury,* undated clipping from the mid-1940s, Social Welfare History Archives, University of Minnesota.

13. The quote is from a study of 1950 census figures reported in *U.S. News and World Report*, September 14, 1956, 8; Hartmann, *The Home Front*, 70.

14. Judith Bake, "Income and Reproductive Motivation," *Population Studies* 21 (November 1967): 185–206.

15. N. Sanford, "Is College Education Wasted on Women?" *Ladies Home Journal*, May 1957, 78–79ff.

16. Marynia Farnham and Ferdinand Lundberg, *The Modern Woman: The Lost Sex* (New York: Harper & Bros., 1947).

17. Cheryl Christina Crane, "Hollywood's Newest Pin-Up Girl," *Photoplay*, December 1943, 32–33 and 70; Joan Crawford, "Fan Experiences with The Stars: Joan Crawford—My Ideal," *Photoplay*, December 1936, 16; "Model Mothers: Family Poses of Some Professional Beauties," *Life*, May 22, 1944, 65–70.

18. "The New American Domesticated Male," *Life*, January 4, 1954, 42–45; *Parents* is quoted in Peter Filene, *Him/Her/Self: Sex Roles in Modern America*, 2nd. ed. (Baltimore, Md.: Johns Hopkins University Press, 1986), 172–73; see also Stephanie Coontz, *The Way We Never Were: American Families and the Nostalgia Trap* (New York: Basic Books, 1992), 27. On the observance of father's day, which was first celebrated in the teens but became a major commercial holiday in the postwar years, see Jane M. Hatch, ed., *The American Book of Days* (New York: Wilson, 1975), 574–75.

19. Maureen O'Hara, "I'm Waiting for My Baby," *Photoplay*, June 1944, 55, 85–86; Peter Biskind, *Seeing Is Believing: How Hollywood Taught Us to Stop Worrying and Love the Fifties* (New York: Pantheon, 1983), 252, 255.

20. Robert L. Griswold, *Fatherhood in America: A History* (New York: Basic Books, 1993), 187.

21. *Penny Serenade* (1941), written by Garson Kanin and Ruth Gordon, videocassette from RSVP Movie Greats. Quotes taken from videocassette, not screenplay.

22. Quoted by David Riesman in "The Found Generation," *American Scholar* 25 (Autumn 1956), 421–36. See also David Riesman, *The Lonely Crowd: A Study of the Changing American Character* (New Haven, Conn.: Yale University Press, 1950); and William H. Whyte, *The Organization Man* (Garden City, N.Y.: Doubleday, 1956).

23. Miriam Bergenicht, "A Build-Up for Dad," *Parents*, June 1948, 19ff; Andre Fontaine, "Are We Staking Our Future on a Crop of Sissies?" *Better Homes and Gardens*, December 1950, 154ff; David R. Mace, "Fathers Are Parents Too," *Woman's Home Companion*, June 1953, 9–11; Andrew Takas, "What Children Need from Dad," *Parents*, May 1953, 44ff; "Dad Takes a Hand," *Woman's Home Companion*, June 1948, 96–97; "The Importance of Father," *Parents*, December 1947, 28ff; Nancy Cleaver, "Are You a Dud as a Dad?" *American Home*, August 1950, 21ff.

24. Quoted in Lillian Ross, "Onward and Upward With the Arts," *New Yorker*, February 1948, 47. On postwar homophobia, see John D'Emilio, *Sexual Politics, Sexual Communities: The Making of a Homosexual Minority in the United States*,

1940–1970 (Chicago: University of Chicago Press, 1983); and Alan Berube, *Coming Out Under Fire: The History of Gay Men and Women in World War II* (New York: Free Press, 1990).

25. Coontz, *The Way We Never Were*, 76–77.

26. See Kenneth Jackson, *Crabgrass Frontier: The Suburbanization of the United States* (New York: Oxford University Press, 1985). Note also that some suburbs, such as Shaker Heights, Ohio, became racially integrated. See Cynthia Richter (Ph.D. diss., American Studies, University of Minnesota, in progress). See also W. Dennis Keating, *The Suburban Racial Dilemma: Housing and Neighborhoods* (Philadelphia: Temple University Press, 1994).

27. Clifford E. Clark, *The American Family Home, 1800–1960* (Chapel Hill: University of North Carolina Press, 1986).

28. For a discussion of family-centered consumerism in the postwar years, see May, *Homeward Bound*, chap. 7.

29. Letty Cottin Pogrebin, "To Tell the Truth," *New York Times Magazine*, November 20, 1992, 22. I am grateful to Judith Smith for sending me this article.

30. Robert L. Boyd, "Childlessness and Social Mobility during the Baby Boom," *Sociological Spectrum* 9 (Fall 1989): 425–38.

31. For an excellent analysis of the *Playboy* ethos, see Barbara Ehrenreich, *The Hearts of Men: American Dreams and the Flight from Commitment* (Garden City, N.Y.: Anchor Press, 1983).

32. "Debut: Janet Leigh's First Baby," *Look*, November 13, 1956, 20–22; and Eleanor Harris, "A Woman At Last," *Look*, July 24, 1956, 43ff. On Monroe, see Alan Levy, "Marilyn Monroe: 'A Good, Long Look At Myself,'" *Redbook*, August 1962, 40ff; Robert J. Levin, "Marilyn Monroe's Marriage," *Redbook*, April 1958, 36ff; Jack Hamilton, "Marilyn Monroe's New Life," *Look*, October 1, 1957, 110–15; and Flora Rheta, "Remembrance of Marilyn," *Good Housekeeping*, January 1963, 30ff.

33. H. David Kirk, "Nonfecund People as Parents—Some Social and Psychological Considerations," *Fertility and Sterility* 14 (1963): 310–19.

34. Julie Berebitsky, "'To Raise as Your Own': The Growth of Legal Adoption in Washington," *Washington History* 6 (Spring–Summer 1994): 5–26.

35. E. Wayne Carp, "The Sealed Adoption Records Controversy in Historical Perspective: The Case of the Children's Home Society of Washington, 1895–1988," *Journal of Sociology and Social Welfare* 19 (June 1992): 27–57; and Helen Louise West, *Adopted Four and Had One More* (St. Louis, Mo.: Bethany Press, 1968), 85.

36. Carp, "The Sealed Adoption Records Controversy"; Barbara Melosh, "Adoption Autobiography and the Construction of Identity," and E. Wayne Carp, "Secrecy Attacked: Social Science, The Media and the Adoption Rights Movement," papers presented at the annual meeting of the Organization of American Historians, April 15, 1994, Atlanta, Ga.

37. Carp, "The Sealed Adoption Records Controversy"; Deutch quoted in Rickie Solinger, *Wake Up Little Susie: Single Pregnancy and Race Before Roe v. Wade*

(New York: Routledge, 1992), 89, 94. See also Barbara Melosh, *Strangers and Kin: A History of Adoption in America* (New York: Basic Books, forthcoming); and E. Wayne Carp, *Secrecy and Adoption in America: A History* (tentative title; in progress).

38. Alice Lake, "Babies for the Brave," *Saturday Evening Post* 227 (July 31, 1954): 27; Carp, "The Sealed Adoption Records Controversy."

39. J. D. Ratcliff, "Clinics for the Childless," *Hygeia* 19 (October 1941): 788ff; Joseph D. Wassersug, "More Help for Childless Couples," Parts I and II, *Hygeia* 25 (November and December, 1947): 834ff, 933; Clarissa Lorenz, "Hope for the Childless," *Today's Health,* October 1951, 20ff; "New Hope for Childless Couples," *Science Digest* (back cover), December 1954; Albert Q. Maisel, "New Hope for Childless Women," *Ladies Home Journal,* August 1957, 46ff; William Engle, "Maybe You CAN Have a Baby," *American Weekly,* November 8, 1953, 8ff; Edward T. Tyler, as told to Roland H. Berg, "Childless Couples Can Have Babies," *Look,* September 17, 1957, 41–50; Agnes S. Wolf, "I Was Sure I Was Sterile," *Cosmopolitan,* December 1954, 8ff; I. C. Rubin, M.D., as told to Margaret Albrecht, "Childlessness and What Can be Done About It," *Parents,* March 1957, 46ff; and Allan F. Guttmacher, M.D., "How To Combat Sterility," *Parents,* July 1962, 50.

40. Rubin,"Childlessness." For a few examples of postwar enthusiasm for expert advice, see Helen G. Sternau, "When Common Sense Is Not Enough," *Parents,* April 1941, 23; Joan Younger, "Mental Illness Begins at Home," *Ladies Home Journal,* May 1949, 40ff; and Robert Mines, "Remember—You're Not a Psychiatrist," *Woman's Home Companion,* June 1951, 42, 159–64.

Chapter 5. Infertility: Freud in the Bedroom, Sex at the Clinic

1. At the end of a long article in *Hygeia,* J. D. Ratcliff wrote, "In a small proportion of cases, when the male is hopelessly sterile, donor fathers represent a possible solution. Despite widespread publicity, remarkably few cases of this are reported in medical literature." J. D. Ratcliff, "Clinics for the Childless," *Hygeia* 19 (October 1941): 788ff, quote on p. 854.

2. Henry B. Stafford, M.D., "Tell Me, Doctor," part 7 and part 8, *Ladies Home Journal,* August and September, 1950, 31ff and 31ff.

3. "Psychological Aspects of Fertility," manuscript draft, dated November 8, 1950, *New York Times,* Stone File, Countway Library of Medicine, Rare Books and Manuscripts, Harvard University, Boston (hereafter Stone File, Countway Library).

4. By 1990, only 20 percent of infertility remained unexplained, yet only half of all infertile couples undergoing medical treatment would achieve pregnancies. See Margarete J. Sandelowski, "Failures of Volition: Female Agency and Infertility in Historical Perspective," *Signs: Journal of Women in Culture and Society* 15 (1990): 475–99.

5. I. C. Rubin, M.D., as told to Margaret Albrecht, "Childlessness and What Can Be Done About It," *Parents*, March 1957, 46ff.

6. Letter to Tyler Clinic from Omaha, Nebraska, undated, Tyler Clinic Archives, Los Angeles.

7. See Edward T. Tyler, M.D., as told to Roland H. Berg, "Childless Couples Can Have Babies," *Look*, September 17, 1957, 41–50.

8. The society changed its name to the American Fertility Society in 1962 and shifted its emphasis "to assist in all matters having to do with reproduction, but also to assist in limiting the number of people who inhabit this planet;" Bruce H. Stewart, M.D., "Reflections of the Growth of the American Fertility Society: The Presidential Address," *Fertility and Sterility* 24 (October 1973): 741–43. See also *Evaluation of the Barren Marriage* (pamphlet) (New York: Paul B. Hoeber, 1956), distributed by the American Society for the Study of Sterility.

9. Abraham Stone, "American Contributions to the Study of Fertility," undated manuscript, Stone Papers, Countway Library.

10. Dr. Abraham Stone, "Further Aid to Childless Urged," press release, 24th Annual Meeting, Planned Parenthood Federation of America, January 23, 24, 1945, in the Stone Papers, Countway Library.

11. Quote is from Edward T. Tyler, M.D., "Practical Medicine: Management of Infertility," *Annals of Western Medicine and Surgery* 5 (May 1951): 491. See also Edward T. Tyler, M.D., and Sheldon Payne, M.D., "Pituitary Gonadotropin in Seminal Inadequacies," *Transactions of the American Society for the Study of Sterility* (1947): 81–87; Edward T. Tyler, M.D., and Sheldon Payne, M.D., "Spermatogenesis and the Therapy of Infertility," *Journal of the American Medical Association* 134 (June 28, 1947): 770–74.

12. Herbert H. Thomas, M.D., "Thirty-Two Years of Fertility Progress," Presidential Address, *Fertility and Sterility* 27 (October 1976): 1125–31.

13. Tyler, "Childless Couples Can Have Babies"; and Willis E. Brown, M.D., "Privilege and Responsibility: Presidential Address," *Fertility and Sterility* 14 (1963): 475–81.

14. Mrs. Gary B., Hurst, Texas, January 14, 1964, to Dr. Rock; reply from Robert E. Wheatley, M.D., March 23, 1964, Rock Papers, Countway Library.

15. Emily Martin, "The Egg and the Sperm: How Science has Constructed a Romance Based on Stereotypical Male-Female Roles," *Signs: Journal of Women in Culture and Society* 16 (1991): 485–501; see also Emily Martin, *The Woman in the Body: A Cultural Analysis of Reproduction* (Boston: Beacon Press, 1987), 45–48.

16. From Norma McKinley letter, relating the story of a friend. McKinley was one of the respondents to the author's query for this book.

17. Genevieve Parkhurst, "Facts About Sterility," *American Mercury* 64 (June 1947): 713–17.

18. Edward T. Tyler, "Evaluation of the Male Factor in Infertility," *Annals of Western Medicine and Surgery* 2 (November 1948): 514–16.

19. Stone, "American Contributions to the Study of Fertility.

20. John Rock correspondence file, Countway Library.

21. Letter to Tyler Clinic, from Santa Ana, CA, no date. Reply, dated May 11, 1954, recommends that she and her husband come in for an exam.

22. Alfred C. Kinsey, W. B. Pomeroy, and C. E. Martin, *Sexual Behavior in the Human Male* (Philadelphia: W. B. Saunders, 1948).

23. Mr. Thomas R., Tulsa, Oklahoma, to John Rock, undated, and reply from Rock, dated January 24, 1964, John Rock correspondence, Rock Papers, Countway Library.

24. Tyler, "Childless Couples Can Have Babies," 41.

25. Stewart, "Reflections." As early as 1929, an article listed deception among the advantages of the Huhner test, "the examination of the spermatozoa as obtained from the cervix and uterine cavity after coitus." In addition to certain diagnostic uses of the test, "in case a woman wishes to check up the cause of a sterility and does not wish her husband to know that she is seeking information as to the condition of the spermatozoa, and if present of not, she can present herself without his knowledge or consent and gain some information." See Clara G. Gottschalk, M.D., "The Huhner Test in the Diagnosis of Sterility," *Medical Woman's Journal* 36 (March 1929): 64–68.

26. Letter to Rock dated January 12, 1964, and reply from Robert E. Wheatley, M.D., in Rock's absence, March 25, 1964, Rock correspondence file, Countway Library. On research efforts in treating male infertility, see, for example, Tyler and Payne, "Spermatogenesis."

27. Mr. Larry L., North Manchester, Indiana, to Dr. Rock, undated, and response from Dr. Rock's secretary, Ann E. Monks, March 9, 1964, in Rock Papers, Countway Library. Perhaps the referral was the result of a hasty reading of the letter, given that so many letters arrived after the television broadcast. Nevertheless, the automatic response is revealing in itself. Another hasty response indicates the difficulty in reading carefully the huge volume of mail. One viewer wrote to Rock outraged at his advocacy of contraception, in opposition to the teachings of his (and the respondent's) Catholic church. She wrote, "It is not for man, but for God to decide whether the natural processes of womanhood should be halted." Rock responded to her scolding with a brief note, "Thanks for your encouraging letter. It set me up considerably." (The secretary added the second sentence. The note Rock scribbled on the top of the received letter simply said, "Thanks for encouraging letter.") The volume of mail is evidence of the huge interest in Rock's appearance, particularly the many responses from Catholics who either agreed or disagreed with his support of the use of oral contraceptives.

28. P. F. C. A. C., Fort Riley, Kansas, to Dr. Abraham Stone, February 9, 1945, and reply from Stone, February 15, 1945, in Stone Papers, Countway Library.

29. Irwin H., Sunnyside, New York, to Dr. Abraham Stone, undated; reply from Dr. Stone, March 21, 1948, Stone Papers, Countway Library.

30. Tyler, "Childless Couples Can Have Babies."

31. Abraham Stone, M.D., "Sexual Factors in Infertility," undated seven-page man-

uscript, Stone Papers, Countway Library; John Rock, manuscript draft on impotence, Rock Papers, Countway Library.

32. Mr. and Mrs. Elwin H., Westfield, Massachusetts, to Dr. John Rock, undated, and reply from Dr. Rock, March 2, 1964, in Rock Papers, Countway Library.

33. Mrs. Elizabeth B., Kent, Ohio, to Dr. Rock, January 16, 1963, and reply from Dr. Rock, January 22, 1964, in Rock Papers, Countway Library.

34. E. B. A., Indianapolis, Indiana, to Dr. Rock (undated), received February 20, 1964, and reply from Dr. Rock, February 25, 1964, Rock Papers, Countway Library.

35. For one such story, see Agnes S. Wolf, "I Was Sure I Was Sterile," *Cosmopolitan*, December 1954, 8–11; see also "Advice to the Childless," *Time*, May 1, 1950, 58–59.

36. Tyler Clinic patient records, Tyler Clinic archives.

37. Stone, "Sexual Factors in Infertility." Comment of the infertility counselor is from a conversation with Lillian B. Tyler, who spent several years counseling patients at the Tyler Clinic.

38. M. Ward, "Survey of 1000 Cases," April 26, 1956, single-page manuscript; and Leonard F. Ciner, M.D., "Is a Complete Infertility Study of Value?" Abstract, New York State Medical Society Meeting, 1956, single-page manuscript, both in Stone Papers, Countway Library.

39. Tyler, "Childless Couples Can Have Babies."

40. For an excellent study of the transformation of psychiatry during the early twentieth century and its cultural significance, see Elizabeth Lunbeck, *The Psychiatric Persuasion: Knowledge, Gender, and Power in Modern America* (Princeton, N.J.: Princeton University Press, 1994).

41. Herbert D. Lamson, Ph.D., Willem J. Pinard, Ph.D., and Samuel R. Meaker, M.D., "Sociologic and Psychological Aspects of Artificial Insemination with Donor Semen," *Journal of the American Medical Association* 145 (April 7, 1951): 1062–63.

42. "Program: American Society for the Study of Sterility, Eighth Annual Conference," June 7 and 8, 1952, Chicago, pp. 10 and 11; and descriptions of papers by Therese Benedek, M.D., "Infertility as a Psychosomatic Defense," and W. S. Kroger, M.D., "The Evaluation of Personality Factors in the Treatment of Infertility," in Tyler Clinic archives.

43. Sandelowski, "Failures of Volition," 475–99.

44. W. S. Kroger, M.D., "Evaluation of Personality Factors in the Treatment of Infertility," *Fertility and Sterility* 3 (November–December 1952): 542–51.

45. Marcel Heiman, M.D., "Reproduction: Emotions and the Hypothalamic-Pituitary Function," *Fertility and Sterility* 10 (1959): 162–76; William S. Kroger, M.D., and S. Charles Freed, M.D., "Psychosomatic Aspects of Frigidity," *Journal of the American Medical Association* 143 (June 10, 1950): 526–32; E. Bergler, M.D., and W. S. Kroger, M.D., "The Dynamic Significance of Vaginal Lubrication to Frigidity," *Western Journal of Surgery, Obstetrics and Gynecology* 61 (December 1953): 711–16; William S. Kroger, M.D., "Psychosomatic Aspects of

Frigidity and Impotence," *International Record of Medicine* (July 1958): 469–78. *Time* magazine reported these findings in 1952, quoting Dr. William Saul Kroger, "a hard-bitten bachelor of 45," as identifying psychological sources of sterility among "neurotic" women. See "Sterility and Neurotics," *Time*, (June 16, 1952), 81–82.

46. E. Wittkower, M.D., and A. T. M. Wilson, M.D., "Dysmenorrhea and Sterility: Personality Studies," *British Medical Journal* 2 (November 2, 1940): 586–90; quote is on p. 587. The authors argued that "tomboy" types and other "maladjusted" children later became sterile. They also stated that "sterile patients . . . display as a main characteristic a self-centredness and lack of warmth in their social and personal relations, clearly seen in a sexual frigidity of which their abnormal reaction to coitus forms an impressive index . . . lack of orgasm through emotional immaturity may interfere with conception by preventing the progress of the spermatozoa" (p. 590).

47. Rickie Solinger, *Wake Up Little Susie: Single Pregnancy and Race Before Roe v. Wade* (New York: Routledge, 1992), 90–91.

48. Vera G. Kinsler, "Sterility Can Be a State of Mind," *Coronet*, April 1953, 109–12.

49. "Family Problems," *American Magazine*, August 1951, 108; William Engle, "Maybe You CAN Have a Baby," *American Weekly*, November 8, 1953, 8; J. D. Ratcliff, "Clinics for the Childless," *Hygeia* 19 (October 1941): 854; Joseph D. Wassersug, "More Help for Childless Couples," *Hygeia* 25 (November 1947): 384–85.

50. Tyler, "Childless Couples Can Have Babies."

Chapter 6. Childfree: The Revolt Against the Baby Boom

1. She described herself as a "casino change person" in her second letter.

2. P. K. Whelpton, A. A. Campbell, and J. E. Patterson, *Fertility and Family Planning in the United States* (Princeton, N.J.: Princeton University Press, 1966), 162–63; and Rick Weiss, "The Kidless Culture," *Health*, July–August 1993, 40.

3. Leslie Miller, "Setting Aside a Day for Non-Parents," *USA Today*, June 5, 1994, 1.

4. Judith Blake, "Is Zero Preferred? American Attitudes toward Childlessness in the 1970s," *Journal of Marriage and the Family* 41 (May 1979): 255.

5. Carroll Lachnit, "No Kids? No Kidding," *Los Angeles Times*, September 15, 1993, E1, E6.

6. In 1940, for example, the rate of childlessness among ever-married White women aged forty-five to forty-nine was 14.8 percent. After a dramatic decline, it rose again to 11.5 in 1990. U.S. Department of Commerce, Economics and Statistics Administration, Bureau of the Census, *Fertility of American Women: June 1990* (Series P-20, No. 454) (Washington, D.C.: U.S. Department of Commerce, Bureau of the Census, 1990), 17, 64. See also Jean E. Veevers, *Childless by*

Choice (Toronto: Butterworth, 1980); and Dudley L. Poston, Jr., and Kathryn Beth Kramer, "Voluntary and Involuntary Childlessness in the U.S., 1955–1973," *Social Biology* 30 (1983): 290–306.

7. Marvin B. Sussman and Suzanne K. Steinmetz, *Handbook of Marriage and the Family* (New York: Plenum Press, 1987), 376. Next in order of frequency of response was an improved marital relationship, female career considerations, monetary advantages, concern about population growth, dislike of children, self-doubts about parenting abilities, concern about the physical aspects of childbirth, and concern about bringing children into a harsh world. The tabulation is on p. 377: "Rationales for voluntary childlessness by occurrence in Studies to Date and by Sex."

8. Although voluntary childlessness was rare and practically invisible, one study found that it was "relatively common" among certain upwardly mobile segments of the population. The researcher concluded, however, that it represented a sacrifice rather than a positive choice: "To overcome obstacles to mobility, couples with the greatest disadvantages must make the greatest sacrifices of child-centered behavior." See Robert L. Boyd, "Childlessness and Social Mobility during the Baby Boom," *Sociological Spectrum* 9 (Fall 1989): 425–38.

9. Roslyn South, "Pity the Childless Couple," *American Mercury* 84 (June 1957): 76–78.

10. Gael Greene, "A Vote Against Motherhood," *Saturday Evening Post*, January 1963, 10–12; Betty Friedan, *The Feminine Mystique* (New York: Norton, 1963).

11. Susan O. Gustavus and James R. Henley, Jr., "Correlates of Voluntary Childlessness in a Select Population," *Social Biology* 18 (September 1971): 277–84; Veevers, *Childless by Choice*; see also Marian Faux, *Childless by Choice: Choosing Childlessness in the Eighties* (Garden City, N.Y.: Anchor Press, 1984), esp. chap. 7.

12. Betty Rollin, "Motherhood, Who Needs It?" *Look*, September 22, 1970, 15–17.

13. Ellen Peck, *The Baby Trap* (New York: Bernard Geis, 1971), 7, 9, 20, 14–15, 98, 100, 141, 204–5, 206–7, 209, 237, 242.

14. *The Baby Trap* was printed in 1971, 1972, 1974, and 1976; figures on sales are from Jeannette Smyth, "Ellen Peck and 'The Baby Trap,'" *Washington Post*, Sunday May 9, 1971, clipping file, Schlesinger Library, Radcliffe College, Cambridge, Mass. See also review by Clarence Petersen, *Washington Post Book World*, May 7, 1972. Critical reviews include Patricia Meyer Spacks, "A Chronicle of Women," *Hudson Review* 25 (Spring 1972): 156–70; and an exceptionally thoughtful negative review from a feminist perspective, Ellen Willis, "To Be or Not To Be a Mother," *Ms.*, October 1974, 28–38.

15. See Ellen Peck and Judith Senderowitz, eds., *Pronatalism: The Myth of Mom and Apple Pie* (New York: Crowell, 1974); Anna and Arnold Silverman, *The Case Against Having Children* (New York: David McKay, 1971); Angela McBride, *The Growth and Development of Mothers* (New York: Harper & Row, 1973); Elizabeth Whelan, *A Baby? . . . Maybe: A Guide to Making the Most Fateful Decision of Your Life* (New York: Bobbs-Merrill, 1975); Ellen M. Nelson, *Voluntarily Childless Couples: The Emergence of a Variant Lifestyle* (Beverly Hills, Calif.:

Sage, 1976); Kate Harper, *The Childfree Alternative* (Brattleboro, Vt.: Stephen Greene, 1980); Diana Burgwyn, *Marriage Without Children* (New York: Harper & Row, 1981); Faux, *Childless by Choice.*

16. Larry D. Barnett and Richard H. MacDonald, "A Study of the Membership of the National Organization for Non-Parents," *Social Biology* 23 (Winter 1976): 297–310.

17. Other support groups for the voluntary childless continued to emerge into the 1990s, including Childless by Choice, based in Leavenworth, Washington, and the Childfree Network, with sixty chapters around the country. See Carroll Lachnit, "No Kids? No Kidding," *Los Angeles Times,* September 15, 1993, E1, E6. For an example of population and personal concerns as issues addressed by these groups, see *Optional Parenthood Today* (the journal of NAOP), 8 (November 1980).

18. One study done in the early 1980s suggested that voluntary childlessness was relatively rare and predicted that following its rise in the 1970s, there would be a long-term downward trend. The increase predicted on the basis of increased education and employment for women had not occurred, in spite of the apparent greater tolerance for the choice. Sharon K. Houseknecht, "Voluntary Childlessness in the 1980s: A Significant Increase?" *Marriage and the Family Review* 5 (Summer 1982): 51–69; E. Pohlman et al., "Changes in Views toward Intentional Childlessness among College Students, 1965–1970," unpublished paper, 1971, cited in Ellen Mara Nason and Margaret M. Poloma, *Voluntary Childless Couples: The Emergence of a Variant Lifestyle* (Beverly Hills, Calif.: Sage, 1976), p. 7.

19. Roper Organization, *1980 Virginia Slims American Women Opinion Poll.* In spite of the growing number of childfree women and men, parenthood still remained the most popular adult status. A Gallop poll in 1980 found that although almost half of all Americans believed that family life had deteriorated since 1965, three out of four women considered marriage with children the "ideal" life, and one out of three wanted to combine marriage, children, and a full-time job. But the poll also revealed that fully one-fourth did not agree with that vision of the "ideal" life, and two-thirds did not think "having it all"—marriage, a job, and children—was a viable possibility. See "Poll Finds People Feel Family Life on Decline," *New York Times,* June 3, 1980, cited in Burgwyn, *Marriage Without Children,* 26; Kristine M. Baber and Patricia Monaghan, "College Women's Career and Motherhood Expectations: New Options, Old Dilemmas," *Sex Roles* 19 (August 1988): 189–203.

20. Harper, *The Childfree Alternative,* 4–8.

21. Quoted in Anne Kirchheimer, "The Couples Who Don't Want Children," *Boston Globe,* October 11, 1979, 57.

22. Faux, *Childless by Choice,* 18; Sussman and Steinmetz, *Handbook of Marriage and the Family,* 377 (see table, note 9).

23. Polls in the mid-1960s indicated that although fewer than 1 percent of White respondents said that they would like to have no children, 5 percent of Black

respondents said that they preferred to be childless, even though these stated preferences do not conform to demographic trends. N. B. Ryder and C. F. West-off, "Relationships Among Intended, Expected, Desired, and Ideal Family Size: United States, 1965" (Washington, D.C.: Center for Population Research, National Institutes of Health, 1969); Whelpton, Campbell, and Patterson, *Fertility and Family Planning in the United States*, both cited in Edward Pohlman, Ph.D., "Childlessness, Intentional and Unintentional: Psychological and Social Aspects," *Journal of Nervous and Mental Disease* 151 (1970): 3. A number of studies have suggested that the privatization of child rearing, by which individual nuclear families or single parents shoulder the entire burden alone, does not prevail in these communities. Whether by economic necessity or preference, or perhaps a combination of both, child rearing is a shared endeavor. See, for example, Carol Stack, *All Our Kin: Strategies for Survival in a Black Community* (New York: Harper & Row, 1974). Childlessness did not correlate neatly with income. The relationship between childlessness and income is complicated, with no clear pattern. See Dudley L. Poston, Jr., "Income and Childlessness in the United States: Is the Relationship Always Inverse?" *Social Biology* 21 (Fall 1974): 296–307. The same issue was explored by Phillip R. Kunz, Merlin B. Brinkerhoff, and Vickie Hundley, "Relationship of Income and Childlessness," *Social Biology* 20 (June 1973): 139–42. They found that 13.1 percent of all White and non-White wives aged thirty-five to fifty-four were childless, but among the very poor, it was 16.1 percent. They also found that a higher percentage of the non-White women than the White women were childless. There is an increase in childlessness as the husband's income rises, except among the lowest occupational categories, suggesting that childlessness among the poor is more likely to be due to infertility and pregnancy loss.

24. A 1977 study found that Whites who reached adulthood after 1965 had a higher rate of childlessness at each age than any other group, probably because of choice. See Dudley L. Poston, Jr., and Erin Gotard, "Trends in Childlessness in the United States, 1910–1975," *Social Biology* 24 (Fall 1977): 212–24. One study noted that the rates converged in the early 1970s and suggested that the convergence indicated that "blacks have made progress into the basic structure of American society." The investigator predicted that the rates of childlessness would continue to converge and increase for both groups. But that did not happen. Instead, the rates for Whites continued to rise, but the rates for Blacks declined. Carl F. Grindstaff, "Trends and Incidence of Childlessness by Race: Indicators of Black Progress over Three Decades," *Sociological Focus* 9 (August 1976): 265–84.

25. Robert L. Boyd, "Minority Status and Childlessness," *Sociological Inquiry* 59 (Summer 1989): 331–42.

26. Quotes are from Burgwyn, *Marriage Without Children*, 20–21.

27. Janet Singleton, "Everything But the Baby," *USA Weekend*, January 21–23, 1994.

28. Paul Popenoe, "Motivation of Childless Marriages," *Journal of Heredity* 27

(1936): 467–72; see also Paul Popenoe, "Childlessness: Voluntary or Involuntary," *Journal of Heredity* 34 (1943): 83–84; J. E. Veevers, "The Lifestyle of Voluntarily Childless Couples," in Lyle Larson, ed., *The Canadian Family in Comparative Perspective* (Toronto: Prentice Hall, 1974). See also Veevers, "The Moral Careers of Voluntarily Childless Wives: Notes on the Defense of a Variant World View," in S. Parvez Wakil, ed., *Marriage and the Family in Canada: A Reader* (Toronto: Capp-Clark, 1974); Veevers, "The Social Meaning of Parenthood," *Psychiatry* 36 (August 1973): 291–310; Veevers, "The Violation of Fertility Mores: Voluntary Childlessness as Deviant Behavior," in Craig L. Boydell, Carl F. Grindstaff, and Paul C. Whitehead, eds., *Deviant Behavior and Societal Reaction* (Toronto: Holt, Rinehart & Winston, 1972); and Veevers, "Childlessness and Age at First Marriage," *Social Biology* 18 (September 1971): 292–95. Her book on the subject is Veevers, *Childless by Choice*.

29. Cardell K. Jacobson and Tim B. Heaton, "Voluntary Childlessness Among American Men and Women in the Late 1980s," *Social Biology* 38 (1991): 79–93. This study noted that of the 47 studies of voluntary childlessness published prior to 1986, only 5 were based on representative samples. Most were small samples, ranging from 18 to 119. Studies done in the late 1970s suggest that the voluntarily childless were less tolerant of deviant behaviors, less politically liberal, but more liberal in lifestyle, more confident about earning a living, and less involved with relatives than were the involuntarily childless.

30. See, for example, "Cribs or Careers? Professionally Employed Married Women's Attitudes toward Motherhood," paper presented at the meeting of the American Sociological Association, August 1971, cited in Ellen Mara Nason and Margaret M. Paloma, *Voluntary Childless Couples: The Emergence of a Variant Lifestyle*, Sage Research Papers in the Social Sciences, 5 (Beverly Hills, Calif.: Sage Publications, 1976).

31. "The Population Boom," *Time*, September 14, 1953, 96; "The Future: Too Many Babies?" *Time*, August 26, 1957, 75; "Population Boom: Too Many Mouths to Feed," *Newsweek*, September 13, 1954, 72; "Few Americans Favor Large Families" (Gallup poll of 1500 adults), *Current Opinion 1* (April 1973): 38–39; Clyde V. Kiser, Wilson H. Grabill, Arthur A. Campbell, *Trends and Variations in Fertility in the U.S.* (Cambridge, Mass.: Harvard University Press, 1968), chap. 1; and Philip Appleman, *The Silent Explosion* (Boston: Beacon Press, 1965), 61.

32. Edward G. Stockwell, *Population and People* (Chicago: Quadrangle Books, 1968), 5–11. See also Margaret O. Hyde, *This Crowded Planet* (New York: McGraw-Hill, 1961), 9: "This population explosion may be the greatest challenge of the present time. Within the next forty years, the world population may double. Can the new frontiers of science meet the needs of the crowded world of tomorrow?" The book calls both for family limitation and for science to solve problems of world hunger and crowding and poverty.

33. Paul R. Ehrlich, *The Population Bomb* (New York: Ballantine Books, 1968), 6; and Paul R. Ehrlich and Anne H. Ehrlich, *The Population Explosion* (New York:

Simon & Schuster, 1990), 9–11; see also Stewart L. Udall, "Our Perilous Population Implosion," *Saturday Review*, September 2, 1967, 10–13.

34. Sandra Barty, "The Synanon Community and its Policy of Childlessness, 1976–1989," paper presented at the International Communal Studies Conference, October 14–17, 1993, New Harmony, Indiana. I am grateful to Sandra Barty for sharing this work in progress with me.

35. Nixon quote is from "The Drive to Stop Population Growth," *U.S. News and World Report*, March 2, 1970, 36ff. Pamela Wasserman, *Planning the Ideal Family: The Small Family Option* (Washington, D.C.: Zero Population Growth, 1990), includes a section on being "Childfree by Choice"; see also Nason and Paloma, *Voluntary Childless Couples*; Gustavus and Henley, "Correlates of Voluntary Childlessness in a Select Population"; Veevers, *Childless by Choice*; quote is from Burgwyn, *Marriage Without Children*, 12; G. N. Ramu and Nicholas Tavuchis, "The Valuation of Children and Parenthood among the Voluntary Childless and Parental Couples in Canada," *Journal of Comparative Family Studies* 17 (Spring 1986): 99–116; and Frances Baum, "Voluntarily Childless Marriages," *International Journal of Sociology and Social Policy* 2, no. 3 (1982): 40–54.

36. Les U. Knight, editorial, *These Exit Times* 1, no. 1 (1991): 3.

37. Sussman and Steinmetz, *Handbook of Marriage and the Family*, 376. Based on a survey of twenty-nine studies, most of them relatively small nonrepresentative samples.

38. Elizabeth M. Armstrong, "'Childless' Women Connect With Our Community's Youth," *San Francisco Chronicle*, May 7, 1993, A23.

39. Catherine S. Chilman, "Major Trends of Families and Their Mental Health in the United States: 1957–1978" *International Journal of Sociology of the Family* 12 (Autumn 1982): 217–27. Rates of joint marital satisfaction were also lower for active parents than for either former parents or childless couples, regardless of how long the couples had been married or the employment status of the wives. Overall, "former parents" were better off than active parents on all indicators, although not as healthy or happy as the childless couples. Karen S. Renne, "Childlessness, Health, and Marital Satisfaction," *Social Biology* 23 (Fall 1976): 183–97.

Chapter 7. Designer Genes: The Baby Quest and the Reproductive Fix

1. See Arthur L. Greil, *Not Yet Pregnant: Infertile Couples in Contemporary America* (New Brunswick, N.J.: Rutgers University Press, 1991), 51.

2. Susan Faludi, *Backlash: The Undeclared War Against American Women* (New York: Crown, 1991), 24–27. On the declining sperm count, see Amy Linn, "Male Infertility: From Taboo to Treatment," *Philadelphia Inquirer*, May 31, 1987, AI, cited in *Backlash*, 31–32. On the new pronatalism, see also Margarete

J. Sandelowski, *With Child In Mind: Studies of the Personal Encounter with Infertility* (Philadelphia: University of Pennsylvania Press, 1993), 9.

3. Articles cited in Faludi, *Backlash*, 104–10.

4. See Mary Ellen Barrett, "Wanted: Baby," *USA Weekend*, October 6–8, 1989, 4–5.

5. James A. Weber, *Grow or Die!* (New Rochelle, NY: Arlington House, 1977), 9–11. Observers noted the trend even earlier. See, for example, "Population Slowdown—What It Means to U.S.," *U.S. News and World Report*, December 25, 1972, 59ff.

6. Ben J. Wattenberg, *The Birth Dearth* (New York: Pharos Books, 1987). See also Art Levine, "The Birth Dearth Debate," *U.S. News and World Report*, June 22, 1987, 64–65.

7. Linda Wolfe, "The Coming Baby Boom," *New York Magazine*, January 10, 1977, 38–42.

8. Cheri Pies and Francine Hornstein, "Baby M and The Gay Family," *Out/Look* 1 (Spring 1988): 79–85.

9. On the proportion of the infertile, see Greil, *Not Yet Pregnant*, 27–28; data on physicians visits from Office of Technology Assessment, in Philip Elmer-Dewitt, "Making Babies," *Time*, September 30, 1991, 56–63; see also David Perlman, "The Art and Science of Conception: Brave New Babies," *San Francisco Chronicle*, March 3, 1990, B3; on the success of IVF, see Nancy Wartik, "Making Babies," *Los Angeles Times Magazine*, March 6, 1994, 18ff.

10. Study cited in Greil, *Not Yet Pregnant*, 11.

11. Most estimates gave infertile couples a 50 percent chance, as they did in the 1950s and 1960s, although some physicians were more conservative. One physician in 1962, for example, gave infertile couples a 40 percent chance of a cure, saying that "more could be helped if husbands would cooperate completely with medical examination and treatment." See Grace Naismith, "Good News for Childless Couples," *Today's Health* 40 (January 1962): 24ff. For 1990 data, see Greil, *Not Yet Pregnant*, 11.

12. Susan Sward, "I Thought Having a Baby Would be Easy," *San Francisco Chronicle*, March 5, 1990, B4. See also Miriam D. Mazor, "Barren Couples," *Psychology Today*, May 1979, 101–12.

13. Greil, *Not Yet Pregnant*, chap. 3, also found this to be true.

14. See Ibid., esp. pp. 51–52.

15. See Lois Wladis Hoffman and Jean Denby Manis, "The Value of Children in the United States: A New Approach to the Study of Fertility," *Journal of Marriage and the Family* 41 (August 1979): 583–96. The exceptions were nonparents, who gave other markers, and Black men, who ranked supporting themselves higher.

16. Tim Carrigan, Bob Connell, and John Lee, "Toward a New Sociology of Masculinity," in Harry Brod, ed., *The Making of Masculinities: The New Men's Studies* (New York: Routledge, 1987), 63–100.

17. See Greil, *Not Yet Pregnant*, esp. chap. 4.

18. The abuse mentioned included psychological or physical abuse that the respondents did not wish to perpetuate or made them feel they would be bad parents. Some said that they had only recently "discovered" their childhood sexual abuse in therapy, by retrieving repressed memories. Although these approaches are highly controversial in the professional therapeutic community, it is noteworthy that several childless people mentioned these "repressed memories" in relation to their childlessness. Other cases, however, like those quoted in this chapter, were not repressed memories. They were well-remembered rapes that continued for years.

19. See Philip Elmer Dewitt, "Making Babies," *Time*, September 30, 1991, 56–62; DES Action and other groups have been formed by and on behalf of women who have been harmed by DES, the Dalkon Shield, and other medical products. See Karen M. Hicks, *Surviving the Dalkon Shield IUD: Women v. The Pharmaceutical Industry* (New York: Teachers College Press, 1994).

20. Lorraine Pascasio, "A Christmas Baby," *Ladies Home Journal*, December 1991, 14–17.

21. Griel, *Not Yet Pregnant*, also found this to be the case.

22. "Infertility: Medical and Social Choices" (Washington, D.C.: U.S. Congress, Office of Technology Assessment, May 1988), 35, quoted in Faludi, *Backlash*, 28. Treated couples have approximately a 50 percent rate of pregnancy, but one study showed that 35 percent of nontreated infertile couples also achieved pregnancy. See Greil, *Not Yet Pregnant*, 32.

23. See, for example, Gena Corea, *The Mother Machine: Reproductive Technologies from Artificial Insemination to Artificial Wombs* (New York: Harper & Row, 1985); Judith Lorber examined why women are likely to subject themselves to treatments, such as IVF, when they are fertile themselves. See Judith Lorber, "Choice, Gift or Patriarchal Bargain? Women's Consent to In-Vitro Fertilization in Male Infertility," *Hypatia* 4 (Fall 1989): 23–36; and Judith Lorber, "In-Vitro Fertilization and Gender Politics," in Elaine Hoffman Baruch, Amadeo F. D'Adamo, Jr., and Joni Seager, eds., *Embryos, Ethics and Women's Rights: Exploring the New Reproductive Technologies* (New York: Hawthorne Press, 1988), 117–33. Griel, *Not Yet Pregnant*, found that women were active participants in their medical care—not passive recipients.

24. Wartik, "Making Babies." See also Jerry Carroll, "Tracing the Causes of Infertility," *San Francisco Chronicle*, March 5, 1990, B3.

25. Sward, "I Thought"; Jerry Carroll, "The Blessed Results," *San Francisco Chronicle*, March 5, 1990, B3.

26. Ellen Hopkins, "Tales from the Baby Factory," *New York Times Magazine*, March 15, 1992, 40ff.

27. For an account of one woman's struggle, see Gilda Radner, *It's Always Something* (New York: Simon & Schuster, 1989), chap. 2.

28. David Hill, M.D., quoted in Wartik, "Making Babies."

29. See, for example, Shelley Levitt and Sue Carswell, "Anchor Aweigh: Dan

Rather's New Sidekick, Connie Chung, Still Hasn't Given Up on Motherhood," *People Weekly*, June 21, 1993, 59–64.

30. "Test Tube Babies," *Newsweek*, December 27, 1954, 48. Commentators at the time claimed that this ruling was out of synch with contemporary practices. See "Test-Tube Test Case," *Time*, December 27, 1954, 52.

31. R. Snowden, G. D. Mitchell, and E. M. Snowden, *Artificial Reproduction: A Social Investigation* (London: Allen & Unwin, 1983).

32. Paul McEnroe, "The Genius Bank," Minneapolis *Star Tribune*, August 28, 1988, 1Aff; Sabra Chartrand, "Parents Recall Ordeal of Prosecuting in Artificial-Insemination Fraud Case," *New York Times*, Sunday, March 15, 1992, 10.

33. Robert Hill quoted in Lynda Richardson, "Adoptions that Lack Papers, Not Purpose," *New York Times*, November 25, 1993, B1ff. See also Carol B. Stack, *All Our Kin: Strategies for Survival in a Black Community* (New York: Harper & Row, 1974), esp. chap. 5.

34. See Elizabeth Bartholet, *Family Bonds: Adoption and the Politics of Parenting* (Boston: Houghton Mifflin, 1993).

35. Greil, *Not Yet Pregnant*, 49.

36. Michael Gold, *And Hannah Wept: Infertility, Adoption, and the Jewish Couple* (Philadelphia: Jewish Publication Society, 1988).

37. Miriam Anne Bourne, *First Family: George Washington and His Intimate Relations* (New York: Norton, 1982), 106. See also discussion in chap. 1.

38. Greil, *Not Yet Pregnant*, 40.

39. Richard J. Herrnstein and Charles Murray, *The Bell Curve: Intelligence and Class Structure in American Life* (New York: Free Press, 1994). See also Stephanie Coontz, *The Way We Never Were: American Families and the Nostalgia Trap* (New York: Basic Books, 1992); and Leila Zenderland, *Measuring Minds: Henry Herbert Goddard and the Origins of American Intelligence Testing* (New York: Cambridge University Press, forthcoming).

40. Many feminist theorists have commented on the implications of the normative connections between womanhood and motherhood. See, for example, Peter Osborne and Lynne Segal, "Gender as Performance: An Interview with Judith Butler," *Radical Philosophy* 67 (Summer 1994): 32–39, for one recent articulation of this phenomenon. See also Carolyn M. Morrell, *Unwomanly Conduct: The Challenges of Intentional Childlessness* (New York: Routledge, 1994).

Index

★☆

Note: Entries followed by *(respondent pseudonym)* refer to respondents to author's query. Material in endnotes is indicated by *n* followed by the note number.